Carolyn Zerbe Enns, PhD

Feminist Theories and Feminist Psychotherapies
Origins, Themes, and Diversity
Second Edition

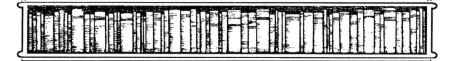

More pre-publication
REVIEWS, COMMENTARIES, EVALUATIONS . . .

"**D**r. Enns demonstrates that thorough, exceptional scholarship can be highly readable and applicable. She engages the reader while reviewing the political history of the women's movement in the United States and the resultant impact on the development of psychological theory, treatment, and assessment. She has successfully interwoven the literature on feminist philosophy with that of feminist therapy. The use of self-assessment inventories helps the reader apply and integrate each of the theoretical concepts presented.

One of the many strengths of this book is Dr. Enns' review of the development and evolution of multicultural theories. Another is her attention to the international women's movement. This new edition is not just a reworking of the previous book. Dr. Enns has added significantly to her original work, especially in terms of bringing the reader up to speed regarding present-day developments. Once again, Dr. Enns has made a major contribution to the field. This second edition is an outstanding update. It is listed first on my must-read and must-own lists for psychology students, mental health professionals, plus students and professionals in women's studies."

Elaine L. Phillips, PhD
Professor and Licensed Psychologist,
University Counseling and Testing Center,
Western Michigan University

"**D**r. Enns seeks to integrate feminist theory with feminist therapeutic practice, not a simple task given the large number and immense complexity of feminist theoretical thinking. In this second edition, within each chapter, she creates clear connections between specific feminist theories and therapeutic practice dimensions consistent with those feminist theories. She teases apart differences and similarities across theories with great care and nuance. Of special interest are her updated and new chapters focused on women-of-color feminisms, global feminisms, postmodern feminisms, lesbian/queer feminisms, and third-wave feminisms. Dr. Enns makes it absolutely clear that the therapist's theoretical orientation 'creates, names, and defines reality' in practice for both the therapist and client. I agree wholeheartedly with Enns' statement that 'becoming fully informed about the intersections of feminist theory and therapy requires significant personal commitment and effort' (p. 2). Such commitment and effort is made much easier because this book exists."

Linda M. Forrest, PhD
Associate Dean,
College of Education,
University of Oregon

More pre-publication
REVIEWS, COMMENTARIES, EVALUATIONS . . .

"**D**r. Enns has outdone herself in this second edition of her important book. It's not unusual today for students of feminist therapy practice to encounter the field without a clear understanding of the roots and heritage of feminist practice, which can lead to misperceptions and misapplications of feminist principles. Dr. Enns gives us an important, invaluable historical overview of feminist practice. Her book allows readers to see the organic processes by which feminist practice developed, and to appreciate the depth and complexity of what is meant by the term 'feminist.' The revision of this book to include sections on global and postmodern feminisms and their impact on feminist practice are particularly valuable to the seasoned reader. Enns' willingness to continue to challenge herself and her readers to expand their definitions of 'feminist' and 'feminist practice' is an important part of keeping the field alive, vital, and responsive to our roots as agents of social justice and social change."

Laura S. Brown, PhD, ABPP
Professor of Psychology,
Argosy University, Seattle

"**F**eminist Theories and Feminist Psychotherapies* is an insider's guide to thirty-five years of North American feminisms and feminist therapies. Dr. Enns' capacious, astute, and inspiring overview of feminist therapies takes us from the rambunctious, rebellious 1960s to the present. Her gracious eclecticism highlights continuities and connections among the diverse therapeutic practices inspired by North American feminism thought. Intended for feminist practitioners, the book steers clear of psychological jargon, high theory, and psychobabble. It invites feminist psychologists to ponder our theoretical, philosophical, and ethical commitments, as well as our practices. It deepens our appreciation of our history and awakens us to vibrant possibilities of a global feminism of the future.

If you enjoyed the first edition of *Feminist Theories and Feminist Psychotherapies,* you'll welcome this expanded and thoroughly updated version."

Jeanne Marecek, PhD
William Rand Kenan Professor,
Swarthmore College

The Haworth Press®
New York • London • Oxford

Feminist Theories and Feminist Psychotherapies
Origins, Themes, and Diversity
Second Edition

HAWORTH Innovations in Feminist Studies
J. Dianne Garner
Senior Editor

Women and AIDS: Negotiating Safer Practices, Care, and Representation edited by Nancy L. Roth and Linda K. Fuller

A Menopausal Memoir: Letters from Another Climate by Anne Herrmann

Women in the Antarctic edited by Esther D. Rothblum, Jacqueline S. Weinstock, and Jessica F. Morris

Breasts: The Women's Perspective on an American Obsession by Carolyn Latteier

Lesbian Stepfamilies: An Ethnography of Love by Janet M. Wright

Women, Families, and Feminist Politics: A Global Exploration by Kate Conway-Turner and Suzanne Cherrin

Women's Work: A Survey of Scholarship by and About Women edited by Donna Musialowski Ashcraft

Love Matters: A Book of Lesbian Romance and Relationships by Linda Sutton

Birth As a Healing Experience: The Emotional Journey of Pregnancy Through Postpartum by Lois Halzel Freedman

Unbroken Homes: Single-Parent Mothers Tell Their Stories by Wendy Anne Paterson

Transforming the Disciplines: A Women's Studies Primer edited by Elizabeth L. MacNabb, Mary Jane Cherry, Susan L. Popham, and René Perry Prys

Women at the Margins: Neglect, Punishment, and Resistance edited by Josephina Figueira-McDonough and Rosemary C. Sarri

Women's Best Friendships: Beyond Betty, Veronica, Thelma, and Louise by Patricia Rind

Women, Power, and Ethnicity: Working Toward Reciprocal Empowerment by Patricia S. E. Darlington and Becky Michele Mulvaney

The Way of the Woman Writer, Second Edition by Janet Lynn Roseman

Feminist Theories and Feminist Psychotherapies: Origins, Themes, and Diversity, Second Edition by Carolyn Zerbe Enns

Lives of Lesbian Elders: Looking Back, Looking Forward by D. Merilee Clunis, Karen I. Fredriksen-Goldsen, Pat A. Freeman, and Nancy Nystrom

Feminist Theories and Feminist Psychotherapies
Origins, Themes, and Diversity
Second Edition

Carolyn Zerbe Enns, PhD

The Haworth Press®
New York • London • Oxford

Second edition of *Feminist Theories and Feminist Psychotherapies: Origins, Themes, and Variations* (Harrington Park Press, 1997).

The Haworth Press, Inc., 10 Alice Street, Binghamton, NY 13904-1580.

Cover design by Marylouise E. Doyle.

Library of Congress Cataloging-in-Publication Data

Enns, Carolyn Zerbe.
    Feminist theories and feminist psychotherapies : origins, themes, and diversity / Carolyn Zerbe Enns—2nd ed.
        p. cm.
    Includes bibliographical references and index.
    ISBN 0-7890-1807-1 (case : alk. paper)—ISBN 0-7890-1808-X (soft : alk. paper)
    1. Feminist therapy. 2. Feminist theory. I. Title.
RC489.F45E56 2004
616.89'14'082—dc22
                                                                                    2003022211

CONTENTS

Acknowledgments

I am grateful to Cornell College for sabbatical leave, which provided me with the necessary time to complete the major revision of this book. The Cornell College McConnell Fellowship also funded my travel and study in Japan, which is reflected in this edition's chapter on global feminist theories and feminist therapy in Japan. I am indebted to many feminist friends, students, mentors, and colleagues who are from my local college community or have been co-participants in various feminist and multicultural mental health, educational, and psychological associations within North America and throughout the world. You are too numerous to name in this brief statement. Thank you for emotional and practical support, helping me clarify and refine my ideas, and facilitating my understanding of lived multicultural feminist practice. Thanks also to my daughters, Larissa and Jessica, who teach me about the challenges facing young adult feminist women today, and to Rich, who has shared (or at least tolerated) my dreams and intellectual curiosities for over thirty years.

ABOUT THE AUTHOR

Carolyn Zerbe Enns, PhD, is Professor of Psychology and co-chair of the Women's Studies program at Cornell College in Mt. Vernon, Iowa. She is a licensed psychologist in the state of Iowa. She teaches a wide range of courses, including Personality Theories, Psychology of Women, Feminist Theories, and Multicultural Psychology. The inclusion of multicultural and feminist content is important in all of her teaching activities. Since 1987, she has published approximately forty articles and chapters on the topic of feminist or multicultural practice in psychology. In 1997, she published the first edition of *Feminist Theories and Psychotherapies: Origins, Themes, and Variations.*

Dr. Enns is the current chair (2002-2004) of the American Psychological Association (APA) Division 17 (Counseling Psychology) Section for the Advancement of Women. She is also a co-chair of the APA Interdivisional Task Force to Develop Guidelines for Counseling/Psychotherapy with Women. This task force recently completed its draft of "Guidelines for Psychological Practice with Girls and Women." She also chaired the APA Division 17 Task Force on Memories of Child Sexual Abuse and the APA Division 35 Psychotherapy with Women Award committee. In 1998, Dr. Enns received the "Woman of the Year" award from the Section for the Advancement of Women of Division 17 of the APA, and was elected to Fellow status in Divisions 35 and 17.

Introduction

This book is the product of a twenty-year journey and my personal desire to integrate the literatures on feminist theory and feminist therapy. I first identified myself as a feminist therapist while I was completing my doctoral degree in counseling psychology during the mid-1980s. During my first semester of doctoral study, I was fortunate to gain exposure to the classic feminist statements on feminist therapy. These commentaries shaped all other aspects of my graduate education. They affirmed my life experiences, influenced my research interests, and played an orienting function throughout my graduate training and subsequent work.

To expand my frame of reference, I gradually immersed myself in various writings associated with feminist interdisciplinary scholarship and theory. I was surprised at the absence of cross-referencing and integration between the two literatures of feminist theory and therapy. I was also impressed with the diversity of feminist thought and conflicting ideas within feminist theory about causes of oppression, goals of feminism, and solutions to problems marked by sexism and the intersecting "isms" of racism, classism, heterosexism, anti-Semitism, ageism, and colonialism. Although authors who discussed feminist therapy noted that their work was informed by feminist theory and philosophy, they rarely discussed how specific theories informed their practice. Ellyn Kaschak's (1981) review of the first decade of feminist therapy was one of the few documents to explicitly note the differences between nonsexist therapy, liberal feminist therapy, grassroots feminist therapy, and radical feminist therapy.

As I became more familiar with feminist therapy and theory literatures, the reasons for the absence of integrated statements on feminist therapy and philosophy became more apparent. First, some feminists resisted defining feminist therapy or connecting it to theory because these activities were seen as "fetishizing a merely intellectual distinction" at a time when "feminist therapy does not need definition so much as decision" (Chase, 1977, p. 22). Consistent with many feminist therapists' goals of participating in social change, early work focused less on "what feminist therapy is but what happens in it" (Lerman, 1976, p. 378). Second, feminist theorists and feminist therapists often come from substantially different academic backgrounds and personal experiences and tend to use different vocabularies or "languages" to communicate their ideas. For example, many feminist theorists have been trained in the humanities whereas many feminist therapists are more comfortable with the methodologies and vocabularies associated with the social sciences. As a result, many writings on feminist theory are not easily digested by feminist therapists, and feminist therapists sometimes remain unfamiliar with many major theoretical and philosophical perspectives on feminism. Furthermore, few opportunities are available during counselor and psychotherapy training programs to participate in the interdisciplinary exploration of feminist thought. Becoming fully informed about the intersections of feminist theory and therapy requires significant personal commitment and effort.

Since the early years of feminist therapy history, authors of feminist counseling and psychotherapy texts have increasingly acknowledged the different feminist theoretical positions that influence the work of feminist therapists (e.g., Worell and Remer, 2003), and feminist psychologists have articulated central features of a feminist theory of psychological practice (Brabeck and Brown, 1997). However, limited attention has been devoted to the specific interdisciplinary feminist theoretical approaches that provide a foundation for a feminist therapy which seeks to be attentive to the complexity and diversity of people's lives. The goal, then, of this book is to provide readers with a brief overview of major feminist theoretical perspectives and to link these theoretical views to applications of feminist therapy that are consistent with these views.

I encourage readers to use this book in combination with a wide range of other books on feminist theory and psychotherapy such as (but not limited to) Laura Brown's (1994) *Subversive Dialogues;* Ellyn Kaschak's (1992) *Engendered Lives;* Lillian Comas-Díaz and Beverly Greene's (1994b) *Women of Color;* Christine Saulnier's (1996) *Feminist Theories and Social Work;* Lucia Gilbert and Murray Scher's (1999) *Gender and Sex in Counseling and Psychotherapy;* Leslie Jackson and Beverly Greene's (2000) edited volume *Psychotherapy with African American Women;* Jeanne Adleman and Gloria Enguídanos' (1995) edited volume *Racism in the Lives of Women;*

Testimony, Theory, and Guides to Antiracist Practice; Jean Baker Miller and Irene Stiver's (1997) *The Healing Connection: How Women Form Relationships in Therapy and in Life;* Judith Worell and Pam Remer's (2003) *Feminist Perspectives in Therapy: Empowering Diverse Women,* Second Edition; Judith Worell and Norine Johnson's (1997) edited volume *Shaping the Future of Feminist Psychology;* Laura Brown and Mary Ballou's (1992) edited volume *Personality and Psychopathology: Feminist Reappraisals* and their most recent edited volume titled *Rethinking Mental Health and Disorder: Feminist Perspectives* (Ballou and Brown, 2002). Each of these books presents rich theoretical bases and practical information about implementing feminist principles of practice.

In contrast to other texts on feminist therapy, this book draws extensively on interdisciplinary scholarship. It focuses on the evolution of feminist therapy and how historical and current feminist practice interconnects with feminist theoretical and political thought. It is not a book about how to implement feminist techniques, which are discussed in many other sources, but represents an effort to provide a brief introduction to feminist thought and to discuss the compatibilities of psychological theories and feminist therapy techniques with the various feminist theories. It also traces the "herstory" of feminist thought and feminist therapy so that practicing feminist therapists can understand the relationship of their work to principles and practices first implemented in the 1960s and 1970s. My hope is that the various overviews and summaries contained herein will provide readers with the background that is necessary to explore connections between feminist theory and therapy in greater depth. In other words, the descriptions provided are brief and cursory. After reading this book, I hope feminist therapists will read many of the original works that are briefly summarized in the following chapters.

The first edition of this book was published in 1997, and I fully expected that it would be both the first and final edition of the book. Within several years of its publication, however, I became convinced that the contents provided a decent but dated overview of the diverse approaches to feminist theory and therapy. As I reviewed the depth and range of new feminist theory, research, and application, it seemed to me that it might be unethical *not* to undertake a new edition. Some of the most impressive growth in feminist conceptual frameworks has appeared in the writings of women of color, lesbian and queer feminists, global/transnational feminists, third-wave feminists, and postmodern feminists. Many of these recent feminisms provide significant insight about the experiences and needs of specific groups of women within North America and around the world. In addition, they have called for more flexible frameworks that emphasize the intersecting social identities, oppressions, and privileges which influence women's and men's experiences. Many of the recent theories have spoken about ways to transcend ethnocentrism and subtle "isms" within feminist thought, and attending to these themes is of critical importance if feminist therapy approaches are to transform psychotherapy practice.

The explosion of theory, research, and applications relevant to the experiences of women can be overwhelming, and it is difficult to stay current about the many exciting theories, models, and research that are relevant to feminist practice. My hope is that this second edition retains important coverage of the foundations and enduring themes on feminist theory and therapy while also providing insight about new models that contribute to a maturing field. I have attempted to accomplish this task without adding substantially to the length of the original book, and this has been a truly daunting task. It has been difficult to eliminate some original material because I have not wanted to contribute to the erasure of formative writings in feminist theory and feminist therapy. I have completed a substantial revision of each chapter of the original book and have included completely new chapters or sections of chapters on postmodern feminism, global feminism, third-wave feminism, lesbian/queer feminism, and women-of-color feminisms. In the first edition of this book, I devoted the first chapters to a review of feminist theory per se, which were followed by a series of chapters on specific approaches to feminist therapy. In this edition, I have summarized feminist theories and their therapeutic connections in a single chapter, and I hope this approach helps readers draw more clear connections between theory and practice.

Chapter 1 describes consensus values of feminist therapy. Although these values and practices are interpreted in diverse ways, the elaboration of shared principles is important as a foundation for later chapters. Chapter 1 is intended to provide an introduction for those with limited or no background in feminist therapy, and a review for those with more extensive background in feminist therapy. Chapter 2 provides a brief summary of liberal feminist therapy and its impact on psychotherapy. Kathleen Crowley-Long (1998) has argued that liberal feminism is the dominant framework in psychology of women, and consistent with its impact on feminist psychology in general, it provides a framework that is consistent with many approaches to counseling and psychotherapy. Chapter 3 provides a summary of the second-wave social change approaches of radical and socialist feminism, and then describes a variety of feminist therapy approaches that have sought to transform the psychotherapy of women. Chapters 4, 5, 6, and 7 follow a similar pattern, focusing on the impact of cultural feminist theory on cultural feminist therapies (Chapter 4); the women-of-color feminisms and their influence on multicultural and inclusive feminist therapy (Chapter 5); global feminisms and their impact on feminist therapy around the world (Chapter 6); and the postmodern, lesbian, and third-wave feminisms and their emphases on rethinking the impact of intersecting social identities in feminist therapy (Chapter 7). Chapter 8 examines methods for thinking in an integrated manner about theory and therapy and for formulating a personal approach to feminist counseling and psychotherapy. Chapters 1 through 7 also include short self-assessment questionnaires that readers may use to reflect on their own orientations to feminist therapy and feminist theory.

I believe that it is important for me to provide brief commentary about my choice to capitalize and not capitalize adjectives or words that refer to women's identities (e.g., white, Black). In general, I followed the lead of previous contributors to feminist theory and therapy. For example, many influential Black feminist authors have capitalized *Black* because it refers to a specific form of theory and identity within women-of-color feminisms. Thus, I chose to capitalize all references to specific identities and specific feminisms of women of color, such as Black feminism and Asian-American feminism. In contrast, I have not capitalized the labels *white* women and *women of color* because they refer to general groups of women or groups of approaches.

It is important to note that the boundaries between the various feminist theories and therapies are not rigid but fluid and continually changing. It is somewhat artificial to divide the various feminisms into the categories and chapters I use in this book. However, for the purpose of helping readers organize their thinking, I have arranged material into specific categories. I hope that readers can view these categories as a work in progress and as flexible, not confining. I have used a "best-fit" approach and embedded the discussion of specific psychotherapy approaches at points where the linkages seemed most logical. Another author with a different set of assumptions and life experiences may organize these connections in a different manner. For example, some of the psychotherapy techniques that I discuss in the chapters on liberal, radical, and socialist feminisms and feminist therapy may be relevant to a variety of other chapters and integrative approaches to theory and therapy.

Postmodern feminisms have warned against creating bipolar categories, and remind us of the fluidity of boundaries and the tentative nature of "truth." In keeping with this principle, I ask readers to view my structure as a tentative framework that is open to modification and change as new advances in theory, research, and application continue to emerge. To encourage feminist therapists to think comprehensively about the frameworks that inform their work, my goal is to show that coherent connections between specific feminist theories and feminist practices can be drawn. However, the specific academic and personal experiences of each person influence the organizational framework that is most meaningful to the individual reader. I encourage readers to maintain a flexible and open frame of references as they think about the most useful intersections between feminist theory and feminist therapy that can inform their work.

Chapter 1

Principles of Feminist Therapy

A carefully articulated and coherent theoretical grounding in feminist theory provides support for purposeful and ethical feminist practice. Feminist theory provides a lens for making one's assumptions visible and transparent, which allows the therapist to practice with assurance as well as evaluate her or his actions on an ongoing basis (Halifax, 1997). In preparation for discussing the diversity of theory and practice in feminist therapy, this chapter describes the complexity of feminist therapy and summarizes the common principles and practices shared by feminist counselors and therapists. These commonalities include (1) a conceptual framework for understanding problems, (2) basic principles of feminist therapy as they relate to the therapeutic relationship and the goals of feminist therapy, and (3) distinctive techniques of feminist therapy. In this chapter, I refer to many of the original definitions of feminist therapy from the 1970s and 1980s in order to preserve the "herstory" and enduring, shared themes of feminist therapy. To demonstrate the continuity of central principles over time as well as emerging themes, I also cite recent definitions that build on original and influential statements about feminist therapy.

THE COMPLEXITY, DIVERSITY, AND VARIATIONS OF FEMINIST THERAPY

Feminist therapy has existed as an approach to psychotherapy since the early 1970s. At its most basic level, feminist therapy represents a conceptual framework for organizing assumptions about counseling and psychotherapy (Ballou and Gabalac, 1985; Ballou and West, 2000; Johnson, 1976; Kaschak, 1981; Marecek, 2001; Worell and Remer, 2003). Feminism, an important foundation of feminist therapy, is defined by bell hooks (2000) as "a movement to end sexism, sexist exploitation, and oppression" (p. 1). Feminist consciousness also includes a commitment to ending all forms of domination, oppression, and privilege that intersect with sexism and gender bias, including (but not limited to) racism, classism, colonialism, heterosexism, ethnocentrism, white supremacy, ageism, and ableism. Feminism empowers all people, including men, to build a world in which equality is experienced at individual, interpersonal, institutional, national, and global levels (hooks, 1981, 2000). This principle of inclusiveness is highlighted by the title of bell hooks' (2000) book *Feminism Is for Everybody.* Mary Ballou and Carolyn West (2000) added that "feminist therapy is unwaveringly rooted in the search for and valuing of ALL women's experiences" (p. 274).

Feminist therapy approaches were initially developed for women in order to correct the negative effects of sexism and bias in psychological theory, diagnosis, and practice, and to ensure that women gained access to gender-aware and gender-sensitive mental health services (Chesler, 1972; Weisstein, [1968] 1993). Because feminist therapy was developed initially by and for women, and because women are more likely than men to identify themselves as feminist therapists and to be consumers of feminist therapy, I often use pronouns that refer to women. However, the principles and practices of feminist psychotherapy are valuable for working with men, members of diverse cultures and racial backgrounds, and all those who view social justice issues as important to counseling and psychotherapy (Enns, 2000; Worell and Remer, 2003).

Feminist therapy was not founded by or connected to any specific person, theoretical position, or set of techniques (Brown and Brodsky, 1992). As stated by Deborah Leupnitz (1988), "Feminism is not a set of therapeutic techniques but a sensibility, a political and aesthetic center that informs a work pervasively" (p. 231). Feminism provides an umbrella framework, or a set of values for evaluating and orienting practice. Feminist counselors integrate complex bodies of knowledge about social structures, counseling methods, feminism, and the diversity of men's and women's lives. A wide variety of personality and counseling theories can be incorporated within a feminist approach (Dutton-Douglas and Walker, 1988; Rawlings and Carter, 1977); the only tools rejected by feminist therapists are techniques which are immersed in sexist theory or which encourage women and men to think in narrow, restricted ways about themselves and their options (Lerman, 1986; Rawlings and Carter, 1977). Thus, multiple forms of feminist counseling exist and are based on the unique combination of the counselor's feminist orientation and counseling approach (Ballou and West, 2000; Dutton-Douglas and Walker, 1988; Worell and Remer, 2003). Although all theories of feminism focus on the importance of equality, beliefs about how equality can be achieved vary substantially; the counselor's personal view of feminism is likely to have a significant impact on how feminist counseling is interpreted and conducted (Enns, 1992b; Kaschak, 1981).

On first glance, it may appear that combining feminist beliefs with feminist counseling is a fairly straightforward and uncomplicated task. Some individuals may conclude that because feminist theory is diverse and because multiple approaches to counseling exist, any mixture of feminism and counseling and psychotherapy theory is acceptable. However, the competent feminist therapist understands that effective feminist counseling is based on an ongoing and continuous examination of personal values, consistency between one's theoretical orientations to feminism and counseling, and an understanding of how intersections of gender, race, class, economic status, and sexual orientation influence women's and men's lives (Ballou, Matsumoto, and Wagner, 2002; Brabeck and Brown, 1997; Feminist Therapy Institute [FTI], 2000; Brown and Brodsky, 1992; Wyche and Rice, 1997). When the "deep" integration of feminist principles and feminist theory occurs, feminist therapy is not just good therapy with gender awareness added; it becomes "a complete transformation of the way in which therapy is understood and practiced" (Hill and Ballou, 1998, p. 5).

In order to develop a fully integrated feminist counseling approach, it is important for the therapist to have working knowledge of a variety of academic and applied fields of study. These disciplines include but are not limited to the psychology of women and gender; women's, gender, and sexuality studies; ethnic, multicultural, and global development studies; counseling and psychotherapy theories; sociological perspectives on gender, race, and class; and political science and social change strategies. Significant knowledge, research, and new theoretical work continue to proliferate within each of the fields that deal with gender issues; the task of staying informed about new developments is an ongoing challenge for persons who integrate feminism with counseling and psychotherapy. Laura Brown's (1994) definition of feminist therapy emphasizes the necessity of depth and breadth of preparation:

> Feminist therapy is the practice of therapy informed by feminist political philosophy and analysis, grounded in multicultural feminist scholarship on the psychology of women and gender, which leads both therapist and client toward strategies and solutions advancing feminist resistance, transformation, and social change in daily personal life, and in relationships with the social, emotional, and political environment. (pp. 21-22)

Therapists and clients are less likely to view feminism as a monolithic, prescriptive, or confining system of "politically correct" or formulaic views when feminist therapists recognize the variations of feminist theory and are able to communicate their complexity. Within feminism, there is room for diversity of practice and the opportunity for individuals to articulate a set of beliefs which are personally meaningful and which guide transformational practice.

A FEMINIST APPROACH
TO UNDERSTANDING PROBLEMS

Feminist therapists hold several distinctive beliefs or assumptions about the problems of living, and these assumptions can be succinctly summarized under the following two themes: (1) the personal is political, and (2) problems and symptoms often arise as methods of coping with and surviving in oppressive circumstances. Consistent with these themes, Bonnie Moradi and colleagues (2000) found that self-labeled feminist therapists were more likely than other therapists to endorse behaviors which reflect the belief that the personal is political. Second, those who most strongly identified themselves as feminist therapists reported greater likelihood of attending to oppressions experienced by clients (e.g., racism, heterosexism, sexism) (Moradi et al., 2000).

The Personal Is Political

The "personal is political" conveys the assumption that personal problems are often connected to or influenced by the political and social climate in which people live. Many feminist therapists prefer to use the phrases *problems in living* or *coping strategies* rather than the term *pathology* to communicate the feminist view that counseling issues are inextricably connected to the social, political, economic, and institutional factors which influence personal choices (Brabeck and Brown, 1997; Butler, 1985; Gilbert, 1980; Wyche and Rice, 1997). Laura Brown (1992a) suggested that many of the problems experienced by persons with limited power in society can be conceptualized as reactions to oppression or "oppression artifact disorders." These disorders reflect the psychological aftermath of stressors that are "embedded in the framework of the culture in which an individual develops" (p. 223) and, as a result, "may be subtle and difficult for either therapist or client to immediately identify" (p. 223). Building initial support for the connection between commonplace discrimination and psychological symptoms, a recent study (Klonoff, Landrine, and Campbell, 2000) found that compared to male respondents and women who indicated they had encountered little sexism, women who conveyed they had experienced frequent sexist discrimination reported significantly more psychological symptoms, such as somatization, interpersonal sensitivity, depression, anxiety, and obsessive-compulsive symptoms.

Intrapsychic explanations of problems and most diagnostic labels based within a medical model tend to decontextualize problems, support gender bias, or promote victim blaming. When counselors and therapists rely solely on traditional diagnostic labels, they are more likely to define problems as a set of internal characteristics and to emphasize goals that focus on overhauling internal deficiencies rather than promote healthy change and the alteration of oppressive environmental conditions. If clients are encouraged to look exclusively inside themselves for clues about the origins and dynamics of their problems, they are also more inclined to blame themselves, and to respond by adjusting to or changing themselves to fit the circumstances around them (Greenspan, 1993; Rawlings and Carter, 1977).

Because most formal diagnoses tend to label individuals without regard to contextual factors, feminist therapists face the challenge of negotiating complicated terrain. Health insurance reimbursement practices often require the use of diagnostic labels as outlined by the most recent edition of the American Psychiatric Association's (2000) *Diagnostic and Statistical Manual of Mental Disorders,* Fourth Edition, Text Revision (DSM-IV-TR). Many feminist therapists believe that such labeling involves "pigeonholing" women's concerns (Lerman, 1996); reducing "a complex set of social, economic, emotional and spiritual dimensions to the terms of a single diagnosis" (Greenspan, 1993, p. xxxi); "pathologizing nonmainstream behaviors and attitudes" (Kupers, 1997, p. 340); or, at a minimum, limiting the therapist's ability to honor the context and personal meaning of a client's concerns. As a result, many feminist therapists view themselves as engaging in "subversive practices" (Beardsley et al., 1998; Brown, 1994), which include using traditional diagnoses for the pragmatic purpose of ensuring that clients receive insurance coverage, but being open and honest with clients about the costs and benefits of such diagnoses, and collaborating with clients in identifying diagnostic categories that the clients view as nonoffensive (Ballou and West, 2000).

In addition to exploring external and contextual factors which contribute to problems is a hallmark of feminist therapy, feminist counselors and therapists attend to physiological, psychological, and intrapsychic factors that interact with external forces (Brown and Brodsky, 1992; Brown, 1994). For example, both the 1990 American Psychological Association Task Force on Women and Depression (McGrath et al., 1990) and the 2000 American Psychiatric Association Summit on Women and Depression (Mazure, Keita, and Blehar, 2002) recommended a biopsychosocial approach to working with depressed women (see also Sprock and Yoder, 1997). Through feminist analysis, clients learn to distinguish between internal/psychological and external/social aspects of the issues they are dealing with, and to identify both personal change and social change strategies that can be used to deal with these respective areas (Brown, 1994; Gilbert, 1980). More recently, Mary Ballou and colleagues Atsushi Matsumoto and Michael Wagner (2002) expanded this approach by proposing a feminist ecological model, which attends to individual dimensions, micro-level concerns (immediate interpersonal themes), exosystem concerns (e.g., those which are influenced by educational, political, religious, cultural, and ethnic systems), and macrosystem themes (e.g., world-views, ideologies, global issues).

In their work with major issues such as depression, many counselors and therapists who are trained in prominent (and dominant) psychotherapy traditions deal primarily with internal cognitive and emotional patterns that reinforce depression; their professional education often prepares them to focus primarily on the psychology of the individual. However, feminist counselors recognize that women who are especially vulnerable to depression include those who have experienced sexual and physical abuse, live in poverty, work in lower status employment positions, or are mothers of young children (Mazure, Keita, and Blehar, 2002; McGrath et al., 1990; Sprock and Yoder, 1997). Some of these factors can be influenced only through legal and social changes. These connections between internal and external worlds illustrate that the personal is clearly political; the cognitive, emotional, and behavioral changes that women make must be matched with institutional changes. As noted by Marcia Hill and Mary Ballou (1998), "the ultimate intention of feminist therapy is to create social change" (p. 3).

Symptoms As Communication and Coping Tools

Feminist counselors view clients as individuals coping with life events to the best of their ability. Many symptoms represent "normal" reactions to a restrictive environment (Greenspan, 1993). In her classic statement on the goals of feminist therapy, Marjorie Klein (1976) noted, "Not all symptoms are neurotic. Pain in response to a bad situation is adaptive, not pathological" (p. 90). Feminist therapists highlight the communication function of symptoms by defining them as behaviors that arise out of a desire to influence an environment that is constricting or oppressive. For example, symptoms may emerge as a consequence of coping with conflicting nontraditional and traditional demands of multiple roles. Alternatively, symptoms often reflect influence strategies that were taught or modeled by others in the environment, such as parents, peers, the media, schools, and intimate others. Coping behaviors that were functional or had survival value at one life stage may become less successful over time and contribute to the person's distress as the client attempts to meet life tasks that require different or new skills (Greenspan, 1993).

For example, a symptom such as dependency may be a reaction to inequality. A person with limited power and influence attempts to vicariously experience some semblance of power by attaching herself or himself to people who hold greater power (Hare-Mustin and Marecek, 1986). If direct forms of power are not available to a person, she or he is likely to rely on "devious" strategies such as dependency, acquiescence, or manipulation (Gannon, 1982). However, the costs of such strategies are high, and they may increase one's vulnerability to a range of problems such as depression and anxiety. When the focus of counseling is to label and remove a symptom without understanding the context in which it was shaped and the current context in which it is reinforced, clients may be deprived of the indirect influence of symptoms, such as dependency. Individuals may, in fact, feel even less powerful after counseling than before counseling (Halleck, 1971). Rather than viewing symptoms such as depression, dependency, anxiety, or passivity as problems to be eliminated, the feminist counselor views these patterns as indirect forms of expression that can be refocused in more direct and productive forms of communication as a client gains a stronger sense of self (Smith and Siegel, 1985; Rawlings and Carter, 1977). It is also helpful to reframe concepts such as dependency as "a process of counting on other people to provide help in coping physically and emotionally with the experiences and tasks encountered in the world when one has not sufficient skill, confidence, energy, and/or time" (Stiver, 1991, p. 160). Redefining dependency in this manner identifies the healthy and normal aspects of this behavior, highlights ways in which it may promote growth rather than stagnation, and frees the individual to try out a wider range of and more flexible behaviors.

The feminist therapist is also aware that symptoms are reinforced by one's environment, and that change is not as simple as "being more assertive." For example, acquiescent individuals may protect partners with more power by providing them with opportunities to play leadership, protector, and hero roles; these roles support and affirm their self-concepts as independent and active persons (Lerner, 1983). One of the counseling strategies that may support greater self-esteem as well as openness to change is the reframing of "dependency" or "passivity" as sensitivity and responsiveness to relational cues. Such redefinition may help clients see these qualities as attributes they may want to modify or redirect rather than those they must reject. It is also helpful for the therapist and client to discuss the connection between the personal and political, or the fact that the culture, which often undervalues relational and responsive qualities, "dangerously strains a woman's ability to meet basic needs for interpersonal relatedness, while maintaining a positive sense of self" (Jack, 1987, p. 44). This type of definition may limit the client's self-blame and may support brainstorming about creative change options.

The feminist counselor also helps the client consider the complexity of negotiating change. For example, change on the part of the relationally oriented ("dependent") person will require that others within her or his social network accept more responsibility for fulfilling socially undervalued roles such as parenting, listening, and other forms of nurturing. The client who makes personal changes and chooses to engage in more independent, assertive, or direct action may experience resistance or the mislabeling of these behaviors as aggressive, selfish, angry, or "bitchy" (Fodor and Rothblum, 1984). In feminist therapy, it is important for therapists and clients to consider the costs, benefits, and consequences of change (Fodor and Rothblum, 1984; Rawlings and Carter, 1977).

A Feminist Framework for Conceptualizing Problems: Two Examples

The following section provides two examples of how feminist therapists incorporate the principles of (1) the personal is political and (2) symptoms as coping mechanisms. The examples apply these principles in conceptualizing problems related to child sexual abuse and eating disorders.

Symptoms Related to Child Sexual Abuse

Feminist researchers Susan Morrow and Mary Lee Smith (1995, p. 25) asked the following question of women who had experienced child sexual abuse: "What were the primary ways in which you survived?" The qualitative analysis of interviews and focus-group interactions revealed two major categories of survival strategies: (1) protecting oneself from becoming overwhelmed by dangerous and threatening feelings related to abuse and (2) managing experiences and feelings of powerlessness, helplessness, and lack of control. The first category included skills of avoiding or decreasing the intensity of feelings through methods such as becoming numb, using alcohol or food to cope, exchanging unmanageable experiences (such as terror) for less intense emotions (such as depression), seeking sex for validation, compartmentalizing emotions and separating them from sensations or thoughts, or excusing perpetrators and minimizing abuse. Strategies for escaping feelings also included a wide range of activities such as physically separating from others through isolation, using dissociation to mentally shut out memories or distance themselves from their bodies, and using self-induced physical pain or self-mutilation to block out or control emotional pain. Although many of these behaviors are labeled as "dysfunctional" ways of coping with stress, they played useful functional survival roles.

Women who had experienced child sexual abuse also developed a wide range of methods for increasing their sense of control by implementing strategies of resistance or rebellion, such as by refusing to eat, or binging and purging; increasing mastery or control over other areas of life, such as by managing the household, excelling in school, or rescuing others; or creating their own pain (e.g., self-cutting), an activity that reinforced the notion that "If I am able to create my own pain, I can manage this pain." In summary, this study found that research participants' symptoms held significant personal meaning and played an important role in coping and survival. However, the success of these strategies was also costly, often leading them to feel fragmented, exhausted, or in a perpetual state of pain (Morrow and Smith, 1995). The goal of feminist therapy is to help women rechannel the energy devoted to these forms of surviving to methods that support a more integrated sense of self, as well as a greater sense of aliveness, wholeness, and health.

Clients who have experienced child sexual abuse often experience a complex array of symptoms and coping skills, such as those described by Sue Morrow and Mary Lee Smith (1995), which may be indicative of a shattered sense of self and which are often labeled as borderline personality disorder. Unfortunately, although several major studies reveal that between 60 and 80 percent of those labeled borderline are victims of abuse (Layton, 1995), this label does not focus on the relationship of symptoms to the "crazy-making" environments that may have fostered the symptoms. Instead, borderline personality disorder has become "a code word for trouble" and "signals a kind of impossible case" (Layton, 1995, p. 36), which may encourage therapists to provide less than empathic treatment. As noted by Laura Brown (1994), "if you call it a skunk, you will assume that it smells" (p. 131). Reflecting her concern for accurate conceptualization, feminist psychologist Dusty Miller (1995) argued that borderline personality disorder is a misdiagnosis for what she believes should be more accurately referred to as *trauma reenactment syndrome*. Molly Layton (1995) added that "viewing borderline traits as the fallout of real suffering ineluctably shifts therapy from a mission impossible with irredeemable clients to a mutually constructed, more empathically demanding task of naming and sizing the effects of trauma" (p. 39). Another alternative to the label *borderline* is *complex post-traumatic stress syndrome*. This conceptualization, proposed by Judith Herman (1992), links long-term trauma in intimate relationships to a complex array of symptoms (many of which could be called borderline) that involve alterations in affect regulation, consciousness, self-perception, meaning systems, and relations to others. It is important to note that feminist therapists hold diverse opinions about diagnosis and about the use of labels such as borderline personality disorder (Becker, 2000, 2001). The philosophical differences underlying conceptualization and diagnosis are discussed in Chapters 2, 3, and 8.

Feminist Perspectives on Eating Disorders

Feminist therapists have viewed eating disorders as related to cultural values and mandates, and over time, a series of feminist models have emerged for understanding how and why these problems develop, and enhancing our understanding of the relationship between culture and distress, as well as culture and coping. The culture-of-thinness perspective suggests that society puts forth thinness as the major precursor to having a happy and successful life; eating disorders become a method for securing this attractive life. A second option, the "weight as power and control" perspective, suggests that controlling one's weight is a method of gaining control in a world in which many things are uncontrollable. Eating disorders may also represent a form of coping that distracts women from difficult issues of major importance in their lives. A third perspective explores how eating disorders may be survival skills for dealing with anxieties about achievement. Achieving the perfect body may be a way to avoid negative stereotypes of high-achieving women as lonely, ruthless, unfeminine, or unattractive. Alternatively, women may try to achieve a small size and take up minimal physical space in order to ensure that men will not be threatened by their power or competence. A fourth hypothesis is the "eating disorders as self-definition" perspective, which proposes that a focus on the physical self may help compensate for having an underdeveloped psychological self (Gilbert and Thompson, 1996; Thompson et al., 1999). A fifth feminist model, objectification theory (Fredrickson and Roberts, 1997), focuses on the way in which society's objectification of women's bodies may increase women's vulnerabilities to a wide range of psychological issues, including eating disorders. According to this view, girls and women absorb the ubiquitous media culture of beauty, internalize this unrealistic perspective, and adopt an observer's view of themselves. This externalized view leads to constant body monitoring and body consciousness, which contributes to body shame and anxiety, the loss of internal signals of hunger and satiation, and the reduction of peak motivational states or "flow." Body objectification may lead to restrained eating and eating disorders, and it may also trigger anxiety, depression, and sexual problems.

Drawing on the lives of diverse women, including women of color and lesbians, Becky Thompson (1994) proposed that eating disorders are not only related to cultural pressures and ideals but often emerge as coping mechanisms at times of significant emotional strain. Thus, eating may allow a woman to "numb out" or shield herself from pain, distract herself, or experience comfort. In other words, eating problems are not only manifestations of conformity to culture but can also be active survival mechanisms when other coping methods are unavailable. Each of the perspectives described in this section has received some research support, and all may be useful for understanding the varied survival roles that eating disorders may play.

In contrast to these feminist models, typical or traditional treatment models of eating disorders emphasize the normalization and monitoring of weight, pharmacotherapy, family dynamics, cognitive-behavioral techniques, or interpersonal psychotherapy (Powers, 2002). Feminist therapists often utilize techniques associated with these models but seek to ensure that medical, family, cognitive, and interpersonal factors are not the only emphases of treatment. Each of these techniques is integrated with a conceptual focus and techniques that address the sociocultural dynamics supporting eating problems.

PRINCIPLES OF FEMINIST COUNSELING

Since the early 1970s, core principles regarding the psychotherapy relationship and goals of feminist counseling have been firmly established. The following summary describes four principles regarding the counseling relationship and six principles related to the goals of counseling. Each guideline is preceded by self-assessment questions that can be used to consider one's level of agreement with basic feminist counseling practices. A goal of this section is to highlight the history and enduring themes associated with feminist therapy. Elizabeth Scarborough and Laurel Furumoto (1987) noted that women's contributions to psychology have often been lost because of the filtering function of recent writings which often overshadow and lead to the invisibility of early contributions. In order to avoid this possibility, I cite both classic and recent sources in order to honor feminist therapy foremothers as well as the rich evolution and continuity of feminist thought.

The following descriptions reflect basic principles of feminist counseling and psychotherapy. Feminist therapists interpret these principles in multiple ways; some counselors place higher priority on some guidelines than others, depending on their theoretical orientations.

THE COUNSELING AND PSYCHOTHERAPY RELATIONSHIP

Relationship Principle One: The Therapist's Values

For all self-assessment items throughout this book, please indicate your level of agreement for each item by using the following scale:

do not agree at all	slightly agree	moderately agree	strongly agree	completely agree
1	2	3	4	5

_____ 1. It is not possible for the counselor to practice value-free or value-neutral counseling.

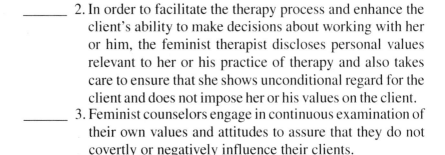

_____ 2. In order to facilitate the therapy process and enhance the client's ability to make decisions about working with her or him, the feminist therapist discloses personal values relevant to her or his practice of therapy and also takes care to ensure that she shows unconditional regard for the client and does not impose her or his values on the client.

_____ 3. Feminist counselors engage in continuous examination of their own values and attitudes to assure that they do not covertly or negatively influence their clients.

Each of these self-assessment items reflects important attitudes and values of feminist counseling and high endorsement reflects agreement with important feminist counseling goals. It is important that the self-disclosure of values (item 2) is based on the client's best interests, such as her or his readiness to hear and use the information effectively.

Feminist therapists believe that it is impossible to practice value-free counseling and, as a result, consider it important for counselors to clarify their values and understand the potential impact of their values on clients (Butler, 1985; FTI, 2000; Gilbert, 1980). At a minimum, feminist counselors monitor their personal behavior in order to ensure that their values do not influence clients in a covert fashion. Feminist counselors do not limit their awareness training to the clarification of personal values but expand their own worldviews by becoming informed about the life experiences of diverse groups of women, such as women in poverty, lesbians, adolescent girls and women, women of color, and older women. In order to expand their frames of reference, feminist counselors read widely about the wide array of political, ideological, sociological, and psychological issues that influence on women's and men's lives.

Many feminist counselors communicate their feminist values to their clients in a direct manner. Others remain hesitant about using the label _feminist_ during the psychotherapy hour because of popular and negative stereotypes about feminism. Several studies suggest that even when one's values remain unstated, potential clients are able to identify important aspects of a counselor's perspectives by observing the counselor's techniques, roles, nonverbal behaviors, and attitudes (Enns and Hackett, 1990, 1993). These studies found that regardless of the implicit or explicit nature of counselors' statements, research participants identified accurately the feminist or traditional goals of videotaped counselors, suggesting that one cannot *not* communicate one's values. The open communication of values, when conveyed in a respectful manner and within a reciprocal conversation, is likely to enhance, rather than detract from, relationship formation. Therapists must remain mindful of the power they hold because of their expert status as therapist, and work toward conveying their values in such a manner that their values are not subtly imposed on the clients.

Relationship Principle Two: Clients As Competent

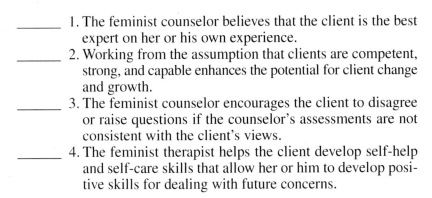

     1. The feminist counselor believes that the client is the best expert on her or his own experience.

     2. Working from the assumption that clients are competent, strong, and capable enhances the potential for client change and growth.

     3. The feminist counselor encourages the client to disagree or raise questions if the counselor's assessments are not consistent with the client's views.

     4. The feminist therapist helps the client develop self-help and self-care skills that allow her or him to develop positive skills for dealing with future concerns.

Since the first definitions of feminist therapy were formulated, feminist therapists have viewed clients as their own best experts (Kaschak, 1981; Laidlaw and Malmo, 1990; Rawlings and Carter, 1977). The four items just listed assess ways in which the client's expertise and competence may be valued. Even when clients' lives are in turmoil, they have developed a great deal of knowledge about coping and survival. It is important to collaborate with clients in discovering how their problems can be best defined and what strategies for change will be effective (Rawlings and Carter, 1977). The counselor shares her or his thinking regarding how clients demonstrate competence; helps clients understand how they have learned to question their competence or believe that they are "crazy"; and renames aspects of a person's behavior, such as helplessness or dependency, as "underground power" (Smith and Siegel, 1985) or indirect forms of influence that can be redirected. Because clients are their own best experts, their opinions and perspectives are sought at each stage of counseling as the counselor and clients brainstorm about alternatives for working through issues and problems (Worell and Remer, 2003).

Valuing and affirming clients' perspectives is especially important because women's views of their own lives have often been discounted by mental health professionals. Phyllis Chesler (1972) described the traditional psychotherapy encounter as "just one more instance of an unequal relationship, just one more opportunity to be rewarded for expressing distress and to be 'helped' by being (expertly) dominated" (p. 140). This relationship mirrored women's experience in the traditional patriarchal family in which they were trained to be helpless, dependent, and "unreasonable." Treating the client as her own best expert is important for undoing a "patient identity" (Greenspan, 1993) and turning perceived weaknesses into strengths.

Relationship Principle Three: Egalitarian Relationships

_____ 1. The feminist counselor knows that the help-seeking situation makes it impossible for the client to experience full equality with the counselor or therapist. Given this knowledge, the feminist counselor works toward sharing power but does not deny power differences inherent in the psychotherapy relationship.

_____ 2. The counselor acts on his or her beliefs about equality by describing the counselor's assessments in clear and jargon-free language.

_____ 3. The open discussion of power differences between the therapist and client exemplifies healthy negotiation skills. The same principles can be used to negotiate issues and relationship concerns outside of counseling.

_____ 4. Well-timed and brief self-disclosures about the counselor's struggles with issues model helpful responses to difficult issues and can help equalize the counselor-client relationship.

Egalitarian relationships are important both as an outcome of counseling and as a condition of the counseling relationship. These four items reflect ways in which feminist counselors attempt to demystify the counseling experience, promote mutuality, and establish egalitarian relationships (Ballou and Gabalac, 1985; Butler, 1985; FTI, 2000; Kaschak, 1981; Worell and Remer, 2003).

The therapist models communication skills such as genuineness, confrontation, self-disclosure, empathy, and congruence as methods for establishing equal relationships. When clients enter counseling, they often feel alone, isolated, and "crazy," and they may believe that the counselor is an all-powerful expert. In such instances, the counselor may use brief self-disclosure statements to communicate that she or he is a human being who must also work to resolve problems and difficulties (Greenspan, 1986). When the client has an opportunity to see the counselor as a coping role model, psychotherapy is demystified, and an egalitarian climate is reinforced (Ballou and West, 2000).

Edna Rawlings and Diane Carter (1977) recommended that feminist therapists adopt a reciprocal model of influence in which counselors share power, avoid making decisions for the client, and communicate confidence in the client's decision-making skills. Both therapist and client seek to share honest feedback with each other about the goals and direction of counseling. The counselor participates as a colleague with clients in order to ensure that clients develop problem-solving skills which will help them become their own therapists in the future (Butler, 1985). Hogie Wykoff (1977b) referred to this process as a "transfer of power and expertise in the process of self-transformation" (p. 394).

Although the counselor and client work toward establishing a relationship of equality, the counselor does not assume that the counseling relationship is one of undifferentiated egalitarianism. Lack of awareness of power differences can result in the blurring of boundaries between counselor and client and inappropriate role reversals (Brown, 1991b). The feminist counselor works toward eliminating artificial boundaries, acknowledges the client's expertise regarding her or his life, and models egalitarian behaviors that help the client negotiate effective relationships across various contexts. However, the feminist counselor also recognizes that she or he brings skills, professional preparation, and the power of expertise and position to the relationship. Assuming the relationship can become fully equal ignores the power relationships that occur throughout life and may allow individuals to rationalize behavior which may lead to unethical practice. The open discussion of power and role differences in the counseling relationship assists the client in becoming aware of how power dynamics influence counseling and other relationships, provides an opening for the counselor and client to explore ways to reduce power differentials when it is appropriate, and helps clients understand how roles can be negotiated effectively in contexts other than counseling (Brown, 1994; FTI, 2000; Ballou and West, 2000).

Relationship Principle Four: The Counseling Contract and Informed/Empowered Consent

_____ 1. The feminist counselor and client should discuss and specify goals in order to ensure that the client and counselor maintain a clear focus in their work and minimize the risk of misunderstandings or that the counselor will manipulate the client.

_____ 2. When goals are specified, clients are able to take greater responsibility for their own change in counseling.

_____ 3. The feminist counselor should provide the client with information about her or his theoretical orientation, competencies, and alternatives to counseling so that the client can make a fully informed choice about whether to enter counseling.

Feminist counselors seek to promote their clients' rights as consumers (Kaschak, 1981). As a result, they may offer low-cost initial decision-making sessions that allow clients to explore the compatibility of the counselor's and client's value systems, and make efforts to inform potential clients of other resources or counseling services available to clients. These procedures help clients arrive at well-informed decisions about participation in counseling or therapy (Brown, 1994; Gannon, 1982; Pope and Brown, 1996).

The feminist therapist informs the client about her or his assumptions about change, theoretical orientation, and other relevant information about her or his approach. The counselor also provides information about the costs and benefits of counseling, what the client can expect from the counselor, and what the therapist expects of the client (FTI, 2000; Hare-Mustin et al., 1979). As a client gains information about how a counselor approaches situations and why the counselor makes specific choices during counseling, she or he is able to take on an active and collaborative role in decision making and is able to take higher levels of responsibility within counseling. Whenever possible, the therapist and client specify the issues and goals they will emphasize. The goals and respective responsibilities of counselor and client can be articulated in written or verbal agreements (Rawlings and Carter, 1977). When clear roles and goals are established, both the counselor and client are able to evaluate progress regularly. Verbal and/or written contracts also lower the risk that either party will attempt to influence the other in a covert fashion. Some feminist counselors also provide their clients with written rights and responsibilities statements, which include descriptions of their orientation to counseling, areas of strength, views about how feminism influences their counseling practice, as well as expectations about the client's role in counseling.

Informed consent is not an "all or nothing" event but an ongoing process of negotiation and discussion (Enns et al., 1998; Rawlings and Carter, 1977). When a client is in crisis, she or he may not be able to concentrate on a counselor's lengthy description about her or his approach. Alternatively, when the client is a child, he or she may be developmentally unprepared to assume an active planning role. Providing the client with relevant information needs to be based on the client's readiness to participate actively in collaborative discussion. Another important element in informed consent involves creating an environment in which the client can feel comfortable asking questions about the direction and focus of counseling.

The concept of informed consent has become incorporated within all major psychotherapy approaches and codes of ethics since being introduced by feminist therapists in the 1970s, pointing to the influence of feminist voices on the general practice of therapy (Brown and Brodsky, 1992). Speaking from an explicitly feminist perspective, Laura Brown (1994) noted that "truly informed consent involves not just information but empowerment" (p. 180), which requires comprehensive collaboration and sharing of information that goes beyond the perfunctory or brief statements used by some therapists. In summary, this form of empowered consent communicates that

> this is their therapy and they have rights and privileges that do not disappear no matter how frightened or vulnerable they feel. ... A corollary aspect of this communication is that the therapist is committed to the protection of those rights and sees the empowerment of the client as integral rather than incidental to the therapy process itself. (Pope and Brown, 1996, p. 166)

THE GOALS, PROCESSES, AND OUTCOMES OF FEMINIST COUNSELING

Goals and Practice Principle One: Valuing and Affirming Diversity

_____ 1. Feminist therapists acknowledge that all clients experience multiple identities which are associated with diverse social locations (e.g., related to class, power, and race) and are interconnected with multiple interpersonal and societal systems. Paying attention to this diversity of meaning and experience is central to the competent practice of feminist therapy.

_____ 2. Feminist counselors who view sexism as the primary or central form of oppression may fail to recognize the significant ways in which racism, classism, religious oppression, ageism, ethnocentrism, nationalism, and homophobia may influence clients.

_____ 3. Learning about the cultures and traditions of diverse groups of women (e.g., women of color, lesbians) is important not only for increasing our understanding of diversity but also for evaluating feminist approaches that have been primarily created by and for Western white women or by and for heterosexual feminists.

_____ 4. White privilege, heterosexual privilege, and/or class privilege represent unconscious, unearned entitlements. To become fully effective as a feminist therapist, the counselor seeks to become aware of how these privileges shape her or his own life and assumptions.

Agreement with the four items just listed suggests that your views are consistent with a multicultural feminist approach to counseling and psychotherapy. Feminist counselors are aware that although women share many common issues, goals, and problems, women's lives are also shaped by multiple issues, sociodemographic variables, and social locations (Ballou, Matsumoto, and Wagner, 2002; Worell and Remer, 2003). As members of multicultural societies, feminist therapists recognize and celebrate the myriad ways in which gender intersects with other aspects of identity such as race, ethnicity, class, and sexual orientation.

Women's lives are influenced by multiple social locations and social identities that interact in complex ways (Ballou, Matsumoto, and Wagner, 2002; Deaux and Stewart, 2001; Worell and Remer, 2003). In many cases, it is impossible to separate one aspect of identity from another. Some aspects of girls' and women's identities may be a part of the foreground in one situation but move to the background in another context. For example, a fifty-year-old woman may be especially conscious of her age when in a classroom with students who are of traditional college age; however, in a group with many fifty-year-old women, her age may become part of the background, and some other aspect of her identity (e.g., race or class) may feel especially salient because they mark her uniqueness in that setting. Although gendered aspects of identity are characteristic of all persons, these identities may be modified substantially by other identities that intersect with gender (e.g., race, sexual orientation, professional status) (Deaux and Stewart, 2001). For some individuals, gender may only rarely become the most significant marker of identity, but may be filtered through other social identities such as race, ethnicity, or class. It is important for counselors to explore how women define themselves in multiple situations and how these constructions influence their daily interactions and self-concepts.

The creation of feminisms that recognize the diversity of experience represents an important priority for the twenty-first century. During the mid-1960s, Betty Friedan's description of the confining role of middle-class homemakers as "the problem with no name" galvanized many women into action and positive change. However, this description referred primarily to the concerns of a select group of women: white, middle-class housewives who were dissatisfied with their stereotyped roles and lack of achievement opportunities. The overgeneralization of this description led to the erasure or invisibility of the experiences of many women who had always worked outside of their homes, struggled to survive economically, and did not have the luxury to claim "the problem with no name." When theorists or activists assume that the issues of one group of women reflect all women's experiences, or claim that all forms of oppression are restrictive in similar or equal ways, the struggles and coping of women who experience multiple forms of disadvantage are minimized. This flawed assumption then allows more privileged persons to ignore the ways in which their analyses are incomplete, racist, classist, ethnocentric, or heterosexist (hooks, 1984; Húrtado, 1989, 1996; Spelman, 1988).

Laura Brown's (1990a) critique of feminist theory and therapy practice represented an important catalyst for growth and change during the past decade. Arguing that feminist therapy was "neither diverse nor complex in the reality it reflects" (p. 3), Brown warned about the dangers of assuming that one woman's context is equivalent to another woman's experience, of subtly imposing one's personal context or worldview on others, and of insisting on the "primacy of gender as *the* issue" or the "ultimate oppression" (p. 13) in the lives of women within and between cultures around the world. Peggy McIntosh (1989) also challenged white, middle-class female feminists to recognize that although they generally hold less power than many men in society, they often resemble men in that they may not recognize the unearned privileges they hold because of their white and middle-class status.

Self-awareness is a key component of competent feminist practice. As a result, feminist therapists educate themselves about the unearned entitlements or status that they may hold on the basis of their class, race, sexual orientation, or ability. Participating in antiracism, antiheterosexism, or anticlassism consciousness-raising groups (Cross et al., 1982) provides excellent opportunities for increasing awareness. Comprehensive training also involves taking personal responsibility for educating oneself about the plurality of human experience and not assuming that clients from diverse backgrounds should provide this education for the therapist. Members of minority or nondominant cultures generally learn a wealth of information about majority or dominant cultures in order to survive and cope effectively, but members of majority cultures often remain ignorant about important aspects of other cultures. Feminist therapists develop awareness about their own backgrounds, strive to learn about the diverse traditions and values of their clients, and seek out experiences and educational opportunities that sensitize them to important themes, issues, and concerns in their clients' lives. The competent feminist counselor seeks to be aware of the ways in which individual differences modify the impact of culture, race, class, religion, and sexual orientation (FTI, 2000).

Learning about women from diverse backgrounds provides an essential foundation for providing optimal treatment, and it also enriches knowledge of women's lives in general. For example, Patricia Romney (1991) proposed that gaining knowledge about women of color can "serve as a springboard to critique and advance our understanding of 'traditional feminism'" (p. 1). Similarly, becoming educated about lesbian concerns "permits us to view woman in her 'purest' form, that is, as untainted by the patriarchy as possible" (Boston Lesbian Psychologies Collective, 1987, p. 12).

In the twenty-first century, the recognition and valuing of diversity has become an important cornerstone of feminist psychological practice (FTI, 2000; Wyche and Rice, 1997). However, practice often lags behind theory and good intentions, and thus vigilance and constant reassessment are essential for ensuring that issues of diversity are recognized and addressed. Although published more than ten years ago, Oliva Espín and Mary Ann Gawelek's (1992) list of core assumptions remains an important feature of a transformative multicultural feminist practice:

1. All women's experiences must be explored valued, and understood.
2. The understanding and appreciation of difference enriches our understanding of women's lives.
3. The principle of egalitarianism includes the understanding that women of diverse statuses can create theory and shape knowledge on their own behalf.
4. The complex intersections of various contexts, cultures, and social locations (e.g., race, class, sexual orientation, age) must be understood for their power in shaping behavior.

Goals and Practice Principle Two: Counseling and Therapy for Change, Not Adjustment

_____ 1. The primary goal of counseling is to eliminate the client's immediate symptoms and suffering.

_____ 2. The client's ability to perform existing family, work, and relationship roles is the primary measure of the success of counseling.

_____ 3. An important aspect of counseling is the client's recognition of how her or his life circumstances, pain, and symptoms are connected.

_____ 4. An important outcome of counseling is the ability to implement new skills and also to identify what problems are not resolvable through individual efforts alone.

_____ 5. Becoming involved in social change activities complements personal growth and helps clients see the connections between their concerns and those of other women.

The five statements just listed are adapted from Marjorie Klein's (1976) early discussion of feminist and traditional goals of counseling. Klein indicated that a strong endorsement of items 1 and 2 suggests an adjustment versus change orientation to counseling, an alternative that may merely reinforce power differentials and the status quo. In contrast, agreement with items 3 to 5 is associated with a change or transformation orientation to counseling.

Traditional models of psychotherapy have emphasized removing pain and helping clients adjust to existing realities (Klein, 1976). Feminist therapists help clients explore the full range of options available to them, especially when their initial statements or presenting problems are shaped by a narrow view of "what is proper for women to complain about" (Klein, 1976, p. 90). Change goals may involve attending to personal development instead of using all of one's energy to adjust to existing relationships, choosing novel responses to difficult circumstances, or developing new attitudes toward circumstances and the realities of women's and men's lives.

One potential change outcome of feminist counseling is involvement in social activism. Individual change should be linked whenever possible to larger social issues because some social problems that are experienced individually will be eradicated only through social change (Greenspan, 1993). Through involvement in feminist therapy, consciousness-raising groups, and community action programs, women often gain experience and confidence for initiating social change (Brodsky, 1976). As noted by Mary Ballou and Carolyn West (2000),

> The goals of feminist therapy are not about achieving a better, a quieter, a more compliant fit within a system that oppresses, but are directed toward helping the individual to recognize the sociopolitical and economic forces, the societal structures and gendered expectations that contribute to pain and discomfort while simultaneously discovering personal resources and healthy resistances as means of empowerment. (p. 275)

Goals and Practice Principle Three: Equality

_____ 1. The counselor helps the client gain freedom from narrowly defined gender roles.

_____ 2. The counselor provides information regarding the unequal status, power, and privilege of women and men of diverse backgrounds in this society.

_____ 3. Counselors should help clients recognize roles that are confining, restrictive, and/or oppressive for both men and women.

_____ 4. Counselors devote time to brainstorming with clients about how to implement more flexible and less gender-bound behavior in relationships with friends, intimate others, and work colleagues.

_____ 5. Counselors encourage clients to negotiate more equality in the distribution of tasks and responsibilities in their private and public roles.

_____ 6. Financial self-sufficiency is important for establishing equal personal relationships.

_____ 7. Feminist therapists help clients consider how factors such as race, class, and sexual orientation influence gender and power relationships.

These seven self-assessment statements articulate values that are consistent with the feminist principle of equality. Feminist therapists have historically encouraged their clients to establish relationships based on equality of personal power (Butler, 1985; Kaschak, 1981; Rawlings and Carter, 1977; Sturdivant, 1980; Worell and Remer, 2003). It is also important for feminist counselors to communicate information about the barriers to and the hard work of achieving egalitarian relationships as an individual male or female in this society. Thus, the following section will outline many of the issues that place limits on equality, as well as its role as a principle in feminist counseling.

One of the reasons that feminists have often emphasized the importance of financial self-sufficiency is that economic power is one of the most powerful ways of establishing equality in relationships (Rawlings and Carter, 1977). However, statistics indicate that equality is still elusive in the arena of women's and men's work. Even with substantial gains in wage equities between 1978 and 1998, women earn approximately 76 percent of men's pay. Furthermore, the wage gap between white women and Black and Hispanic women has widened during the past twenty years (Costello and Stone, 2001). Women are more frequently seen in professions and high-status jobs than in the past, but most women remain clustered in lower-status jobs that bring fewer financial benefits (Yoder, 2003). Even when women's incomes at the early stages of their careers approach the income levels of men, institutional power structures, values, and promotion policies still limit the likelihood that they will achieve equal power with men over the course of a career (Crawford and Unger, 2004). Women between the ages of twenty-five and twenty-nine earn eighty-five cents for every dollar earned by men, and women between the ages of fifty and fifty-nine earn sixty-nine cents for every dollar earned by men. Within nontraditional work contexts, women often experience token status, which is associated with high visibility and performance pressure, isolation, and the tendency for co-workers to view them as representative of all women (Crawford and Unger, 2004; Yoder, 2003). Women are more similar to than different from men with respect to internal qualities such as achievement motivation, but they often work within environments that treat women and men differently. In comparison to men, women generally hold less earning power, experience more devaluation of their performance and different attributions for their success, and encounter work-related hazards such as sexual harassment or discrimination (Crawford and Unger, 2004; Gutek, 2001).

Despite these realities and problems, employment is an important factor in women's satisfaction and provides positive experiences of feedback, self-esteem, social connections, control, and challenge (Steil, 1997, 2001). Egalitarian roles in heterosexual relationships are more likely to occur when the financial power of partners is similar. However, Mary Crawford and Rhoda Unger (2004) concluded that "even when wives earn more money than their husbands, beliefs about the appropriate roles of women and men still influence the balance of power in favor of men" (p. 293). Although combining paid work and caregiving is the most common pattern of adult women's lives, it is also important to value the work of women who choose to pursue nonpaid work in their homes, as volunteers, and as caregivers, and whose work often remains invisible and underappreciated.

Egalitarian personal relationships are difficult to achieve within current social structures. Janice Steil (2001) concluded that although there is greater endorsement of egalitarian intimate relationships than in the past, and although those who share household responsibilities report fewer feelings of dysphoria, less stress, and a higher sense of fairness, "relationships remain unequal" (Steil, 2001, p. 350). Although men have increased their participation in household work and women have decreased the amount of time they devote to household responsibilities, women continue to perform roughly two times as much housework as their spouses and approximately 80 percent of the time-consuming and ongoing tasks associated with food preparation, house cleaning, and laundry (Chadwick and Heaton, 1999; Steil, 2001). In addition, although economic power increases a woman's influence within a household, Janice Steil (2001) noted that "as a wife's income surpasses her husband's, the proportion of housework she performs again increases while that of her husband decreases" (p. 351). This reality points to the enduring hold of traditional gender expectations on private life, even among those who have moved beyond traditional role definitions in other areas of their lives. After reviewing the literature on intimate relationships, Mary Crawford and Rhoda Unger (2004) concluded that egalitarian marriage between heterosexual partners is relatively uncommon and represents an ideal rather than reality both in single-earner and dual-career families. These realities point to the complexity of and importance of dealing with these issues in feminist therapy.

It is also essential to recognize the diversity among women with regard to home-career issues. Most research on multiple roles and home-career issues has focused on role distributions in white, middle-class households (Crawford and Unger, 2004), which limits the generalizability of conclusions about partner role definitions in non-heterosexual relationships and various cultural settings. In contrast to research on heterosexual partners, research on lesbian couples reveals that partners typically reject traditional roles, achieve more egalitarianism in relationships, believe that both partners should work for pay, and share more social/leisure interests. Thus, despite few cultural supports and social disapproval, lesbian couples may be well prepared to experience the satisfactions associated with egalitarian relationships (Kurdek, 1998; Patterson, 1995; Savin-Williams and Esterberg, 2000; Steil, 2001). Finally, despite the tendency to see pairings between people as normative human behavior, the lifestyles of single women who do not have intimate partners must also be recognized and valued. Single women generally experience less serious psychological distress than their married counterparts, and they enjoy higher levels of education and occupational status, suggesting some significant benefits associated with this lifestyle choice (Crawford and Unger, 2004).

As U.S. society has recognized the costs of gender inequity, gender-neutral policies have been enacted and have often treated women and men as though their life situations were identical. Carol Tavris (1992) indicated that providing equality should not be confused with providing identical treatment. A substantial body of research demonstrates that differences between men and women on measures of personality and ability are minimal; differences within each gender group overshadow differences between men and women. However, women and men face dramatically different reproductive events, life experiences, employment opportunities, and responsibilities at home and at work. When men and women are treated identically, social inequities and power imbalances are often perpetuated. Although work is considered a gender-neutral environment where sex discrimination is illegal, the potential for men's and women's achievement of real equality is still limited because the success of workers is "so thoroughly organized around a male worker with a wife at home to take care of the needs of the household—including childcare—that it transforms what is intrinsically just a male-female difference into a massive female disadvantage" (Bem, 1993, p. 184). Another example of equal treatment with unequal consequences is the "no fault," gender-neutral divorce laws which were intended to secure the equitable allocation of assets but have resulted in greater disparities between men's and women's standards of living (Crawford and Unger, 2004). Furthermore, the poverty rate for female-headed families with children (divorced and never married) stands at 41 percent (Costello and Stone, 2001).

When women enter feminist therapy, they may be overwhelmed by myriad life tasks and may have difficulty conceptualizing the complexities of gender equality. Within feminist therapy, the counselor helps the client to carefully explore relationships in public and employment contexts, as well as in more private and relational spheres. Some clients may engage in self-blame for their lack of progress in achieving goals because they do not understand how institutions with gender-neutral policies often perpetuate traditional power relations and status quo arrangements. When clients explore their personal experiences in light of social structures, they are more likely to release themselves from self-criticism, self-blame, and discouragement.

Women often feel less entitled to the same rewards as men or engage in a variety of mental gymnastics or "modest delusional systems" (Hochschild, 1989) to minimize the hard realities of unequal work distribution. For example, the myth of equality may be maintained by beliefs or justificatory beliefs that the individual man contributes more to the household than most other men, or that the woman is more organized or compulsive than her partner (Major, 1993). As women become more aware of these dynamics, they may become more confident about their rights and more determined to ask for the rewards they have earned. Finally, individuals in feminist counseling often recognize that isolated personal efforts often result in limited change within the environment. Support groups may help women maintain motivation and energy for negotiating the ongoing issues of establishing egalitarian intimate relationships. Seeking the assistance of advocacy groups may help women negotiate complex institutional and legal issues. In light of the reality that social change supports egalitarianism in social and personal relationships, some clients will experience renewed energy by staying informed about political and legal issues, and by becoming involved in grassroots or community organizations that focus on achieving social justice.

Goals and Practice Principle Four: Balancing Instrumental and Relational Strengths

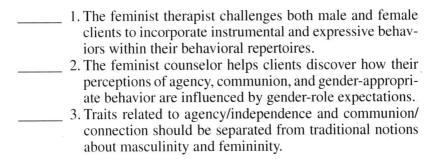

_____ 1. The feminist therapist challenges both male and female clients to incorporate instrumental and expressive behaviors within their behavioral repertoires.

_____ 2. The feminist counselor helps clients discover how their perceptions of agency, communion, and gender-appropriate behavior are influenced by gender-role expectations.

_____ 3. Traits related to agency/independence and communion/connection should be separated from traditional notions about masculinity and femininity.

_____ 4. The feminist therapist helps clients explore how their gender schemas influence their perceptions of the behavior of others.

_____ 5. The counselor is interested not only in the client's ability to enact new or nontraditional behaviors but also in educating clients about how contexts elicit certain behaviors and how other people may misperceive or distort behaviors.

_____ 6. Androgyny, or the incorporation of both "masculine" and "feminine" characteristics within the person, should be a primary goal of counseling.

_____ 7. One of the most important goals of counseling is to help women identify and value their relational selves.

Feminist psychologists have proposed a variety of models for balancing instrumental and expressive skills. Many of the early statements on feminist counseling promoted the goal of androgyny, or the systematic integration of both traditional masculine and feminine characteristics as an ideal model of mental health (e.g., Kaplan, 1976; Rawlings and Carter, 1977). During the 1980s, emerging models of women's identity focused on the importance of revaluing the underappreciated relational skills of women rather than viewing psychological health as synonymous with independence, autonomy, and agency (e.g., Gilligan, 1982; Jordan et al., 1991; Miller and Stiver, 1997). Both approaches to integrating agency and communion have provided useful tools for helping individuals explore expanded personal options.

Items 6 and 7 inquire about personal reactions to the androgyny and relational approaches for balancing interdependence and independence. Consistent with controversies within the psychology of women, feminist counselors may disagree about the relative importance of androgyny, autonomy, and/or relational skills. High endorsement of the first five items is consistent with assumptions that the qualities of connectedness and autonomy should be balanced in flexible ways and should be removed from traditional notions of gender. The feminist therapist's emphasis on the relative merits of agency and communion will depend on the specific feminist philosophical position she or he endorses. These themes are discussed in Chapters 2 and 4 on liberal and cultural feminist themes in feminist therapy.

Feminist therapists have also become more aware in recent years that the qualities of agency and communion are best represented not as traits that describe permanent internal characteristics but as verbs that involve "doing" or engaging in behavior (West and Zimmerman, 1987) and that are manifested differently in a variety of social encounters (Deaux and Stewart, 2001). At home, for example, a woman may show executive authority (agency); however, in close relationships with other women, her behaviors may be marked primarily by empathy, caring, and a love for fun (communion). In her secretarial role at work, a woman may smile and facilitate positive relationships (communion); as a community volunteer, she may implement her organizational and advocacy skills (agency). Individual decisions to display communal or agentic qualities are socially constructed and arise from efforts to fulfill specific social roles.

Goals and Practice Principle Five: Empowerment and Social Change

_____ 1. The feminist counselor should help clients discover assertive and productive ways of expressing power and strong emotions such as anger.

_____ 2. The feminist therapist should support competence in women and men in both traditional and nontraditional roles.

_____ 3. The feminist counselor should help women experience increased self-esteem by pointing out their unique contributions, strengths, and achievements.

_____ 4. The feminist therapist should encourage the client to evaluate her or his own change and growth.

_____ 5. The feminist counselor should be willing to act as an advocate on behalf of clients and should contribute time and support to projects that initiate social change.

_____ 6. The feminist counselor should help the client find productive ways of contributing to social change and the empowerment of other women.

_____ 7. The feminist therapist should help clients become aware of external forces that limit their freedom so that clients can release self-blame and focus their energy on circumstances that they can influence.

High levels of endorsement of the seven items just listed suggest high levels of agreement with the feminist principle of empowerment. A major goal of feminist counseling is to help individuals see themselves as active agents on their own behalf and on behalf of other people. Ellen McWhirter (1991) defined empowerment as

> the process by which people, organizations, or groups who are powerless: (a) become aware of the power dynamics at work in their life context, (b) develop the skills and capacity for gaining some reasonable control over their lives, (c) exercise this control without infringing upon the rights of others, and (d) support the empowerment of others in their community. (p. 224)

Within feminist therapy, empowerment involves

1. an analysis of power structures in society;
2. discussion and awareness of how women are socialized to feel powerless;
3. discovery of how women can achieve power in personal, interpersonal, and institutional domains; and
4. the use of advocacy skills on behalf of women (Hawxhurst and Morrow, 1984).

Susan Morrow and Donna Hawxhurst (1998) also noted that empowerment involves three dimensions: personal, interpersonal, and sociopolitical. The integration of all three levels of intervention is necessary in order to connect the personal and political in an optimal fashion.

Many of women's presenting problems emerge directly from their less powerful position in society, and these problems include rape, abuse, battering, and sexual harassment. Furthermore, problems such as eating disorders, agoraphobia, post-traumatic stress disorder, and depression often emerge from women's efforts to deal with the aftermath of traumatic events and thus represent the internalization of issues related to violation and unequal power relationships. Some women experience powerlessness not only because of their gender status but also because of the intersecting impacts of racism, homophobia, classism, or ableism. As a result, a social analysis of power helps educate clients about the contextual frameworks that support and reinforce their problems. The foundation for empowerment is based on this knowledge.

After clients become aware how gender-role socialization, violence, or other forms of oppression have limited their options, it is important for them to develop "response-ability" to dynamics that have constricted their life sphere or focus. As a method of reaching this goal, clients may need to gain awareness of denied, buried, or distorted emotions. Anger is a frequent outcome of this exploration. As a part of counseling, clients learn to channel their anger effectively so that it is not expressed haphazardly or indiscriminately but is stated in direct, constructive, assertive expressions which facilitate personal efficacy (Van Velsor and Cox, 2001). As clients gain confidence in describing their feelings directly, they may also need new methods to respond effectively to individuals who express negative reactions to the changes they have made (Fodor and Rothblum, 1984). Empowerment is most likely to occur when clients are fully aware of both the benefits and the costs of personal change, and base their choices on knowledge of both positive outcomes and risks.

Within a culture in which women's overt power is often denied, women often learn to

exercise power while denying it; to reach toward a goal while pretending, to oneself and others, not to want it; to act upon others without knowledge that one's actions have any effect; and, in general, to be manipulative, sneaky, underhanded, and devious. (Smith and Siegel, 1985, p. 17)

Women often express discomfort with the term *power* because of their limited experience with power or their exposure to only aggressive or forceful aspects of power. An important role of the counselor is to help the client understand the differences between "power over," which implies dominance, coercion, and oppression; "power within," which involves feeling that one has the inner strength to enable one to make sound decisions; and "power to," which signifies the enactment of goal-directed behaviors that respect the rights of all parties in an interaction (Gannon, 1982; Smith and Douglas, 1990). Differentiating between coercive power and the power of information, expertise, reciprocal influence, encouragement, and reward is also a useful task for helping the client discover positive manifestations of power (Douglas, 1985).

As a part of recognizing clients' competence and coping skills, the feminist counselor helps clients explore how they currently use power and how they desire to redirect efforts in line with new behavioral goals. Empowerment often involves a complex resocialization process in which women gain permission to see themselves in new ways and gain skills to enact new knowledge of themselves. It is difficult to relearn behaviors that have been practiced and reinforced for many years or decades. Relearning, then, must include opportunities for practice, confidence building, and systematic, gradual change.

Based on her extensive study of markers of mental health in women, Judith Worell (2001) developed a list of ten components of personal empowerment:

1. Self-esteem and self-affirmation
2. A positive comfort-distress ratio as exhibited in daily functioning
3. Self-sustaining behaviors informed by knowledge of gender, culture, and power issues
4. Personal efficacy and control beliefs
5. The ability to engage in self-nurturance
6. Access to problem-solving skills
7. Flexibility of gender-related behaviors and thinking
8. Assertiveness
9. The ability to access and use community and personal resources
10. The ability to engage in social justice activity

Several research studies of the goals of feminist therapists and self-ratings of clients have provided initial support for this model, which emphasizes personal competence rather than symptom removal.

As noted previously in this section, empowerment involves individual, interpersonal, and sociopolitical levels of intervention. Feminist conceptualizations of ethics emphasize the importance of a therapist's commitment to social action directed toward establishing social justice within health and mental health, political, religious, economic, legal, and educational institutions (Brabeck and Brown, 1997; Brabeck and Ting, 2000; FTI, 2000). Social activism may be viewed along a continuum that encompasses microlevels to macrolevels of social change (Worell and Remer, 2003). For example, feminist therapists' microlevel activism may involve serving as an expert witness on battered woman syndrome, helping a client negotiate the complexities of a local social service network, or advocating for a client when institutional policies are blocking her movement (Laidlaw and Malmo, 1990; Rosewater, 1990). In contrast, macrolevel activism may involve challenging unjust rape or sexual harassment policies at the national level. Feminist therapists' social change efforts may occur at the local community level, at the state or national legislative level, within professional organizations, or at the international level.

As clients gain confidence, they may also take on advocacy roles by becoming involved in grassroots community organizations, local sexual assault coalitions, and volunteer organizations that support the empowerment of those with limited power. Involvement in community action groups can expand a client's outlook, build confidence in skills, increase awareness of both the commonalities and differences among women, and help the client transcend personal pain.

Goals and Practice Principle Six: Self-Nurturance

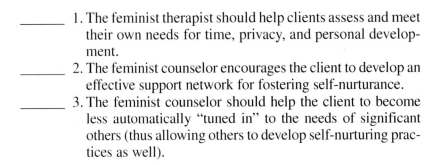

_____ 1. The feminist therapist should help clients assess and meet their own needs for time, privacy, and personal development.

_____ 2. The feminist counselor encourages the client to develop an effective support network for fostering self-nurturance.

_____ 3. The feminist counselor should help the client to become less automatically "tuned in" to the needs of significant others (thus allowing others to develop self-nurturing practices as well).

Helen Collier (1982) indicated that women often bring the following issues or characteristics to counseling:

1. Limited emotional and behavioral options
2. Difficulties expressing their needs and wants
3. Lack of trust in their own abilities and self-direction
4. Blurred boundaries between the self and others
5. A diffused sense of self and "who am I?" questions

6. Difficulties making choices

7. Concerns about fulfilling obligations, rules, and "shoulds"

Each of these characteristics is related to the consequences of caregiving and lack of attention to self-care.

The socialization of women encourages them to nurture others effectively but to view self-nurturing activities as "selfish" (Eichenbaum and Orbach, 1983). As a result, many women lose touch with their own emotions, desires, identity, and goals. Carol Gilligan (1982) suggested that the outlook of many women is based on a morality of self-sacrifice that leads them to define the "good woman" as one who pleases others, denies her own needs, and gives of herself to others with no limits. Many women also believe that anger or strong emotions jeopardize closeness, which leads them to negate their emotions or to view interpersonal conflict as their fault. The "good woman" gains the love and acceptance of others in her environment but may lose her authentic self (Jack, 1991).

Self-nurturance involves gaining awareness of personal goals and desires, considering new options, and transcending old roles. It involves balancing concerns for oneself with concern for others. Caring for oneself involves recognizing oneself as a valuable person and setting priorities that will contribute to personal well-being (Gilbert, 1980). Self-nurturing activities often help a person experience a sense of pleasure and/or mastery. These experiences may include fantasy and goal-setting exercises, physical exercise, personal care, stress-management techniques, or classes that increase career options or allow the individual to experience the joy of learning. Activities that contribute to an increased knowledge of values and goals, a wider perspective or frame of reference, or an expanded sense of personal options represent important forms of self-care.

Self-nurturing is useful not only for helping clients engage in self-care but also for providing a buffer against future stressful events. This principle is embedded in the assumption that the skills clients learn in counseling should be applicable to multiple aspects of their lives. This principle builds on the belief that clients are their own best experts because they will use the tools learned in counseling for the enhancement of functioning and the prevention of future difficulty.

A BRIEF SAMPLER OF FEMINIST THERAPY TECHNIQUES

As noted at the outset of this chapter, feminist therapy is a philosophical perspective for organizing one's counseling practice. Feminist therapists use a wide variety of techniques associated with humanistic, cognitive, existential, family, and psychodynamic schools of therapy. Nevertheless, several techniques are distinctive to feminist therapy and represent important methods for enacting the principles described in earlier sections of this chapter. The following descriptions of these techniques are brief; these techniques are discussed in greater detail in later sections of this book. For more extensive descriptions of these and other feminist therapy techniques, I encourage readers to refer to Judith Worell and Pamela Remer's (2003) book, *Feminist Perspectives in Therapy*.

Gender Role or Social Identity Analysis

Ellyn Kaschak (1981) noted that although feminist therapists use diverse theories to inform their work, a hallmark of feminist therapy is gender- or social-role analysis. Gender-role or social-identity analysis represents an important component of assessment, and involves exploring the impact of gender and other identity statuses (e.g., age, sexual orientation, race) on psychological well-being. It also involves exploring the costs and benefits of role-related behaviors and engaging in decision making about future behaviors that the client hopes to enact. Laura Brown (1990b) indicated that comprehensive gender role analysis includes the following:

- Exploration of gender in light of personal values, family dynamics, life stage, cultural/ethnic background, and current environment
- Clarification of the rewards and costs for social role conformity or nonconformity
- Discussion of the manner in which the therapy relationship mirrors gendered relationships in the "real world" or provides insight about the client's gender and other social roles
- Exploration of the client's experience with regard to oppression and victimization

A history regarding victimization may include discussion of sexual harassment, interpersonal violence, assault and abuse, racism, sexism, heterosexism, and other injustices that have contributed to an individual's internalized gender-role rules. The goals of gender-role or social-identity analysis are to increase understanding regarding how the client learned and absorbed rules associated with gender and other social locations, what functional and dysfunctional roles they have played, and how the client can use new information to increase her or his mental health.

Social identity analysis can be conducted by helping clients (1) identify expectations associated with the various social identities one enacts, (2) clarify the ways in which these messages and associated behaviors are reinforced or punished, and (3) consider the costs and benefits of expectations associated with various social identities and gender roles. This reflection phase is followed by decision making about whether change is desired, and the construction of new expectations and behaviors that are less restrictive and more empowering. The final phase of gender and social-identity analysis focuses on developing strategies for enacting changes. Throughout the restructuring process, it is important for clients and counselors to consider the impact of multiple aspects of identity and oppression (e.g., class, gender, race, sexual orientation, age) on her or his social role identity (Worell and Remer, 2003).

Feminist Power Analysis

Feminist power analysis refers to the range of methods designed to help clients understand how unequal access to power and resources can influence personal choices and distress. Therapists and clients explore how inequities or institutional and cultural barriers may limit self-definitions, achievements, and well-being. Therapists may suggest readings or provide information about dynamics or statistics associated with problems related to the unequal distribution of power (e.g., family violence, workplace issues, sexual abuse). Feminist counselors may also use open-ended questions to help clients explore these issues and assist them in developing positive approaches to power that facilitate the self-esteem and mental health of themselves and others. Bibliotherapy, well-timed self-disclosure, and psychoeducational groups and classes also enhance feminist analysis.

Assertive Expression of Emotion, Thoughts, Intentions, and Behaviors

Feminist therapists help clients increase the flexibility and range of their expressive and behavioral repertoires in order to develop "response-ability." A major challenge is helping clients develop skills that are often considered inappropriate for either men or women. The expression of vulnerability and tender emotions is often a major affective issue for men. In parallel fashion, assertiveness and permission to express feelings of anger often represent important affective and expressive issues for women. Although anger is often described as a negative emotion, it can be an important tool for working with clients, such as sexual abuse survivors, who have used numbing or suppression as coping tools (Van Velsor and Cox, 2001). Learning to express themselves assertively and use anger effectively may help clients increase personal efficacy, facilitate active and direct coping, and reattribute responsibility for abusive and oppressive events.

Self-Disclosure

Feminist therapists may use self-disclosure to equalize the psychotherapy relationship, promote the client's feminist consciousness and empowerment, build connections between personal and political issues, convey feminist values, validate clients' feelings, decrease client self-blame and shame, and foster solidarity with the client (Mahalik, Ormer, and Simi, 2000; Peterson, 2002; Simi and Mahalik, 1997). Nicole Simi and James Mahalik (1997) found that feminist therapists expressed greater willingness than other therapists to share information about personal background and were more likely to be open to client requests for self-disclosure. Compared to psychoanalytic/ dynamic therapists, feminist therapists were more likely to believe that self-disclosure decreases power differentials, is useful for validating clients' feelings, and can be liberating and empowering for clients. Self-disclosure is also a method for making linkages between political and personal issues.

Feminist therapists strive to use self-disclosure in the best interests of the client. As a result the timing, nature, and length of self-disclosure must be carefully considered with regard to its potential to support the needs of the client (Brown and Walker, 1990; FTI, 2000;

Wyche and Rice, 1997). Karen Wyche and Joy Rice (1997) recommended that therapists engage in "constant self scrutiny" (p. 64) when considering and using self-disclosure. Self-disclosure has a high likelihood of being harmful when the counselor self-discloses to meet her or his own needs for closeness and validation, holds assumptions that her or his personal experiences are indicative of the experiences of most women or men, or discloses inappropriate information about current stresses or problems (e.g., those about which the counselor has limited closure) (Peterson, 2002).

Group Work

The earliest forms of feminist therapy were modeled after consciousness-raising groups (see Chapter 3), and groups remain an important context for feminist therapy practice. Group work helps decrease feelings of isolation among participants and provides an atmosphere in which individuals learn to trust one another. Group work, which includes self-disclosure by multiple individuals, facilitates mutuality and the awareness of common issues facing group members. The individual concerns of participants are often legitimized and validated when members discuss the similar issues they confront. Members are encouraged to connect abstract concepts about gender issues to real-life concerns experienced by real people.

Group work is also an effective antidote to restrictive socialization. Groups empower individuals through participation: Members are able to practice new skills, develop confidence, and make new choices in a safe environment. Members of groups, including consciousness-raising groups, support and therapy groups, and psychoeducational groups, learn to use power effectively by providing support to one another, practicing new skills, and taking interpersonal risks in a safe environment. Groups may also decrease power imbalances between therapists and clients because members are not only receiving but also giving emotional and practical support.

SUMMARY

Despite the reality that feminist counselors apply diverse theoretical perspectives to their work, several common themes permeate the discussions of feminist counseling as applied to women. First, some form of unequal power, victimization, or abuse often underlies the issues that women bring to counseling. Furthermore, many women experience abuse or unequal power over a long period of time, and they often enter counseling with intense feelings of guilt, isolation, and self-blame. Clients may use denial or minimization as a way of coping with the long-term, insidious effects of unequal power and abuse in relationships and often find it difficult to identify and name the problems they are experiencing. As clients disclose information, the therapist and client examine how problems exist in a both a personal and social context, confront personal myths that lead to self-blame, and identify ways in which symptoms serve as survival mechanisms. It is often difficult and time-consuming to work through these problems, which have often been influenced by many years of restrictive socialization and relationships of unequal power.

As clients focus on these issues, it is often important for them to express feelings of anger, pain, grief, or sorrow that have been internalized or "swallowed." The discovery of personal methods for experiencing strength, capability, and power as a person is also crucial. Training in coping skills, cognitive restructuring, communication skills, imagery, self-nurturing, and decision making represent some of the tools for helping clients reach their goals. Given the reality that many individuals feel isolated as they enter counseling, the development of new support systems that reinforce the goals of counseling is often crucial. These systems may include self-help or consciousness-raising groups, new family and social relationships, volunteer activities, group counseling, or groups that support social activism.

In this chapter, I have identified shared understandings of feminist therapy as described in the literature which has emerged since 1970. These themes have also been explored in research studies that focus on the attitudes and behaviors of feminist therapists. Bonnie Moradi and colleagues (2000) completed a factor analysis of the Feminist Therapy Behaviors instrument and identified three major themes or clusters of behaviors. The first cluster was the personal is political, and included items such as educating the client regarding the inequality of status and power, raising gender-role issues, and reframing definitions of problems to include the impact of socialization. The empowerment factor or cluster included items such as focusing on strengths; helping clients balance their own and others' needs; paying attention to race, ethnicity, class, and culture issues; and developing collaborative roles in psychotherapy. The final factor, assertiveness and autonomy, emphasized using assertion and anger in functional ways, developing personal support networks, and balancing instrumental and expressive/relational behaviors.

The study conducted by Moradi and colleagues (2000) also explored the top-five self-reported behaviors of therapists, and found that both feminist and other therapists identified one of their top-five behaviors as displaying empathy and unconditional positive regard toward clients. However, feminist therapists differed from other therapists in their rankings of other top-five behaviors. Compared to other therapists, feminist therapists were significantly more likely to rank the following behaviors as consistent with their most strongly endorsed behaviors:

1. Paying attention to clients' experiences of discrimination
2. Adopting a collaborative role with clients
3. Reframing problems to include an emphasis on socialization
4. Enhancing self-esteem by emphasizing clients' unique and positive qualities

In addition to the quantitative study just described, Marcia Hill and Mary Ballou's 1998 open-ended survey of thirty-five feminist therapists revealed similar themes:

1. Attention to power differences, overlapping relationships, and therapist accountability
2. An emphasis on the sociocultural causes of distress
3. The valuing of women's experience
4. An integrated analysis of the multifaceted and interlocking aspects of oppression
5. An emphasis on social change

The perspectives summarized in this chapter reveal that the basic principles of feminist therapy are well established. The remainder of this book will focus on the diverse ways in which these principles are interpreted and enacted, describing many of the prominent perspectives that have influenced feminist theory and how these philosophical views have been incorporated within feminist therapy.

The next seven chapters review specific forms of feminism and their implications for feminist therapy. These chapters discuss historical ideas and foundations, provide brief overviews of current thought and emerging trends, and discuss specific applications of respective feminisms for feminist therapy. Whenever possible, I use direct quotes to illustrate the creative and original ways in which feminist theorists and therapists have expressed themselves over time. Sections summarizing each of the feminisms are preceded with a brief set of statements that can be used to assess the degree to which one's personal assumptions are consistent with specific theoretical perspectives.

Chapter 2

Liberal Feminist Theory and Therapy

Liberal feminism has focused on destroying stereotypes about differences between men and women and providing men and women with a more level playing field. Liberal feminists have historically viewed restrictive gender socialization and nonrational prejudice as the primary causes of sexism. According to this view, sexist thinking and behavior can be eradicated through rational debate, resocialization of men and women, and the application of gender-neutral policies that allow men and women to achieve individual aspirations. Liberal feminism is sometimes referred to as conservative or mainstream feminism because its assumptions are embedded in traditions associated with individualism and personal freedom, and the implementation of liberal feminism does not require the rethinking of widely accepted Western social values. Similarly, the goal of liberal feminist therapy is to eliminate aspects of psychotherapy practice that have supported traditional socialization, are based on biased views about men and women, or include assumptions about gender difference that are not supported by empirical research.

Mary Ballou and Nancy Gabalac (1985) named two early strands in feminist therapy as a *questioning* approach and a *radical* approach. Liberal feminist therapy, which can also be referred to as nonsexist therapy, is consistent with a questioning approach. Feminist therapists raised questions about bias within psychology and other mental health systems, provided recommendations for revising existing theory, and created new models for supporting equitable treatment of men and women. Rather than proposing new approaches to therapy, liberal feminist therapists have generally focused on ways of reshaping "mainstream" therapies (e.g., cognitive-behavioral or humanistic therapy) in ways that are consistent with liberal feminist principles.

51

LIBERAL FEMINISM

To use the following items as a form of self-assessment, respond to each statement with a "yes" or "no."

_____ 1. Passage of the Equal Rights Amendment, which guarantees equal rights for men and women under the law, is essential for furthering women's rights.

_____ 2. Equal employment must be guaranteed to all women by ensuring that prohibitions against gender discrimination are enforced.

_____ 3. Maternity leaves of absence should be granted by all institutions and supported by guarantees that women will retain job security and seniority upon their return to work.

_____ 4. Laws should guarantee that tax deductions for home and child care expenses are available to working parents.

_____ 5. Child care facilities should be established on the same basis as parks, libraries, and schools, and should be available to citizens from all income levels.

_____ 6. Women must be guaranteed the same educational opportunities as men.

_____ 7. Welfare and antipoverty programs should ensure women dignity, privacy, and self-respect. Women experiencing poverty should have the right to housing, job training, and family allowances that are equal to those of men. Women in poverty should also have the right to remain at home to care for children.

_____ 8. Women have the right to control their reproductive lives and must have access to contraceptive information, effective contraceptive methods, and abortion.

The preceding statements are based on the eight major points of the National Organization for Women (NOW) Bill of Rights (1967/ 1970), and they represent the foundational rights that contemporary liberal feminists demanded in the mid-1960s. Endorsement of these items suggests a correspondence between your views and liberal feminist goals.

Early Liberal Feminist Thought

Liberal feminism has its roots in the eighteenth- and nineteenth-century enlightenment and natural rights philosophies, and significant contributors included Mary Wollstonecraft ([1792] 1972), Elizabeth Cady Stanton, Susan B. Anthony (Stanton, Anthony, and Gage, 1881), and Sarah Grimké ([1838] 1972). These early feminists built their ideas on the foundation provided by liberal male theorists who proposed that as rational beings, men are entitled to exercise certain "natural" or inherent rights to impose order on the world. Feminists argued that women are also rational beings with the same capacities as men, and liberal feminism arose out of efforts to grant women the same rights that had been granted only to men (Freedman, 2002). Josephine Donovan (2000) noted that although early-enlightenment liberal feminists conveyed diverse views in their writings, they shared five major beliefs:

1. Faith in the power of rationality
2. The belief that women and men share the same basic rational qualities
3. The conviction that education, with an emphasis on critical thinking, is the most productive, efficient way to change individuals and society
4. The assumption that individuals are independent beings who seek truth in isolation, and that the rational and independent nature of persons is central to human dignity
5. The endorsement of a natural rights doctrine, which conveyed that humans hold certain inalienable rights by virtue of their rational abilities

Early liberal feminists identified ways in which men oppressed women in order to preserve their superior roles, and how women's socialization hampered their ability to claim their natural rights. Mary Wollstonecraft ([1792] 1972) described women's conditioning in ways that are remarkably similar to contemporary feminist descriptions:

> Women are told from their infancy, and taught by the example of their mothers, that a little knowledge of human weakness, justly termed cunning, softness of temper, *outward* obedience, and a scrupulous attention to a puerile kind of propriety, will obtain

for them the protection of man; and should they be beautiful, everything else is needless, for, at least, twenty years of their lives. (p. 6)

Wollstonecraft also declared that women had been "stripped of the virtues that should clothe humanity" (p. 13) and deluded to follow "artificial graces" and values such as love, sentiment, gentleness, docility, and "spaniel-like affection" (p. 12). These virtues "raise emotion instead of inspiring respect" and destroy "all strength of character" (p. 13). Wollstonecraft ([1792] 1972) argued that women must be given the opportunity to "cultivate their minds" (p. 12). She proposed that education "in common with man" (p. 12) and training in critical thinking would allow women to think clearly about their own situations, make women less vulnerable to deception, and enable women to transcend selfishness and self-interest (Freedman, 2002).

Sarah Grimké's ([1838] 1972) "Letters on the Equality of the Sexes and the Condition of Women" stated that "our powers of mind have been crushed" (p. 42) and that "man has exercised the most unlimited and brutal power over woman" (p. 47). Grimké wrote that it was especially through woman's union with man in marriage that her position was lowered and her sense of individuality and independence was lost. However, "Men and women were CREATED EQUAL; they are both moral and accountable beings, and whatever is *right* for man to do, is *right* for woman" (Grimké, [1838] 1972, p. 40). Grimké asked "no favors for my sex" (p. 38) but requested that men "take their feet from off our necks" (p. 38), reinstate the rights that have been "wrested from us" (p. 38), and allow women to gain education and nurture their intellectual potential.

The Declaration of Sentiments and Resolutions ([1848] 1972), which was drafted at the Seneca Falls Convention, became an important marker for organized feminism in the United States and reflected many liberal feminist ideals. It stated, "We hold these truths to be self-evident; that all men and women are created equal; that they are endowed by their Creator with certain inalienable rights" (p. 77). The declaration stated that "the history of mankind is a history of repeated injuries and usurpations on the part of man toward woman" (p. 78). These usurpations resulted in the denial of education and profitable employment, rights to property, and rights to vote. The declaration concluded with a series of resolutions that were designed to rectify these wrongs.

Elizabeth Cady Stanton worked toward changing basic attitudes about men and women, gaining educational and coeducational opportunities for women, and securing liberalized divorce laws on behalf of women. Emphasizing men's and women's basic similarity, she used liberal biblical scholarship to argue that God contained both masculine and feminine characteristics (Stanton, 1895/1898). She based her arguments on the principles of feminist individualism and the importance of personal freedom, personal merit, self-reliance, and self-control (Banner, 1980; DuBois, 1981), stating that "nothing strengthens the judgment and quickens the conscience like individual responsibility" (Stanton, [1892] 1972, p. 159). Woman must "rely on herself" and "make the voyage of life alone" (p. 159). In light of her belief in men's and women's similarity and individual responsibility, Stanton asked that legislators "strike out all special legislation for us; strike the words 'white male' from all your constitutions, and then, with fair sailing, let us sink or swim, live or die, survive or perish together" (Stanton, [1860] 1972, p. 121).

Stanton stressed the importance of women having sovereignty over their own bodies and sexuality (DuBois, 1981). She stated that the "aristocracy of sex" within marriage allowed men to dominate and tyrannize women; she characterized marriage as a form of licensed prostitution, and stated that all women were kept in slavery by their constant fear of rape. Later, radical feminists of the 1970s described the sexual oppression of women in similar ways.

Susan B. Anthony, who often worked closely with Stanton, is known less for her theoretical work and more for her pragmatic applications and ability to organize women on behalf of suffrage issues and other legal reforms (DuBois, 1981). In her discussion of the tenacity of tradition and the difficulties of gaining equality, she noted,

> Even when man's intellectual convictions shall be sincerely and fully of the side of freedom and equality to women, the force of long existing customs and laws will impel him to exert authority over her, which be distasteful to the self-sustained, self-respectful women. The habit of the ages cannot, at once, be changed. (Anthony, [1877] 1981, p. 148)

Susan Anthony noted that laws and amendments would not necessarily transform relationships. She speculated that during the transition from inequality to equality, women might need to opt for single-ness as an alternative to the subjugation of women inherent in marriage; singleness would ensure that women could maintain self-respect and equality. Unmarried women "are not halves, needing complements, as are the masses of women, but evenly balanced well rounded characters" (Anthony, [1877] 1981, p. 151).

One of Anthony's strategies was to propose that the constitution had already granted women the right to vote, arguing that the constitution makes "explicit assertions of the equal right of the whole people." The "omission of the adjective 'female' should not be construed into a denial; but instead should be considered as of no effect" (Anthony [1872] 1981, p. 155). She proposed that if women's rights were denied on constitutional grounds, women should also be exempt for taxation and from the obligation to support the government. In a series of actions that resembled the feminist sit-ins and activism that occurred a full a century later, Anthony organized women to cast ballots illegally. Her arrest and later trial provided an opportunity to further disseminate the argument that women were already entitled to vote (DuBois, 1981; Schneir, 1972). Although interested in a wide range of issues such as equal pay for equal work, labor exploitation, international peace, and temperance, Anthony concluded that the ballot would provide women with the necessary power to secure a place of equality. She asked, "Now what do women want? Simply the same ballot" (Anthony, [1871] 1981, p. 143).

Many early feminists were involved in antislavery and abolition activities, which increased their awareness of their own oppressed status and led them to adopt a feminist platform. They often linked the plight of women and slaves, noting that both male slaves and women were expected to take on the name of their masters, were denied the ownership of property, had no legal rights, and could be physically punished by their husbands or owners. Anthony ([1872] 1981) stated,

> There is and can be but one safe principle of government—equal rights to all. Discrimination against any class on account of color, race, nativity, sex, property, culture, can but embitter and disaffect that class, and thereby endanger the safety of the whole people. (p. 161)

Women of color were also actively involved in the women's movement, with Sojourner Truth ([1867] 1972) noting the following about the concerns of Black women:

> There is a great stir about colored men getting their rights, but not a word about the colored women; and if colored men get their rights, and not colored women theirs, you see the colored men will be masters over the women, and it will be just as bad as it was before. (p. 129)

Unfortunately, as it became apparent that Black men would gain the vote following the Civil War and women would not gain this right, white feminists became embittered, conveniently forgot their concern for all women, and resorted to racist rhetoric in their fight for the vote (Banner, 1980; Donovan, 2000). This issue and its impact on contemporary feminism will be discussed further in Chapter 5.

Roughly three-quarters of a century after the Seneca Falls Convention, women in the United States eventually won the right to vote in 1920. Feminists engaged in a wide array of causes, including abolitionist endeavors, issues of working women, and divorce and property rights reform (Banner, 1980). Only rarely did liberal feminist theorists connect the battle for public rights with the private world of women. They focused primarily on how men as a class oppressed women and believed that legal changes would lead to equality for women. They did not attend to ways in which women's domestic roles could limit women's ability to claim their rights as well as interfere with gaining equal economic status (Donovan, 2000). Although early liberal feminists often viewed marriage as a primary form of oppression, they did not challenge the basic structure of marriage; women were encouraged not only to take on increased economic roles but also to practice "enlightened motherhood" (Banner, 1980).

Contemporary Liberal Feminism

Liberal Feminism During the Twentieth Century

After winning the right to vote, liberal feminist ideas were less influential between the 1920s and the 1960s. However, most of the early ideas of liberal feminism remained intact when they were revived during the feminist movement of the late 1960s and early

1970s. Betty Friedan ([1963] 1983) described the ways in which women were manipulated by various social institutions to organize their lives around the "feminine mystique," the belief that "the highest value and the only commitment for women is the fulfillment of their own femininity" (p. 43). Friedan ([1963] 1983) argued that women had been falsely deluded into believing that "the root of women's troubles in the past is that women envied men, women tried to be like men, instead of accepting their own nature, which can find fulfillment only in sexual passivity, male domination, and nurturing maternal love" (p. 43).

As women began talking about their malaise, "the problem that has no name burst like a boil through the image of the happy American housewife" (Friedan, [1963] 1983, p. 22). Friedan asserted that this problem, which she defined as any way in which women are blocked from reaching their full potential, was likely to exact a greater toll on the mental and physical health of the country than any other disease. However, the creation of new social norms, educational options, and definitions of femininity would allow women to achieve a sense of identity, completeness, and maturity. Once individual women constructed life plans based on their own abilities and gained access to supportive services such as child care and maternity leave, they would not have to "sacrifice the right to honorable competition and contribution anymore than they will have to sacrifice marriage and motherhood" (p. 375). Women would be able to integrate professional and mothering roles without conflict and would "carry more of the burden of the battle with the world, instead of being a burden themselves" (p. 377).

Betty Friedan invested energy in various women's rights causes that focused on helping women fulfill their individual potential. She was also active in establishing and providing direction for the National Organization for Women, which identified individual rights that would allow women to make responsible choices about their own lives. In ensuing years, affirmative action, reproductive rights legislation, educational reforms, and equal opportunity legislation represented important liberal feminist programs designed to ensure that women and other minority groups are not systematically disadvantaged. Liberal feminists have been active in many organizations and legal efforts to secure equal rights including the Women's Equity Action League, the Equal Employment Opportunity Commission

(EEOC), the Equal Pay Act, the Family and Medical Leave Act, the Education Amendments Act of 1972, and Title IX (which prohibited discrimination in higher education institutions), and abortion rights legislation. Liberal feminists also endorsed legal programs designed to break up power structures that have limited women's actual access to many social roles (Berkeley, 1999; Donovan, 2000; Ferree and Hess, 1995; Jaggar, 1983).

Feminist Empiricism and Liberal Feminism

Feminist empiricism has been and remains an important strategy for those who hold a liberal feminist worldview. From a liberal feminist perspective, social policy and legal changes designed to decrease sexism and increase less privileged persons' access to resources and opportunity need to be based on empirical research that refutes myths about gender, race, ability, and other "isms," and careful documentation of the impact of various "isms" on the lives of those with limited access to opportunity and power. Consistent with the values of liberal feminism, feminist empiricism represents an approach to research and seeking knowledge that does not challenge the basic values of traditional science, provides methods for applying rules of science fairly and objectively, and provides a rational basis for supporting social change efforts. Feminist empiricism is attentive to the ways in which unspoken biases or gender privilege lead to "badly done science" (Harding, 1990, p. 90).

Feminist empiricism challenges the incomplete way in which scientific inquiry is conducted and has sought to eliminate sexism by adhering more strictly to rules of good research design and the scientific method. It does not question the basic norms or tenets of science and utilizes respected and accepted methods of the natural and social sciences. By asking unbiased questions, using representative samples and appropriate explanatory models, interpreting data objectively, and attending to complex interactions that are influenced by culture, feminist empirical researchers seek to produce evidence that meets respected standards within science. Feminists who rely primarily on empiricism assume that when research is free of bias, accurate observations can be made and equitable policies for men and women can be implemented.

Feminist empiricism subverts traditional scientific inquiry or traditional "objectivism" by suggesting that feminists (men and women) are more likely than nonfeminists to bring a critical consciousness about injustice or bias to the research process and, as a result, are more likely to identify and eliminate problems that lead to biased outcomes. Feminist researchers who rely on empirical methods expand on the range of topics studied, pay careful attention to context in which findings emerge, and apply interpretive frameworks embedded within feminist beliefs about equality. Feminist empiricism also challenges the traditional assumption that politics and science must remain separate from each other (Harding, 1986, 1990). Feminist empiricism has been an important strategy for supporting liberal feminist claims and has been especially useful for conveying information and evidence to individuals who value the traditional scientific method in the search for answers to gender issues.

Summary of Liberal Feminist Themes

Liberal feminists have emphasized how the subordination of women is embedded in legal, economic, and cultural constraints that have blocked women's access to many opportunities which are available to men. They have argued that women should be entitled to the same civil rights and economic opportunities as men. Liberal feminists have consistently promoted the ideals of human dignity, equality, self-fulfillment, autonomy, and rationality, and have sought to reform existing legal and political systems that limit individual freedom. According to most classic liberal feminist thought, oppression is caused by rigid sex-role conditioning and irrational prejudices which lead people to believe that women are less intellectually or physically capable than men. Solutions to these gender-related problems are likely to be achieved through rational argument, the transcendence of cultural conditions, and the legislation of laws that allow for equal opportunity for all individuals. Legal reforms and the guarantee of civil rights are seen as providing opportunities for personal initiative and choices that will permit individuals to advance as far as their talents permit. Within the realm of personal relationships, nontraditional behaviors are considered appropriate for both men and women, but behavioral choices must be based on personal preferences and should not be externally imposed (Donovan, 2000; Jaggar, 1983; Tong, 1998).

The goal of liberal feminism is to preserve individual dignity and establish individual freedom, autonomy, self-fulfillment, and equality; liberal feminist programs promote equality through reform, education, equal opportunity, gender-fair policies, and the legislation of personal rights (Donovan, 2000; Freedman, 2002; Jaggar, 1983; Jaggar and Rothenberg, 1984). Liberal feminist activists have generally focused on redistributing persons within power structures and have not questioned the basic assumptions of major social institutions. As a result, liberal feminism is often referred to as conservative or mainstream feminism. Ellen Willis (1975) declared that this "self-improvement, individual-liberation philosophy is relevant only to an elite" (p. 170). Despite its image as conservative, liberal feminists have gradually moved away from the belief that individual efforts alone will liberate women and have often adopted more radical politics at points when the struggle for women's emancipation has intensified (Eisenstein, 1981; Tong, 1998).

LIBERAL FEMINISM AND THERAPY

The remaining sections of this chapter discuss liberal feminist themes as they are reflected in feminist approaches to counseling and psychotherapy. The following sections describe critiques of traditional therapy which are consistent with liberal feminist perspectives as well as approaches to feminist therapy which are consistent with liberal feminism.

As noted at the beginning of this chapter, Mary Ballou and Nancy Gabalac (1985) identified early forms of feminist therapy as reflecting either a questioning or radical approach. These two forms of feminist therapy were associated with two major strands of second-wave feminism: (1) a liberal feminist tradition that reflected the values of women's rights organizations such as the National Organization for Women and (2) a more "radical" branch of feminism, sometimes labeled the women's liberation movement, whose leaders created antihierarchical experimental structures and chose to work outside of established institutions to instigate social change (Carden, 1974;

Hole and Levine, 1971). Feminist themes linked to the women's liberation movement are discussed in Chapter 3.

Women's rights organizations operated in ways that were generally consistent with the values of traditional psychology and mental health systems. Liberal women's rights organizations did not call for radical alteration of social or institutional systems but worked for equality of opportunity for men and women. Likewise, feminists within mental health professions raised important questions about biases in research, diagnosis, and treatment; and they provided suggestions for altering the practice of psychotherapy (Ballou and Gabalac, 1985). This chapter reviews many of these significant contributions as well as discusses the strengths and limitations of liberal feminist approaches.

Revealing Gender Bias

Some of the strongest feminist critiques of psychology came from within the profession of psychology. In 1968, Naomi Weisstein presented a paper titled "Psychology Constructs the Female," which has since been reprinted at least thirty times and continues to be applauded for its far-reaching insights (Marecek, 2001; Unger, 1993). Naomi Weisstein ([1968] 1993) charged that "Psychology has nothing to say about what women are really like, what they need and what they want, especially because psychology does not know" (p. 197). She criticized psychology for creating views of women based on subjective theories and clinical impressions rather than on empirical evidence, for ignoring the impact of context on women's lives, and for adhering to flawed biologically based theories. Most of Weisstein's arguments were consistent with aspects of liberal feminist thought but also contained radical themes that called for a reconstruction regarding how psychology examines women's lives.

Bias in Therapist Attitudes

Numerous articles that were critical of psychology's treatment of women appeared in academic and professional journals during the 1970s. These articles elaborated on how therapeutic practices replicated hierarchical therapist-client relationships, and outlined how therapeutic goals, psychological theories, and diagnostic practices encouraged adherence to masculine or biased criteria of psychological health and adjustment to traditional, stereotyped roles (e.g., Barrett et al., 1974; Chesler, 1971; Holroyd, 1976; Klein, 1976; Marecek and Kravetz, 1977; Rice and Rice, 1973; Tennov, 1973).

Consistent with the values of feminist empiricism described previously in this chapter, empirical studies about sexism and bias in psychotherapy provided support for the claims of feminist critics. One of the earliest and most widely cited studies on bias against women reported that psychotherapists rated a hypothetical healthy woman as more submissive, less adventurous, more easily influenced, less competitive, more emotional, and less objective than a hypothetical healthy man or a hypothetical healthy adult whose gender was not specified (Broverman et al., 1970). This study served as a catalyst for numerous studies that were conducted by academic researchers with many different orientations, assumptions, and political perspectives. By the mid-1980s, over 150 studies on sex or gender bias had been conducted (Richardson and Johnson, 1984), and approximately a dozen reviews of the body of research had been written (e.g., Abramowitz and Dockeki, 1977; Brodsky, 1980; Richardson and Johnson, 1984; Sherman, 1980; Zeldow, 1984).

The conclusions of reviewers were diverse, suggesting that gender-related bias occurs in complex contexts which are difficult to study through contrived laboratory or analog studies that are often transparent and provide minimal cues for participants (Brodsky, 1980; Lopez, 1989; Marecek, 2001; Zeldow, 1984). Gender effects are also more likely to appear when studies examine interactions between clients and therapists, when clients engage in gender-discrepant or role-discrepant behaviors, or when gender interacts with other variables such as sexual orientation, diagnostic category, race, or class (Enns, 2000; Garb, 1997; Landrine, 1989; Lopez, 1989; Zeldow, 1984).

The body of research regarding mental health professionals' judgments of clients served as a consciousness-raising experience for mental health professionals. Replications of the original Broverman et al. (1970) study during the mid-1980s suggested that although some double standards for men and women still existed, clinicians had moved closer to adopting a single, more androgynous standard of mental health for men and women (e.g., Phillips and Gilroy, 1985; Thomas, 1985). The data suggest that the dramatic social changes which occurred during the 1960s and 1970s were associated with the liberalization of therapists' values as well as a decrease in negative attitudes toward women in the general public (Campbell, Schellenberg, and Senn, 1997).

In recent years, psychologists have explored sexist and racist attitudes that are more automatic, subtle, clandestine, and "kinder and gentler justifications of male dominance and prescribed gender roles" (Glick and Fiske, 1997, p. 121). Janet Swim and Laurie Cohen (1997) defined subtle sexism as "unequal and harmful treatment of women that goes unnoticed because it is perceived to be customary or normal behavior" (p. 104). Therapists are not immune from holding these biases, which can be unintentional or nonconscious. Those who treat others in subtly racist or sexist ways may be unaware of their behaviors, and they are also likely to endorse values associated with gender equality and to rate attitudes toward and characteristics of men and women in ways that are consistent with gender-neutral attitudes.

Biased Personality Theories

During the early 1970s, feminists identified the ways in which traditional personality theories contributed to the skewed or narrowly defined worldviews of clinicians. Psychologists were critical of many Freudian concepts as well as Freud's descriptions of women as passive, masochistic, and narcissistic. Feminist psychologists also labeled these views as blatantly biased (Barrett et al., 1974; Caplan, 1984; Holroyd, 1976; Lerman, 1986; Marecek and Kravetz, 1977; Rawlings and Carter, 1977; Rice and Rice, 1973). Nathan Hurvitz (1973) stated,

> Psychodynamic psychology with concepts such as "Electra complex," "penis envy," "vaginal orgasm," etc., has fostered a view of women as appendages to men, as less developed human beings, and as "natural" or "instinctive" mothers and homemakers, fostering conditions and attitudes that create problems for many women. Psychotherapy thus presumes to help these women overcome their problems by inducing them to accept the very conditions that give rise to their complaints. (p. 235)

Although psychoanalytic concepts of personality received the earliest attention, critics also described ways in which a variety of developmental and personality theories based on men's lives were presumed to be automatically relevant to both men and women (e.g.,

Erikson, 1968; Kohlberg, 1981; Perry, 1970). Doherty (1973) argued that any theory of personality which treats female development as a pathway that diverges from the male norm should not be considered a theory of personality.

Bias in Diagnosis

In general, liberal feminist practitioners do not question the value of formal diagnosis but believe that diagnostic categories may reflect gender stereotypes and may be applied in gender-biased ways. Eliminating bias is central to gender-fair treatment. The primary contributions of liberal feminism to the study of bias in diagnosis focused on the relationship of diagnostic categories to gender-role stereotypes. In her groundbreaking book *Women and Madness,* Phyllis Chesler (1972) stated that women are diagnosed for overconforming and underconforming to gender-role stereotypes. A decade later, Marcie Kaplan (1983) noted that biased assumptions about healthy behavior are codified within diagnostic nomenclature. For example, the *Diagnostic and Statistical Manual of Mental Disorders* (American Psychiatric Association, 1980, 1987, 1994, 2000) devotes attention to the ways in which many women express dependency or emotionality in the form of "dependent personality disorder" or "histrionic personality disorder." It does not mention, however, the dependency of people, often men, who rely on others to take care of their children and maintain their households, nor does it label the emotional restrictiveness that often characterizes men's behavior. Marcie Kaplan (1983) concluded that the description of histrionic personality disorder parallels adjectives that were ascribed to healthy women in the Broverman et al. (1970) study. Kaplan (1983) stated, "It appears then that via assumptions about sex roles made by clinicians, a healthy woman automatically earns the diagnosis of Histrionic Personality Disorder or, to help female clients, clinicians encourage them to get sick" (p. 789).

A decade later Dana Becker and Sharon Lamb (1994) examined clinicians' reactions to a male or female version of vignettes depicting a person who met the criteria of both borderline personality disorder (BPD) and post-traumatic stress disorder (PTSD). The person in the female version was more likely than the person in the male version to be categorized as borderline. Further exploration revealed that male versions were also more likely to be rated as antisocial and female versions as histrionic. Becker and Lamb concluded that gender bias may "inhere in the current system of diagnostic classification itself, at times in association with sex of client, sex of clinician, and professional affiliation" (p. 59).

Due to efforts to decrease bias in diagnosis and to pay closer attention to the role of culture in shaping symptoms, the most recent versions of the DSM (American Psychiatric Association, 1994, 2000) have been characterized as substantial improvements over previous manuals. However, Terry Kupers (1997) argued that despite efforts to base diagnostic categories on empirical data and rigorous evaluation, even the DSM-IV, published in 1994, can be used as a "more rigorous rationalization for pathologizing nonmainstream behaviors and attitudes" (p. 340). Another review of the gender and diagnosis literature (Hartung and Widiger, 1998) concluded that subtle forms of bias in assessment may be supported by sampling biases in research studies and subtle biases within diagnostic criteria. Many gender prevalence rates cited in the DSM-IV may be inaccurate due to the differential help-seeking behaviors and referral patterns of men and women, which may result in inaccurate prevalence statistics. The inclusion of only men or women in research on specific problems (e.g., conduct disorder, eating disorders) may result in an incomplete representation of relationships between gender and distress. Diagnostic criteria that are designed to be gender neutral "may disproportionately favor the manner in which the disorder appears in one gender relative to the other" (Hartung and Widiger, 1998, p. 267) because it is difficult to create gender-neutral descriptions of problems when the symptoms of these problems are influenced by gender socialization (e.g., some personality disorders, conduct disorder, somatization disorder, sexual disorders). Some disorders described in gender-neutral terms may actually be expressed differently in men and women or in subcultures of men and women. Limited efforts to consider how gender may influence the expression of distress "is likely to result in the development of diagnostic criteria that are not equally valid for the two sexes" (p. 272).

In summary, feminist practitioners have pointed out ways in which the symptoms displayed by men and women are often consistent with gender-role stereotypes and that women's efforts to conform more closely to feminine gender-role stereotypes have been more likely to be labeled as forms of pathology than are exaggerations of men's stereotypes (e.g., Franks and Rothblum, 1983; Kaplan, 1983). Violet Franks and Esther Rothblum (1983) also indicated that although some women may be inappropriately labeled for merely subscribing to traditional feminine roles, the demands of these gender roles also increase women's vulnerability to disorders such as depression, agoraphobia, eating disorders, and sexual dysfunction. The following warning summarizes this reality: "Sex-role stereotypes may be hazardous to your health" (Franks and Rothblum, 1983, p. 3).

In her twenty-five-year reassessment of *Women and Madness,* Phyllis Chesler (1997) proposed that clinical bias has decreased but continues to be evident in a number of domains. More specifically, therapists need to be cautious about subtle ways in which biased assessment and diagnosis can lead to the mislabeling of some medical illnesses as psychological problems; the pathologizing of victims of sex discrimination and violence within both clinical and legal systems; and a lack of sensitivity to issues of diversity and concerns of people of color. Over time, feminist psychologists and therapists have continued to express concern about subtle gender bias in assessment and diagnosis, including the tendency for therapists to pay minimal attention to the impact of environmental factors on behavior, the presence of gender bias in assessment instruments, the use of different labels for similar behaviors in men and women, and therapist misjudgments about appropriate diagnoses due to stereotyped beliefs about gender and its intersections with other aspects of identity (Santos de Barona and Dutton, 1997; Worell and Remer, 2003).

LIBERAL FEMINIST ALTERNATIVES TO GENDER-BIASED THEORIES

Feminist mental health practitioners have proposed a wide range of gender-fair theories and approaches designed to overcome the biases of past mental health practices. The results of these efforts and the impact of liberal feminism on feminist therapy can be seen in the following applications and approaches:

1. Androgyny therapy
2. Feminist humanistic therapy

3. Feminist cognitive-behavioral interventions and assertiveness training
4. Feminist family therapy
5. Feminist career counseling
6. Gender aware therapy with men

Each of these approaches emerged from efforts to reform practices within the academic or psychotherapy community and each application carried with it the endorsement of a professional community of psychotherapists or academics. Each of these models is also consistent with nonsexist therapy (Marecek and Kravetz, 1977; Rawlings and Carter, 1977). Though not labeled "feminist," nonsexist therapy is based on liberal feminist principles of gender-fair treatment and efforts to ensure that men and women are accorded equal treatment in psychotherapy. Major assumptions of nonsexist therapy include

1. a belief in the importance of therapist awareness of values and power and the potential impact of these values on the psychotherapy relationship;
2. the view that variations from "normative" gender roles are appropriate and potentially healthy;
3. the assumption that women and men have similar capacities for assertiveness and autonomy as well as for expressiveness and tenderness; and
4. the rejection of theories that are biased or posit biological sex and gender differences.

The nonsexist therapist creates a bias-free counseling environment, facilitates clients' awareness of their options, and trusts clients to make personally relevant choices based on their values and preferences.

The liberal feminist or nonsexist therapist works primarily within existing mental health systems in order to create the conditions that allow for equality of treatment. Gender differences are minimized, and the individual man or woman is viewed as capable of autonomy and self-determination. Although the nonsexist or liberal feminist therapist encourages clients to develop understanding of gender-role socialization and the impact of social forces on personal problems, the individual preferences and choices of the client are always of paramount importance in the formulation of therapeutic goals. The ther-

apist does not assume that certain outcomes, such as economic autonomy, are better than others, but believes that men and women will
choose a variety of lifestyle, family, and economic options, and that
whatever "works" for clients constitutes an appropriate goal. One of
the most clear recent descriptions of a nonsexist framework for working with men and women can be found in Lucia Gilbert and Murray
Scher's (1999) book on gender and sex in counseling.

The Promise and Limitations of Androgyny Therapy

As information about sex bias in mental health professions emerged
during the early 1970s, studies heralded the "promise" of androgyny,
or the value of combining masculine and feminine characteristics to
create a new model of mental health (Bem, 1976). Numerous studies
focused on defining androgyny and its characteristics, creating methods of measuring this construct, and demonstrating its relationship to
mental health (Cook, 1985). Lucia Gilbert (1981) suggested that
practitioners who adopted a personal value system based on androgyny would be less likely to view healthy men and women differently,
thus counteracting the double standard of mental health which was
demonstrated in a variety of studies. Alexandra Kaplan (1976) added
that the model of androgyny would help the individual woman "broaden
her sense of what is appropriate and acceptable for her, enlarging the
scope of her self-definition" (p. 355). Sandra Bem (1976), who introduced the benefits of androgyny to self-development, noted that

> the major purpose of my research has always been a political
> one: to help free the human personality from the restricting
> prison of sex-role stereotyping and to develop a conception of
> mental health that is free from culturally imposed definitions of
> masculinity and femininity. (p. 59)

Each of these viewpoints is consistent with the primary goal of liberal
feminism: to free the individual person from negative conditioning so
that she or he can achieve important personal goals.

Although androgyny was identified as an important goal for therapy with women during the mid-1970s, questions about and criticisms of androgyny also emerged. Susan Vogel (1979) noted that although androgyny provided the possibility for greater behavioral
flexibility and less rigid gender roles, an androgynous score is not "an

automatic stamp of psychological health" (p. 255), nor will it "immediately undo the social inequities of sexism" (p. 256). Later research revealed that androgyny was not consistently related to self-esteem or the behaviors of competence, flexibility, and adaptability. Furthermore, although the masculinity component of androgyny was related to mental health in men and women, the femininity component was not associated with mental health. Androgyny researchers had not considered the extent to which so-called gender-neutral ideals are contaminated by notions of masculinity or "the appropriate ingredients for successful action in a male-centered world" (Morawski, 1987, p. 57). The concept of androgyny was also criticized for implying a false dichotomy between connectedness and autonomy, two sets of traits that already coexist at some level in all humans. Furthermore, approaches that define androgyny as a high endorsement of both masculinity and femininity create a prescription that one must incorporate double the number of characteristics within the personality than is required by traditional role expectations. This represents an unrealistic, unattractive, or unattainable goal for many people.

Jill Morawski (1987) indicated that androgyny research represented a liberal feminist agenda which presumed that many "differences" between men and women were superficial and that the reduction of these imposed differences would lead to equal and gender-neutral treatment. Early concepts and research on androgyny did not question or critically analyze the nature of masculine and feminine values, nor did they consider the context in which these values arise and are sustained (Morawski, 1987); they presumed that "androgynous individuals seem to operate (effortlessly) in a social vacuum where expectations for gender-related behavior or gender-based constraints on choice of action are noticeably absent" (p. 55). Researchers and therapists failed to consider the differential power structures, contexts in which men and women live, as well as the differential rewards and consequences that are accorded to men and women. Jill Morawski (1987) concluded that in their efforts to increase women's options, feminist psychologists had adopted male language, symbols, and research styles, but that women had not realized any real increase in power.

Although androgyny therapy holds less promise than early commentators suggested (e.g., Kaplan, 1976, 1979), it represents an important liberal feminist legacy within feminist psychology and therapy. For example, the goal of integrating instrumental and expressive characteristics apart from gender-role stereotypes remains an important principle of feminist therapy (see Brown and Brodsky, 1992). In her later assessment of androgyny theory, Sandra Bem (1993) articulated a more comprehensive perspective and concluded that the original conceptualizations of androgyny were "theorized at too private and too personal a level to be of any value politically. The elimination of gender inequality will require institutional change, not just personal change" (p. 123). Sandra Bem (1987) indicated that gender should not be considered primarily as a set of internal characteristics but as a method by which a culture transmits stereotypes and encourages individuals to internalize gender-polarized visions of reality. Her alternative to androgyny, which she named *gender schema theory,* describes how beliefs about gender become organized around the culture's stereotypes and how these cognitive structures are used by individuals to anticipate, perceive, encode, and interpret information according to the culture's polarized images of gender. These cognitive structures not only influence one's judgments about personal behavior but also one's perceptions of the behavior of others. Gender schemas are powerful and forge "a cultural connection between sex and virtually every other aspect of human experience, including modes of dress, social roles, and even ways of expressing emotion and experiencing sexual desire" (Bem, 1993, p. 192).

The concept of gender schemas moves beyond a liberal feminist perspective in several ways. First, it acknowledges the complexity and tenacity of gender stereotypes and notes how power structures perpetuate stereotypes. The biased lenses of individuals and institutions encourage selective attention, recall, and interpretation of men's and women's behaviors; these biases have a significant impact on women's ability to realize their full potential (Deaux and Major, 1987; Deaux and Stewart, 2001). Gender schema theory is built on the assumption that gender operates on multiple levels: as a set of personal attributes at the individual level, as a set of relational cues at the interpersonal level, and as a system of power relations at the social level. Second, gender schema theory does not prescribe any particular combination of agency and communion as an ideal of mental health. It acknowledges the diversity of healthy human behavior and rejects the labeling of expressive traits as "feminine" and instrumental traits as "masculine." Ideal mental health is associated with the organization of the personality around some combination of personally relevant characteristics other than masculinity or femininity. Cultural relativism schemas, sexism schemas, and individual differences schemas represent some of the cognitive structures that can help the person combat gender stereotypes (Bem, 1983). Compared to androgyny theory, gender schema theory presents a more complete understanding of how context shapes and elicits behavior. It focuses less on the *content* of gender stereotypes and more on the *process* of how gender stereotypes arise and are perpetuated despite individual change (Bem, 1987).

Recent discussions of gender-role identity speak to the limitations of thinking about gender in isolation from other aspects of identity. Kay Deaux and Abigail Stewart (2001) spoke about the importance of considering the "multiplicity of identities—their variety, shifting salience or importance, intersection, and mutual influence" (p. 94). Gender roles and gender schemas are influenced by multiple aspects of identity including ethnicity, religious background, immigration status, socioeconomic class, race, sexual orientation, age, and privilege.

Humanistic Therapy

Susan Sturdivant (1980) posed the following rhetorical question: If humans have the capacity for autonomy and self-actualization, why have women been thwarted in their efforts to achieve this goal? She answered this question by proposing that feminist humanism, the modification of traditional humanism, views women as "competent and independent and as intellectually and morally equal to men; in other words, as autonomous and fully human" (p. 89). Feminist humanistic counselors "expose the myths about women for what they are" (p. 89) and pave the way for new and accurate images of women's potential. Sturdivant's conclusion is consistent with a liberal feminist view that new information will enlighten individuals, replace mythology and stereotypes, and pave the way for egalitarian relationships.

In one of the earliest descriptions of feminist therapy, Hannah Lerman (1976) indicated that feminist therapy is "an outgrowth of eclectic humanistic thought and represents a logical extension of humanistic thinking into the awareness of sex-role issues" (p. 378). Although she noted that feminist therapists come from various theoretical persuasions, she also stated, "I don't think I have met a feminist therapist, however, who has not been influenced by humanistic principles" (p. 378). The following sections discusses the use of person-centered and Gestalt approaches and their modifications from a liberal feminist perspective.

Person-Centered Therapy

Early feminist psychotherapists viewed humanistic psychology as consistent with their goals because of

1. its emphasis on each person's uniqueness, human potential, and capacity for autonomy and self-directedness;
2. its assumption that the phenomenological world of the individual should be trusted and viewed as the most important frame of reference;
3. its emphasis on the capacity of individuals to be self-actualizing, self-determining, and capable of making productive choices for their own lives; and
4. the belief that symptoms are not signs of pathology but represent growing pains, and that painful feelings and behaviors can be redirected and refocused in positive directions.

Furthermore, the core conditions of empathy, congruence, and unconditional positive regard proposed by Carl Rogers (1951) provide the foundation for an egalitarian relationship and for trusting clients as their own best experts (Lerman, 1992; Waterhouse, 1993). Feminist therapists often borrowed from the concepts of humanistic therapy because its relatively limited number of concepts did not contain overtly sexist features. Therapists working with women did not need to subtract or eliminate negative aspects of humanism in order to make it viable; they merely added elements to the theory so that women would be included as a focal point (Lerman, 1992).

In her early statement on feminist therapy, Hannah Lerman (1976) identified three principles of feminist therapy: (1) the therapist views the client as competent and knowledgeable about her experience, (2) the therapist helps the client acknowledge personal power, and (3) the personal is political. Although the first two principles were highly consistent with the feminist modifications of person-centered therapy, the third principle was not easily incorporated into person-centered approaches. In contrast to the notion that the personal is political, person-centered theory does not acknowledge the ways in which the external world influences the private self.

Ruth Waterhouse (1993) criticized Carl Rogers for overemphasizing the American tradition of "vigorous self-reliance," adding that person-centered therapy lacks "a sensitivity to people's 'real suffering' and an understanding that personal troubles come not only from within the self, but also from the real world" (p. 58). In addition, the emphasis of person-centered therapy on individualism, autonomy, and an internal locus of control may be potentially disempowering if it leads clients to blame themselves for factors outside of themselves such as racism, sexism, or violence. In summary, "the woman must change her 'self' for a society that basically remains the same. Furthermore, she must do this ultimately *by* and *for* herself" (Waterhouse, 1993, p. 63). Building on the concerns of Waterhouse, many feminist therapists have noted the limitations of humanistic therapy for connecting personal themes with the political implications of private concerns. They believe that optimism about the power of the individual to effect personal change must be matched with efforts to address the external oppression which may limit a person's efforts to reach his or her potential.

If one operates strictly from a liberal feminist worldview, humanistic liberal feminism may seem relatively complete. However, many feminist therapists note its inadequacy for connecting personal themes with the political implications of private concerns. The person-centered approach provides counselors with powerful relational tools which are necessary but not sufficient for feminist therapy that connects the personal and the political.

Gestalt Therapy

Gestalt therapy emphasizes the importance of self-awareness and self-responsibility, and shares many of the strengths and limitations of person-centered therapy. From this perspective, persons with problems in living live in a "what if" or fantasy world, are limited by stereotyped behaviors and attitudes, throw roadblocks in their own paths, and leave little room for realizing personal potential. In contrast, fully functioning persons are self-supporting, autonomous, and spontaneous. They make choices, take risks, and assume responsibility for the results of personal decisions (Polster, 1974).

Women often enter counseling with a sense of powerlessness, lack of trust in self-direction, and permeable "I" boundaries (Collier, 1982). They may adhere to numerous "shoulds," fail to engage in self-care, and have difficulty communicating suppressed emotions. Gestalt therapy provides useful tools for addressing these issues, especially as they pertain to expanding women's self-definitions and self-perceptions, developing the courage to express strong emotion, and expanding behavioral alternatives (Enns, 1987). Through the use of Gestalt techniques, women can become more aware of their personal power and can learn to take greater responsibility for their communication patterns and feelings by using the pronoun "I" rather than "we," "it," and "they." Instead of using soft language and qualifiers (e.g., "I guess" and "maybe"), women learn to use more powerful and assertive language. When women learn to change verbs, such as "need" to "want" and "should" to "choose," they become more aware of inner feelings and choices and experience greater courage to take risks.

Second, Gestalt therapy focuses on the importance of recognizing a full range of human emotions, gives women permission to recognize and express reactions that they have previously discounted or repressed, and encourages women to use those feelings to motivate action. Anger is expressed directly: "I'm angry" rather than "It makes me angry." Through techniques such as the "empty chair" that are designed to complete unfinished business, women can safely express feelings of disappointment, anger, or guilt toward significant people in their past or present (Polster, 1974). Through the use of nonverbal exercises, clients can focus on areas of body tension and learn how strong feelings may be internalized in the form of physical constriction. Women learn "response-ability" by experiencing and expressing a full range of emotions (Enns, 1987). Through guided fantasy, the empty chair, and many verbal techniques, women learn to accept and integrate polarities associated with their emotions, behaviors, or perceptions of others (Brien and Sheldon, 1977; Collier, 1982; Polster, 1974).

In addition to helping women develop higher self-esteem and expressiveness, Gestalt approaches have been applied to a variety of significant women's issues including sexual abuse (Reichert, 1994) and intimate violence (Little, 1990). Despite the usefulness of Gestalt tools for increasing one's sense of self as a powerful person, the traditional practice of Gestalt therapy is associated with some limitations. Similar to person-centered therapy, Gestalt therapy can magnify the belief that people are masters of their own fates. There are many events, external realities, and experiences of discrimination over which clients have little control, no matter how aware and self-responsible they become. From a traditional Gestalt perspective, identifying biases or sociopolitical factors that influence personal experience may be labeled as rationalizing, making excuses, projecting personal inadequacy on the external world, or evading responsibility (Mander and Rush, 1974). The Gestalt focus on taking responsibility may increase women's feelings of self-blame, guilt, and inadequacy, thus minimizing or discounting the toxic nature of oppressive social conditions. However, from a traditional Gestalt perspective, identifying biases or sociopolitical factors that influence personal experience may be labeled as rationalizing, making excuses, projecting personal inadequacy on the external world, or evading responsibility (Mander and Rush, 1974). Counselors who hold a feminist worldview believe that the recognition of external constrictions often completes women's awareness and releases them from self-depreciation. Analysis of external factors does not encourage women to avoid responsibility by blaming boredom or pain on others; instead, it frees them to engage in realistic action (Rawlings and Carter, 1977).

Another issue is that Gestalt therapy emphasizes the importance of personal autonomy and gives inadequate attention to the interrelatedness and interdependence of all persons. Many women seek goals other than autonomy, such as the ability to participate in relationships with others while also pursuing self-development. Therapists who use Gestalt tools benefit from remaining aware that the consequences of autonomy are different for women and men. Autonomy and assertion in women may not be met with acceptance but with skepticism and rejection. Thus, counselors who use a Gestalt approach must also recognize that a comprehensive approach must also attend to the barriers that women face as they work toward becoming more spontaneous and "response-able."

The tools of Gestalt therapy are relatively compatible with liberal feminism, especially as they relate to emphasizing personal awareness and choice. Like person-centered therapy, this model does not adequately address environmental factors that limit the free choice of individuals. Feminist therapists who use Gestalt techniques may need to seek creative ways to balance attention to internal choices with the realities of the sociocultural world in which the client and therapist live.

Cognitive-Behavioral Therapies

In the wake of early critiques offered by individuals such as Weisstein ([1968] 1993) and Chesler (1972), counselors often adopted cognitive-behavioral therapy (CBT) interventions as resocialization tools to help women become aware of their interpersonal rights, alter negative self-beliefs, transcend gender stereotypes, use direct forms of personal power to influence their environments, and reframe and redirect "underground power" in productive ways (Jakubowski, 1977; Moore, 1981). Over time, cognitive-behavioral approaches for working with women have become more specialized and have been applied to numerous problems including post-traumatic stress disorder, eating disorders, depression, and borderline personality disorder.

Many general concepts of cognitive-behavioral therapy are compatible with the counseling needs of women, including the assumptions that problematic behavior is learned and can be modified; the therapist plays a consulting and collaborative role rather than an expert role; and clients should be encouraged to establish their own goals and take charge of their own lives. Furthermore, cognitive-behavioral methods are based on an optimistic view about change (Fodor, 1988; Mohlman, 2000; Worell and Remer, 2003; Wolfe, 1995). Many CBT tools, such as modeling, contracting, functional analysis, self-monitoring and reinforcement, stress inoculation, assertiveness training, and cognitive restructuring, can be integrated with efforts to increase women's confidence and repertoire of skills for pursuing their goals (Worell and Remer, 2003).

However, several general cautions are also important. Cognitive-behavioral interventions focus primarily on individual change and do not suggest methods for addressing larger environmental issues that limit personal choice (Kantrowitz and Ballou, 1992). In her assessment of cognitive-behavioral methods, Iris Fodor (1988) stated that narrowly defined programs place the burden of change on individuals and imply that through individual change alone one can eliminate poor parenting, negative conditioning, and sexist socialization. In the real world, women are more frequently sexually harassed, interrupted in conversation, and addressed with inappropriate forms of familiarity than are men, and cognitive-behavioral methods alone may not challenge the social conditions that support these behaviors. Second, traditional cognitive-behavioral approaches do not critically examine androcentric or culturally normative assumptions about mental health, such as those that place greater value on rationality than emotional sensitivity. Potentially pathologizing labels such as "distortion" and "irrationality" may deny a client's view of reality and thus should be relabeled. For example, some beliefs that have been presumed to be irrational (e.g., "I will be punished if . . .") are based on occasions when women's assertive responses have been rejected rather than rewarded. Finally, cognitive-behavioral techniques can be combined with techniques which explore the client's affective experiences (e.g., Gestalt therapy) in order to decrease the likelihood that rationality is overvalued and emotion is undervalued (Kantrowitz and Ballou, 1992; Worell and Remer, 2003).

Assertiveness Training

Assertiveness training was one of the first CBT methods that was used for working with women, and it has been used as a tool to help women overcome internalized restrictive beliefs about gender and build skills for achieving their goals. Janet Wolfe and Iris Fodor (1975) hypothesized that the combination of assertiveness training and rational emotive therapy concepts would help women combat harmful "shoulds" and irrational beliefs that are embedded in gender role stereotypes, such as the ideas that

1. one should be loved by everyone,
2. others' needs are more important than one's own,
3. it is easier to avoid than to face difficulties,
4. women need a strong person to rely on, and
5. women have no control over their emotions.

Through "depropagandization," women learn to identify irrational beliefs and the ways in which they are reinforced, test these beliefs against objective reality, and replace them with more adaptive beliefs and behaviors (Wolfe, 1995; Wolfe and Fodor, 1975).

A variety of studies also compared the outcomes of consciousness-raising groups with those that included both a consciousness-raising and a skills component, such as assertiveness training or communication skills training (e.g., Ballou, Reuter, and Dinero, 1979; Gulanick, Howard, and Moreland, 1979; Wolfe and Fodor, 1977). The results suggested that consciousness-raising groups represented effective tools for changing attitudes and building personal self-esteem, but behavioral change is more likely to occur in groups that emphasize a skills component.

After a period of initial optimism, feminist therapists raised questions about the exclusive use of cognitive-behavioral interventions for women. First, appropriate assertive behavior may be misperceived or punished because it is inconsistent with expectations of how women *should* behave. A recent study (Rudman and Glick, 2001) found, for example, that an agentic female was perceived as "insufficiently nice" (p. 743) for a job that was described in feminized terms, the authors concluded that women may be penalized "unless they temper their agency with niceness" (p. 743). Mary Wade (2001) also indicated that self-advocacy, a form of assertiveness on the part of women, may result in personal costs. Although women do not appear to incur significant costs when advocating for others, women who engage in self-advocacy may be rendered ineffective because they are seen as drawing attention to themselves and acting in a manner that is inconsistent with gendered norms of likeability, modesty, and selflessness.

These findings are consistent with Laura Solomon and Esther Rothblum's (1985) conclusion that "there are sometimes harsh contingencies in the natural environment for women behaving in nontraditional ways" (p. 318). The adage that states, "He's aggressive, she's pushy; he's firm, she's stubborn; he exercises his authority, she's tyrannical" (Muehlenhard, 1983, p. 163) still appears to reflect social attitudes in at least some circumstances. Feminist therapists face the challenge of helping clients deal with the "intermittent success" of assertiveness (Solomon and Rothblum, 1985, p. 318).

Although assertion training remains an important tool for empowering women in the twenty-first century, some feminists have also critiqued this approach and recommended some modifications of its early characteristics. Traditional assertiveness training includes an overly narrow definition of "correct" assertive responses, presumes that assertiveness will naturally lead to successful interpersonal interactions, promotes techniques that encourage the use of traditional power tactics, and defines human rights as existing apart from an understanding of complex gender-role injunctions (Stere, 1985). The greater value placed on instrumental, rational problem-solving skills implies that women must eschew and devalue traditional relational skills or merely use these relational skills to increase the likelihood that their assertive responses will be successful. Prescriptions for assertive speech closely resemble positive stereotypes of masculine behavior, and assertiveness training can also promote "masculine stereotypes as implicit norms" (Gervasio and Crawford, 1989, p. 9) and imply that individualism is more important than interdependence.

To transcend the problems of traditional assertion training, Amy Gervasio and Mary Crawford (1989) proposed that "ecologically valid" (p. 11) assertion training must communicate the benefits, costs, and risks of assertive communication, and acknowledge that women and men experience different social contexts with different types of personal infringements and rewards. In addition, assertiveness training may be balanced with self-confidence training that includes four major components or goals, including

1. learning to accept personal feelings as valid and based on one's responses to something real;
2. developing the capacity to please oneself and engage in self-nurturing behavior;
3. identifying and developing strengths; and
4. developing realistic expectations and accepting shortcomings, as well as acknowledging that perfection is not necessary or desirable (Stere, 1985).

Such training is based on an understanding of the complex relationship between women's social status and personal esteem and attitudes, and encourages women to develop self-defined strengths that incorporate but also move beyond the restrictions of cognitive-behavioral assumptions (Enns, 1992a; Stere, 1985). Finally, consciousness-raising principles can be integrated with assertiveness concepts in order to more consistently connect political with personal change issues (e.g., Enns, 1992a) and to encourage women to become involved in social activism.

CBT for Depression, Eating Disorders,
and Coping with Trauma

During recent years, CBT applications have been applied to high prevalence problems experienced by women, including depression, eating disorders, and trauma. The rates of depression and PTSD are twice as high for women than men (Foa and Street, 2001; Mazure, Keita, and Blehar, 2002), and roughly 90 percent of those experiencing severe eating disorders are women (Barlow and Durand, 2002). Thus the examination of specific approaches designed to deal with these issues is important.

Cognitive-behavioral therapy for depression consists of

1. education about depression from a CBT perspective,
2. behavioral methods and experiments for increasing active coping,
3. self-monitoring techniques designed to provide information about and challenge the client's feelings and dysfunctional thoughts,
4. examination and alteration of negative schemas or belief systems that support depression, and
5. education about strategies for preventing relapse (Craighead, Craighead, and Ilardi, 1998).

Susan Nolen-Hoeksema's (2000) research found that women's greater tendency to employ ruminative cognitive styles in response to negative events places them at increased risk for depression. Rumination is defined as "a repetitive and passive mental focus on symptoms of distress and their possible causes and consequences" (Mazure, Keita, and Blehar, 2002, p. 8). Examining and challenging this pattern may be especially important for CBT with depressed women.

Studies reveal that CBT is as effective as antidepressant medication in relieving symptoms of depression, and at least in some studies, is shown to be superior to antidepressant medication for preventing relapse (Craighead, Craighead, and Ilardi, 1998; Elkin et al., 1989; Evans et al., 1992; Mazure, Keita, and Blehar, 2002). A comparison of men's and women's responses to CBT revealed similar levels of improvement, with the exception of severely depressed women, who showed a poorer response to CBT than severely depressed men (Thase et al., 1994).

Cognitive-behavioral therapy has also been well established as an efficacious treatment for bulimia nervosa. It is based on the assumption that social pressures lead to the overvaluation of thinness and trigger dysfunctional cognitive distortions and emotions about attaining and maintaining a perfect body type. Treatment typically includes educational components about bulimia, behavioral and nutritional education designed to help clients establish normal eating habits, and cognitive procedures that help clients challenge dysfunctional cognitions about weight and shape. Counseling often follows two major phases; the first focuses on interrupting a cycle of overeating and vomiting and gaining control over one's food intake, and the second focuses on identifying and challenging the circumstances and cognitions that contribute to loss of control and block behavior change. Self-monitoring, problem-solving procedures, and exposure therapies are also incorporated in this therapy (Williamson and Netemeyer, 2000; Wilson et al., 2002).

Research demonstrates that the treatment effects of CBT for bulimia are rapid (Wilson et al., 1999) and more effective than antidepressant medication (Wilfley and Cohen, 1997) or other treatments to which it has been compared (Wilson and Fairburn, 1998). Terence Wilson and Christopher Fairburn (1998) concluded, "CBT is the most effective means of eliminating the core features of the eating disorder [bulimia] and is often accompanied by improvement in comorbid psychological problems such as low self-esteem and depression" (p. 501). A recent study found that CBT clients experienced more rapid improvements than did individuals experiencing interpersonal psychotherapy (IPT, reviewed later in this chapter). However, posttreatment differences between CBT and IPT were no longer evident at a one-year follow-up (Agras et al., 2000; Wilson et al., 2002).

Cognitive-behavioral treatments also represent prominent methods for working with those experiencing PTSD effects of traumas such as rape and child sexual abuse (e.g., Foa and Rothbaum, 1998; Foa and Street, 2001; Foa and Zoellner, 1998; Resick and Schnicke, 1993). Cognitive-behavioral treatments are designed to help clients work through and normalize the following aspects associated with trauma: emotional processing of memories, the organization and narrative associated with trauma, and basic beliefs and schemas about oneself and the world (Foa and Zoellner, 1998). The major CBT approaches for treating PTSD include exposure therapy, stress inoculation, and cognitive restructuring (Foa and Street, 2001). Exposure therapy typically includes education about trauma reactions, repeated exposure to memories of trauma, and exposure to situations that the client avoids. Stress inoculation training, which emphasizes anxiety management, includes relaxation, guided self-dialogue, thought stopping, cognitive restructuring, modeling, and role-playing components. Cognitive restructuring focuses primarily on relieving symptoms by identifying, challenging, and replacing unrealistic or dysfunctional thoughts with more functional cognitions. A variation of CBT, cognitive processing therapy (CPT) for rape victims (Resick and Schnicke, 1993), uses successive writing assignments as a form of exposure. Cognitive restructuring components emphasize the five themes of safety, trust, power, esteem, and intimacy.

A study that compared group CPT for rape victims with a wait list control condition found that CPT clients experienced more reductions in depression and PTSD symptoms. More specifically, the mean symptom reduction for CPT clients was 40 percent, but only 1.5 percent for wait-list controls (Resick and Schnicke, 1992). Another study compared the outcomes of female clients who had experienced rape, child sexual abuse, or nonsexual assault and were randomly assigned to prolonged exposure, stress inoculation, a combination of exposure and inoculation, or a wait-list group (Foa et al., 1999). Women in the three active cognitive-behavioral treatment groups experienced significantly higher reductions of PTSD symptoms and depression than did wait-list controls, and these gains were maintained over a follow-up period. No significant differences occurred between the three cognitive-behavioral treatment groups. Patricia Resick's (2001) review of seven outcome studies with at least some component of CBT (e.g., cognitive processing therapy, CBT plus exposure) concluded that therapies with a cognitive component were more effective than supportive counseling, relaxation alone, or no treatment. Outcomes for cognitively oriented therapies were similar to those of exposure therapy.

Dialectical Behavior Therapy and Borderline
Personality Disorder

Seventy-five percent of those who receive the controversial label of borderline personality disorder are women; in addition, roughly three-fourths of those with this label have experienced child sexual abuse (Butler, 2001). Marcia Linehan (1993) described persons with BPD as having experienced invalidating environments in which "communication of private experiences is met by erratic, inappropriate, and extreme responses" (p. 49). Persons with borderline symptoms exhibit emotional, interpersonal, and behavioral dysregulation, reactivity, and instability, and often demonstrate a pattern of suicidal and self-harming behaviors.

Marcia Linehan's (1993) dialectical behavior therapy (DBT) was first developed with women and is built on cognitive-behavioral treatment methods and an emphasis on "dialectics," or the reconciliation of tensions and opposites. One dialectic involves efforts to reconcile polarities in the client's behavior; another dialectic involves integrating cognitive-behavioral change and Zenlike acceptance (Butler, 2001). The therapist reframes the client's symptoms as aspects of the client's learned problem-solving repertoire and emphasizes the importance of active change. Systematic problem solving is balanced with a "corresponding emphasis on validating the patient's current emotional, cognitive, and behavioral responses just as they are" (Linehan, 1993, p. 19). During treatment, the therapist balances "technologies of change" or cognitive-behavioral therapies with "technologies of acceptance" (p. 110), represented by more humanistic and client-centered alternatives. To operate effectively, the therapist must show a "stance of centeredness" or certainty in her or his direction while also showing "compassionate flexibility," marked by the therapist's ability to modify her or his approach based on new information. Centeredness involves "keeping one's feet on the ground" while flexibility involves "moving your shoulders to the side to let the patient by" (p. 110).

Dialectical behavior therapy includes four treatment components, including individual psychotherapy, group skills training, between-session telephone consultation (client and therapist), and consultations groups for all team members who are working with the client. DBT consists of four stages, beginning with the stabilization of behavior and daily functioning. Phase two, referred to as posttraumatic stress reduction, involves exposure to and the processing of past trauma. Phase three emphasizes the development of independent problem-solving and self-soothing skills, and phase four is designed to foster optimal functioning (Butler, 2001; Linehan, 1993; Scheel, 2000).

Marsha Linehan (1993) believes that her approach is different from other cognitive-behavioral methods because of its acceptance of clients' behavior, integration of cognitive and emotion-focused interventions, emphasis on the centrality of the client-therapist relationship, integration of perspectives influenced by meditation and Eastern spirituality, and emphasis on interrelatedness and wholeness. The holistic perspective recognizes that relationships with others as well as one's access to social power represent larger contexts which may facilitate or limit individual change. Unlike some feminist mental health practitioners (e.g., Becker, 2001), Marsha Linehan does not question the validity of the label *borderline.* However, she challenges "blame the victim" traditions associated with this disorder and the stereotype of "borderline" women as manipulative (Butler, 2001; Scheel, 2000). She has also "reconfigured the borderline diagnosis in behaviorist terms, stripping it of judgment and shame and posing an explicit feminist challenge" to "damning and pessimistic views of it" (Butler, 2001, p. 30).

A major study explored the therapeutic outcomes of women with BPD who exhibited parasuicidal behaviors (intentional self-injurious behaviors not associated with suicidal intent) (Linehan et al., 1991). Compared to women who received "treatment as usual in the community," women in DBT were more likely to stay in therapy with a single therapist for a year, were hospitalized for fewer inpatient days, and experienced fewer parasuicidal behaviors. Although DBT clients remained in the impaired category with regard to social adjustment and global functioning (rated by interviewers) and trait anger (rated by clients), their outcomes in these areas were superior to those in the control condition. Based on these findings and those from three other studies, Karen Scheel (2000) described the research base for DBT as "broadly promising"; however, a variety of questions about the reliability and generalizability of these findings remain.

Family Systems Therapy

The family systems therapies escaped early criticism by feminists because these approaches were characterized by their neutral views on gender, emphasis on problem solving, recognition of family environments that shape behavior, and refusal to use traditional diagnostic labels with the potential for blaming individuals (Ault-Riché, 1986). From a systems view, interpersonal sequences that contribute to relationship problems are explained in terms of circular causality, which defines each action and/or individual as influencing every other aspect of a system as a part of a complex, reciprocal process of reinforcement. No specific situation or person is considered the antecedent, cause, or effect of problematic interactions.

Despite their strengths, Rachel Hare-Mustin (1978) noted that family systems models virtually ignored the powerful impact of gender on family relationships. Although they appeared to offer an "equal opportunity" for understanding many daily interactions, family systems models did not adequately address issues related to power differences, gendered family roles, or the pain associated with physical, sexual, and emotional abuse. Hoffman (1981), for example, described battering as a relational pattern between an overadequate woman and an underadequate man that serves a functional role in the maintenance of the family system. Second, although family therapy systems approaches define most issues in neutral terms, many basic terms have been based on "prototypically male attributes and sometimes define them as standards of healthy family functioning" (Bograd, 1988, p. 122). In traditional family systems therapy, terms such as *hierarchy, complementarity, autonomy,* and *differentiation* are often used to signify the degree of health within the family and are often associated with role definitions along traditional lines. In contrast, terms such as *enmeshment, fusion,* and *symbiosis* are used to label overinvestment in relationships, and these terms can be used to pathologize women's relational qualities (Avis, 1988; Bograd, 1988; Enns, 1988; Goodrich et al., 1988).

The "neutral" concepts of mainstream family systems therapy can also contribute to mother blaming. Although all family members are viewed as contributing to the family climate, women are often more actively involved in their children's lives than men, and they are often allotted more than their share of blame for family problems (Caplan,

1989). When women play counterstereotypical roles, their behavior may be described in pejorative terms, and the family therapist may attempt to "restore" power to the father (Minuchin, 1984). Michele Bograd (1988) argued that "many formulations draw on stereotypical, culture-bound ideals of men and women that, in very subtle ways, denigrate women and perpetuate traditional assumptions about male-female interactions" (pp. 122-123). Finally, traditional family systems approaches have typically focused on the nuclear family alone and imply that gender-role stereotypes and the larger social context are disconnected from family dynamics.

Lois Braverman (1988) proposed that although the assumptions underlying traditional family systems therapies are flawed, many of the techniques can be reformulated to support nonsexist practice. The nonsexist family therapist strives to model behavior that is not constrained by gender stereotypes and helps families explore gender patterns and the manner in which gender stereotypes may influence the allocation of power, rewards, and labor. The family therapist also helps family members transcend restrictive gender roles, increase their behavioral options, and create greater reciprocity and symmetry among family members. Out of respect for the diverse choices that individuals make, the nonsexist family therapist affirms the value of roles that women have traditionally played, such as nurturing and caring for others, while also supporting women's desires and choices to experience rewarding achievement roles in various work and social institutions.

In contrast to the ease of combining family therapy with liberal feminism, it was initially more difficult for therapists to integrate traditional family systems concepts with more radical theories that highlight diversity. Family systems thinking was not based on a critical or historical analysis of the family but typically represented middle-class views of the family.

In recent years, feminist family therapy approaches have continued to mature and have transcended definitions of the traditional family as well as the boundaries of liberal feminist theory. For example, Louise Silverstein and Thelma Goodrich's (2003) edited volume contributes to the transformation of family therapy by speaking to the intersections of class, gender, and race as they influence family structures and by focusing on themes such as migration, lesbian families, stepfamilies, violence, and AIDS. New developments in feminist family therapy are discussed further in Chapter 7.

Feminist Career Counseling

Career feminism is concerned primarily with helping women achieve equality in the labor force. Important strategies include encouraging women to enter nontraditional careers, fighting sexual harassment on the job, and increasing the proportion of women in well-paying jobs. Interventions designed to help women achieve their personal career goals include mentoring, networking, and creating support networks. Career feminism emphasizes "the need for individual women to take their lives into their own hands and dare to be what they can become, to fight back if men try to stop or limit them, and to help other women" (Ferree and Hess, 1985, p. 42).

Psychological theory and research on women's achievement, career choice, and professional advancement provide a foundation for a variety of models that seek to explain how personal, family, contextual, racial, ethnic, and cultural factors influence the career paths of women (e.g., Betz and Hackett, 1981, 1997; Byars and Hackett, 1998; Eccles, 1994; Farmer, 1997; Fassinger, 1990; Fassinger and O'Brien, 2000; O'Brien and Fassinger, 1993; Weitzman, 1994). Feminist psychological theories of career development have also explored the intersections between women's paid work and family responsibilities (e.g., Barnett and Hyde, 2001; Gilbert, 1993; Gilbert and Rader, 2001; Weitzman, 1994; Worell and Remer, 2003). Lucia Gilbert and Jill Rader (2001) described models of women's career and family roles as moving from an emphasis on career expansion (1974-1984), to concern with women's multiple and competing roles (mid-1980s to mid-1990s), to an emphasis on work-family role convergence that identifies both family and work roles as compatible, interrelated, and integral to women's adult lives.

During the mid-1990s, Linda Brooks and Linda Forrest (1994) concluded that although many career models identified the negative impact of stereotypes and cultural prescriptions on women's careers, "many authors still conceptualized internal barriers as the primary source of women's career development problems" (p. 116). Since that time, models of career development have increasingly acknowledged the role of institutionalized oppression, educational barriers, stereotyping, and occupational discrimination in career choice (e.g., Byars and Hackett, 1998; Fassinger and O'Brien, 2000; Lent, Brown, and Hackett, 2000; Worell and Remer, 2003). Feminist models of career counseling have tended to focus primarily on women's socialization and methods for creating gender-fair environments in which women can make the best possible choices about their personal and work lives. Much of the literature emphasizes the relevance of socialized patterns associated with women's attributions regarding success, self-efficacy beliefs, self-confidence, fear of failure, fear of success, the imposter phenomenon, stereotype threats, limited assertiveness, and home-career conflict (Eccles, 1994; Farmer, 1997; Worell and Remer, 2003). An expanding literature on mentoring also emphasizes the role that individual sponsorship and guidance play in career development and advancement (Gutek, 2001).

Feminist career counseling emphasizes the importance of an egalitarian relationship, which validates the clients' expertise about their own lives and models the types of active and interactive roles that are important to women as they choose and pursue challenging career goals (Brooks and Forrest, 1994). In addition, gender- and social-role analysis is an important tool for helping women gain awareness of the subtle ways in which social contexts influence personal aspirations. Clients are encouraged to identify family and social messages about careers, become acquainted with the experiences of women who have defied traditional career roles, and clarify the meaning of gender as it relates to career and the meaning of career success or failure as a woman or man. Feminist career exploration provides a foundation for helping women combat internalized limited expectations and potential fears about success, and also increases their awareness of career options. Fantasy and role-playing exercises augment exploration by helping individuals imagine attractive career goals and prepare them for the potential rewards and conflicts they may encounter in pursuing goals (Brooks and Forrest, 1994; Hackett and Lonborg, 1994). Feminist career counseling also assists women in identifying and choosing appropriate mentors and role models and developing career skills. These skills include communication, interpersonal, political/ organizational, and adaptive cognitive skills.

One of the most influential theories in the women's career counseling literature has emphasized the role of self-efficacy in career choice (Betz and Hackett, 1981, 1997). Self-efficacy approaches, which are often referred to as social cognitive career theory, are supported by substantial research that identifies significant predictive linkages between self-efficacy beliefs and career decision making and achievement (Betz, 2002; Juntunen, 1996). In its present form, social cognitive career theory addresses

1. the social identities and social context of the individual such as race, ethnicity, gender, class, sexual orientation, acculturation, feminist attitudes, and the mother's education and occupational traditionality;
2. the learning experiences of the person;
3. self-efficacy beliefs, interests, and outcome expectations;
4. perceived support from family members and society; and
5. occupational barriers (Flores and O'Brien, 2002; Lent, Brown, and Hackett, 2000).

Applications of this model to diverse groups and women of color have been promising (e.g., Byars and Hackett, 1998; McWhirter, Hackett, and Bandalos, 1998).

Although career counseling has often placed central emphasis on women's socialized patterns and individual choices, contextual variables and structural factors are some of the most powerful determinants of work adjustment (Fitzgerald and Rounds, 1994). One example of structural factors is the null environment, which "neither encourages nor discourages individuals—it simply ignores them" (Betz, 1994, p. 17). The consequence of the null environment is that women have little opportunity to receive feedback about themselves as competent people and thus have few opportunities to develop self-images that sustain the self through difficult times. Women are left at the mercy of the specific environmental forces that are present at any point in time. Second, the devaluation of women's performance is often an issue when women are employed in nontraditional fields in which they are the "wrong" sex or when evaluation criteria are ambiguous or unclear (Crawford and Unger, 2004). Third, workplace discrimination because of one's lesbian identity or ethnic/racial identity poses substantial barriers and may also influence one's identity development (e.g., about whether one should be "out" in the workplace) (Fassinger, 1996). Fourth, sexual harassment remains a major problem encountered by women in the workplace (Gutek, 2001). It is important for feminist counseling to help women become aware of political and social structures that have shaped or limited their aspirations and to assist women as they face challenges and barriers. Counselor self-disclosure, occupational power analysis, educational interventions, and bibliotherapy (e.g., popular and current articles about sexual harassment and/or discrimination) represent some of the tools that facilitate the exploration of external barriers and methods for counteracting these barriers and challenges. Finally, a promising development in the career counselor literature is recent emphasis on the career counselor's role as a social change agent (e.g., Fassinger and O'Brien, 2000; Heppner, Davidson, and Scott, 2003; Worell and Remer, 2003).

Counseling Men About Restrictive Gender Roles

During the 1980s, profeminist male psychologists identified the inadequacy of traditional androcentric models for understanding men's lives, noting that traditional masculine gender roles are associated with substantial conflict and stress (e.g., O'Neil, 1981; Pleck, 1984). During the 1980s and 1990s, profeminist approaches to the psychology and counseling of men became increasingly visible and influential (Brooks, 1998; Brooks and Good, 2001). The most well-known and widely studied conceptualization of men's gender-role issues is referred to as male gender-role conflict (GRC) (O'Neil, Good, and Holmes, 1995). Male GRC has been studied extensively and the literature on male gender-role conflict has become even more substantial than research on women's experience of these issues (Enns, 2000).

Male gender-role conflict most typically occurs when men violate masculine role norms, when they attempt but fail to meet masculine gender-role rules, or when they encounter lack of congruence between their self-concepts and an ideal self-concept that is influenced by traditional masculine ideology. Male GRC consists of four major components:

1. Restrictive emotionality, which is reflected in cautiousness about expressing emotion, or the tendency to use anger to mask other emotions
2. Success, power, and competition, or the tendency to subscribe to traditional masculine ideals of personal achievement, excel

through the use of power and competition, and evaluate oneself on the basis of comparison to others
3. Restricted affectionate behavior with men, which reflects men's difficulty expressing emotions toward other men
4. Work-family conflict, or difficulties balancing work and family as well as prioritizing career over personal life and family (O'Neil, Good, and Holmes, 1995)

Research studies have linked male gender-role conflict to depression (Good and Mintz, 1990; Good et al., 1996; Mahalik and Cournoyer, 2000; Sharpe and Heppner, 1991; Shepard, 2002); physical strain marked by physical illness or poor self-care (Stillson, O'Neil, and Owen, 1991); sexually aggressive attitudes (Rando, Rogers, and Brittan-Powell, 1998); fear of intimacy and alexithymia (lack of words for emotion) (Fischer and Good, 1997); and the use of immature psychological defenses such as turning against others (Mahalik et al., 1998). Jeffrey Hayes and James Mahalik's (2000) research identified a variety of relationships between distress and GRC. Success, power, and competition were associated with hostility; restrictive affectionate behavior to men with social discomfort; and conflict between work and family with hostility, social discomfort, and obsessive qualities. Of the four aspects of GRC, restrictive emotionality has been identified as the most significant predictor of psychological distress levels (Good et al., 1995).

Compared to men with lower levels of GRC, men with higher levels are more likely to hold negative attitudes about counseling (Blazina and Marks, 2001), state lower levels of willingness to seek psychological health (Wisch et al., 1995), and experience greater stigma about participating in career counseling (Rochlen and O'Brien, 2002). Stephen Wester and David Vogel (2002) proposed that the most acceptable and useful counseling interventions are likely to incorporate an action orientation, emphasize instrumentality, and focus on solutions. James Mahalik (1999) recommended the use of interpersonal therapy, which seeks to help men balance the interpersonal motivations of control needs and affiliation needs. A number of authors have also noted that male therapists who experience GRC may have difficulty displaying empathy and warmth, and may feel pressured to "perform" for their clients rather than work collaboratively with clients (Scher, 2001; Wester and Vogel, 2002; Wisch and Mahalik, 1999). As a result, it is important for those who provide counseling for men to examine and resolve their own experiences of GRC.

Feminist therapy principles that are embedded in a liberal feminist framework are highly appropriate for working with men. Anne Ganley (1988) articulated the following feminist therapy goals for men:

1. Learning to balance and integrate relational and achievement values
2. Taking risks in establishing healthy intimate relationships of shared power
3. Increasing listening skills, empathy for others, and the ability to disclose emotions and reactions that are often kept as "secrets"
4. Developing collaborative and noncoercive working and relationship practices
5. Increasing the capacity for self-nurturance rather than expecting women to play this role
6. Developing positive models of consensual sexuality
7. Accepting and interpreting "no" responses as disappointments rather than as rejections or the removal of those things to which one feels entitled

Glenn Good, Lucia Gilbert, and Murray Scher (1990) presented a similar model and labeled it *gender aware therapy*. The concepts of gender aware therapy resemble the principles of nonsexist therapy as defined by Edna Rawlings and Diane Carter (1977) and are designed to be equally applicable to work with men and women. The key components and goals of gender aware therapy include viewing men's and women's problems within the social context, working toward changing gender injustices, and implementing collaborative therapeutic relationships. Gender sensitive therapy (Philpot et al., 1997) is a variant of gender aware therapy designed for work with couples and includes the phases of

1. reflection, which consists of the therapist's demonstration of empathy for both partners' positions;
2. psychoeducation about the social construction of gender;
3. confrontation of the couple's gender-related issues; and
4. brainstorming about solutions.

Key components of this approach include the validation and normalization of gender-role conflicts; reframing individual communication problems as products of socialization; and encouraging partners to unite against the enemy, which is referred to as the "gender ecosystem" (Philpot et al., 1997, p. 179).

Although some feminist therapists have declared that only female therapists can practice feminist therapy, feminists who espouse a liberal feminist position are likely to believe that men who have examined their own gender behavior, have developed sensitivity to and awareness of gender-role issues, and endorse egalitarian roles can work effectively as feminist or gender aware therapists. Anne Ganley (1988) encouraged male therapists who use feminist analyses to refer to themselves as "profeminist" therapists. This title acknowledges the value of men's contributions as therapists but also recognizes that the phenomenological experiences of female and male therapists are often different. Principles of profeminist practice call for men to confront sexist behavior; redefine masculinity according to values other than power, prestige, and privilege; and actively support women's efforts to seek justice. Profeminist therapists actively interrupt men's efforts to devalue women, confront their controlling behaviors, and help men and women establish egalitarian relationships (Adams, 1988; Tolman et al., 1986).

One of the limitations of liberal feminist approaches that emphasize gender conflict issues alone is that they focus almost exclusively on personal components of psychological distress and are not linked adequately to knowledge of power dynamics, especially as they are manifested in abuse or violence (Brooks and Silverstein, 1995). A focus on gender conflict alone provides limited insight about the social change implications of men's and women's problems because analyses of gender roles and gender-role conflict tend to focus on individual manifestations of gender-related issues rather than on institutional and cultural analyses of gender and power (Messner, 1998). Second, the fact that the literature on male GRC is not integrated with work on women's gender-role conflicts may subtly support the exaggeration of differences between women's and men's role-related conflicts. Third, although discussions about gender roles and gender-role conflict help explain how roles are reinforced and reproduced, they do not provide insight about large-scale social change. An emphasis on individual gender roles alone "implies a false symmetry between the male role and the female role, thus masking the oppressive relationship between women and men" (Messner, 1998, p. 258). These concerns point to the importance of developing more complex models that attend to gender-role conflict as well as social structural changes for supporting gender equality.

CONCLUDING COMMENTS

This chapter has described the many ways in which mainstream psychological approaches can be combined with liberal feminist assumptions. Given the centrality of values such as personal choice, autonomy, independence, and individual freedom to both liberal feminism and many psychotherapy traditions, the integration of these models is relatively straightforward and uncomplicated.

Liberal feminist therapists work toward creating environments in which both men and women have equal opportunity to define and choose personal goals. Deviations from socially prescribed gender roles are seen as normal, and the liberal feminist therapist conveys that a wide range of behaviors should be available to both men and women. The liberal feminist therapist encourages the client to become aware of the impact of gender-role socialization and the social environment on personal problems. The therapist hopes that this awareness will contribute to flexible gender-related behaviors but is careful to avoid imposing his or her perceptions of reality on the client. The liberal feminist therapist is particularly concerned with respecting and trusting the client's ability to make personally satisfying choices for her or his own life. As a result, the therapist does not assume that certain outcomes, such as economic autonomy, are better than others, but that men and women will choose a wide array of lifestyle, family, and economic options. In general, whatever works for the individual constitutes an appropriate goal for psychotherapy.

From a liberal feminist perspective, symptoms related to depression, eating disorders, or fear of success are seen as outcomes of socialization and overly rigid adherence to stereotyped feminine roles. Therapeutic solutions emphasize the building of skills to overcome individual deficits in functioning. From this perspective, "the personal is political" means that once individuals are free from gender-role constructions, they are likely to adopt flexible, nonstereotyped behaviors that will lead to personal changes and fulfillment, which will lead to changes in the social environment.

It is important to note that the use of the modified and revised mainstream or nonsexist therapies described in this chapter is not limited to those therapists who define themselves as feminist therapists. The approaches and techniques described in this chapter may also be incorporated within the frameworks described in later chapters.

In general, feminist therapists who endorse more radical social change traditions in feminism argue that a liberal feminist perspective may merely reinforce status quo Western values and devotes inadequate attention to intersections of gender and other social identities, such as race, class, culture, and sexual orientation. Therapists with radical orientations to feminism emphasize the importance of transforming psychotherapy and society through social activism as well as individual change. The major themes associated with these therapies are the focus of Chapters 3, 5, 6, and 7.

Chapter 3

Radical Social Change Feminisms in Feminist Theory and Therapy

Many of the second-wave feminisms, including radical and social-ist feminisms, are based on the assumption that if gender equality is to be realized, society must be changed at its very roots. A logical extension of this assumption is that psychotherapies which have mirrored unequal relationships must be replaced with new alternatives. The institution of psychotherapy must be altered radically. Many social change and liberation themes in feminist therapy are linked to the activities and values of consciousness-raising groups, radical and socialist feminist theory, and the radical therapy movement. It is important to note that although social change is a major emphasis in radical and socialist feminisms, social change themes are not limited to these feminisms. This chapter begins with a summary of radical and social-ist feminisms, which is followed by an overview of social change themes in feminist therapy.

RADICAL FEMINISM

To use the following items as a form of self-assessment, respond to each statement with a "yes" or "no."

_____ 1. In order for liberation to be achieved, gender relation-ships must be transformed and people must be free of all gender-role distinctions.

_____ 2. Marriage, as it is traditionally defined, prevents the full development of women by establishing a pattern of life-long servitude and encouraging women to direct all of their energy toward fulfilling the interests of others.

_____ 3. Sexism categorizes women as an inferior class on the basis of sex and represents the fundamental form of political oppression.

_____ 4. Personal choices related to the "private" world are not just matters of personal taste but hold political significance.

_____ 5. Fundamental social and political change is necessary in order to eradicate the oppression of women and establish full equality.

_____ 6. Traditional male-female relationships promote men's dominance and women's dependence, vulnerability, and submission.

_____ 7. The major causes of sexism and oppression are male domination, patriarchal values that permeate the culture, and men's control over women's bodies.

_____ 8. Many of the major issues facing women are consequences of violence against women (e.g., battering, pornography, incest, and rape).

Emergence of Radical Feminism

Agreement with the items in this list indicates endorsement of views consistent with radical feminist views that rose to prominence during the late 1960s and early 1970s. Many radical women found inspiration in the writings of the French feminist existential author Simone de Beauvoir (1952), who articulated ways in which women have historically been understood only in comparison to men rather than as autonomous beings: "She is defined and differentiated with reference to man and not he with reference to her; she is the incidental, the inessential as opposed to the essential. He is the Subject, he is the Absolute—she is the Other" (p. xvi).

At the level of life experience, many contributors to radical and socialist feminism became aware of gender oppression through involvement in "New Left" and civil rights organizations that emphasized "human rights" but gave token or no support to women's concerns (Berkeley, 1999; Brownmiller, 1999; DuPlessis and Snitow, 1998). When women introduced issues related to sexism, they were often ignored or labeled as frivolous for being concerned with issues that were deemed insignificant in comparison to race and class oppression. At times, women were also subjected to sarcastic, demeaning remarks, or exploitive catcalls which defined women as sexual objects (Deckard, 1979; Echols, 1989; Hole and Levine, 1971). The authors of a Canadian radical feminist manifesto (Bernstein et al., 1969) described their roles as "servicing the organization's men" (p. 252) by providing the "stable, homey atmosphere which the radical man needs to survive" (p. 252) and engaging in financial and emotional support roles that allowed men to "run around being political, creative—writing, thinking, and oozing charisma" (p. 252). When women sought leadership roles, they were often named "castrating females." One manifesto stated, "It is our contention that until the male chauvinists of the movement (North American and world-wide) understand the concept of Liberation in relation to us, the most exploited members of *any* society, the Women, they will be voicing political lies" (Bernstein et al., 1969, p. 253).

Some of the first radical feminists participated in NOW during its early years, but reacted negatively to its hierarchical structure, use of traditional democratic methods for making decisions and organizing change, and willingness to cooperate with existing political institutions that radical feminists hoped to eradicate (Berkeley, 1999; Brownmiller, 1999). Radical feminist activist Ti-Grace Atkinson (1974) resigned from NOW, stating, "you cannot destroy oppression by filling the position of the oppressor. I don't think you can fight oppression 'from the inside'" (p. 11). Most radical feminists participated in small, loosely organized units that arose spontaneously in various parts of the country and focused on creating cultures of active resistance to mainstream society. Decision making was based on consensus and equal participation, and all members engaged in both support and leadership roles. In contrast to liberal feminist messages that called for equality with men within existing power structures, Jo Freeman argued that "women's liberation does not mean equality with men" because "equality in an unjust society is meaningless" (quoted in Echols, 1989, p. 60). Bonnie Kreps (1973) added:

> We, in this segment of the movement, do not believe that the oppression of women will be ended by giving them a bigger piece of the pie, as Betty Friedan would have it. We believe that the pie itself is rotten. (p. 239)

Radical Feminist Manifestos and Practice

Some of the most active radical feminist groups included the Redstockings, The Feminists, the New York Radical Feminists, the Furies, and the Radicalesbians. These groups demonstrated enormous energy, using a wide variety of tactics, speak-outs, and demonstrations to raise public awareness; and creating an extensive literature of pamphlets, manifestos, journals, articles, books, and creative works (Brownmiller, 1999; DuPlessis and Snitow, 1998). From the start, women in these groups expressed diverse opinions, and conflict between groups was sometimes extensive and divisive (Echols, 1989; Willis, 1984).

Four fundamental beliefs are shared by classical radical feminists:

1. Women represent the first oppressed group.
2. Women's oppression occurs in all cultures and is the most widespread of all oppressions.
3. Gender oppression is the most virulent and difficult form of oppression to eliminate.
4. Gender oppression cannot be abolished through other social changes, such as the erasure of class differences (Jaggar and Rothenberg, 1984).

Radical feminists believe that women share roles as members of a sex class, that these oppressive roles need to be understood in political terms, and that these roles must be completely eradicated. Some of the most provocative works of radical feminists have critiqued the institutions of the family, love, marriage, and normative heterosexuality (Echols, 1989). During the 1960s and 1970s, radical feminist groups emphasized the importance of defining a shared voice, and their consensus values were often communicated in manifestos. Following is a sample of some of the ideas of prominent manifestos.

The Redstockings

The goal of the Redstockings was to achieve "final liberation from male supremacy" for all women. The Redstockings Manifesto (Redstockings, 1969) declared, "Our oppression is total, affecting every facet of our lives" (p. 272). The agents of oppression were defined as men:

All other forms of exploitation and oppression (racism, capitalism, imperialism, etc.) are extensions of male supremacy: men
dominate women, a few men dominate the rest. All power structures throughout history have been male-dominated and male-
oriented. Men have controlled all political, economic and cultural
institutions and backed up this control with physical force. They
have used their power to keep women in an inferior position. *All
men* receive economic, sexual, and psychological benefits from
male supremacy. *All men* have oppressed women. (p. 273)

The Redstockings developed the "pro-woman" line, which conceptualized women's submission as a product of unequal power and
daily pressures from men. They rejected any internal and psychological explanations for women's behavior, stating that women's acquiescence and apparent collaboration in their own oppression are the consequences of powerlessness and not passivity. Furthermore, rebellion
against "proper" roles is punished, further reinforcing women's acquiescence. Women's submission is based on necessity and not choice
(Echols, 1989). Carol Hanisch (1971) defined the pro-woman line as
meaning that

> women are really neat people. The bad things that are said about
> us as women are either myths (women are stupid), tactics women
> use to struggle individually (women are bitches), or are actually
> things that we want to carry into the new society and want men to
> share too (women are sensitive, emotional). (p. 155)

Judith Brown (1971) argued that women's behaviors such as "con-
niving, vamping, and flirting" (p. 165) are skills of survival. By using
these behaviors "we either avoid material danger (loss of a job or a
man) or gain material advantage (a promotion, a man)" (p. 165). Consistent with this perspective, the Redstockings did not criticize
women for maintaining intimate relationships within the flawed institution of marriage but noted that marriage often represents the best
option or bargain available to women in an oppressive world.

The literature of the Redstockings emphasized the relevance of
feminism for women of all economic, racial, and educational statuses, and called on all women to unite in the struggle for liberation.
They opposed the antimarriage position taken by some radical feminist groups, noting the classist bias of this position and the reality that

many women must remain in marriages to survive economically. The Redstockings also noted that oppression varies by class and culture, and recommended that white women become aware of their privileges, renounce their privileges, and identify with less privileged women (Echols, 1989; Redstockings, 1969).

The Redstockings highlighted the value of consciousness raising (CR) as the basis for analyzing women's common situation (Redstockings, 1969). Through CR, women defined a program of liberation based on the daily and subjective realities of women's lives. Carol Hanisch (1971, p. 153) noted, "One of the first things we discover in these groups is that personal problems are political problems. There are no personal solutions at this time. There is only collective action for a collective solution." The "genius" of this strategy was its relevance and concreteness; it asked women to explore and respond to issues that created the most pain in their own lives (Willis, 1984).

New York Radical Feminists

The manifesto of the New York Radical Feminists stated, "We believe that the purpose of male supremacy is primarily to obtain psychological ego satisfaction, and that only secondarily does this manifest itself in economic relationships" (New York Radical Feminists, 1973, p. 379). Their analysis of "male ego identity" stated, "It is not out of a desire to hurt the woman that man dominates and destroys her; it is out of a need for a sense of power that he necessarily must destroy her ego and make it subservient to him" (p. 380). The more powerless a man feels in relationship to other men, the more likely he is to oppress women (Echols, 1989; New York Radical Feminists, 1973). The New York Radical Feminists argued that women's behavior is enforced by external constraints but also internalized through socialization experiences which teach women to conform to social expectations and to accept these limitations as natural.

In their analysis of sexual institutions, the New York Radical Feminists (1973) stated that positive heterosexual relationships could occur when "the need to control the growth of another is replaced by love for the growth of another" (p. 381). One of the influential members of the New York Radical Feminists was Shulamith Firestone, whose book titled *The Dialectic of Sex* (1970) proposed that male supremacy is rooted in inequities associated with the reproductive roles of women. Firestone encouraged women to gain control of reproduction as a way of abolishing sexual class oppression. By renouncing biological reproduction, which leads to possessiveness and jealousy, and relying on technological reproductive advances, traditional sex roles and the biological family could be eliminated and replaced with new forms of childbearing and child rearing that would be shared by society as a whole. Women would no longer be confined to the home but would be free to enter the workplace unencumbered by reproductive and family roles. Women would experience the freedom to engage in sex voluntarily and as a free expression of themselves.

The Feminists

The Feminists developed a more psychological analysis of gender roles than did the Redstockings, and they believed that men oppress primarily because of their psychological needs rather than their greater access to power (Echols, 1989). They declared that the male-female role system "distorts the humanity of the Oppressor and denies the humanity of the Oppressed" (The Feminists, 1973, p. 369). Men justify their existence by denying the humanity of women, and women's roles represent a form of "self-defense" against men's impositions over women. The Feminists declared that both male and female roles must be annihilated because they stabilize a flawed male-female system: "If any part of these role definitions is left, the disease of oppression remains and will reassert itself again in new, or the same old, variations throughout society" (p. 370).

The Feminists were critical of the Redstockings' emphasis on external forces as the primary sources of women's oppression and believed that it is important for women to identify ways in which women internalized traditional gender roles, which then distorted their self-definitions. The Feminists also criticized women who "collaborated" with their oppressors by participating in sexist institutions, and they viewed the Redstockings' pro-woman line as leading to self-deception or excuses for avoiding personal and social change (Echols, 1989).

According to The Feminists, "the personal is political" means that one's personal life must clearly reflect a commitment to feminism and radicalism. Ti-Grace Atkinson (1974, p. 118) stated, "Only when all people, *each* of us, refuse to submit, will oppression disappear." To facilitate transformation, The Feminists focused on setting standards of appropriate feminist behavior and proposed the destruction of all institutions that reinforce women's traditional roles, including love, childbearing, and heterosexual sex (Echols, 1989; The Feminists, 1973; Willis, 1984). The Feminists' views of oppression generally reflected the views of Ti-Grace Atkinson, who considered marriage inherently unequal, debilitating for women, and an easy retreat from the radical demands of feminism. Atkinson (1974) stated that "marriage and the family are as corrupt as institutions as slavery ever was. They must be abolished as slavery was" (p. 5).

The Feminists eventually adopted a standard that no more than one-third of its members could live with a man in a formal or informal relationship, and they advocated separatism as a method for altering social structures and for organizing a "counter power block to that of men" (Atkinson, 1974, p. 105). Whereas The Feminists viewed ongoing association with men as undermining the liberation movement, the Redstockings viewed separatism as impractical, unappealing, and as an ineffective means for challenging male power. They believed that it is possible to work toward equality while remaining within heterosexual relationships (Willis, 1984).

The Feminists directed efforts toward eradicating sexual exploitation as manifested in rape, prostitution, and marriage, and suggested that women needed to be liberated from sex. Heterosexual sex was seen as reinforcing roles of dominance and passivity: "Sex, because it is genitally determined, is in the interests of the male and against the interests of the female" (Atkinson, 1974, p. 67). Thus, The Feminists encouraged women to love one another but to avoid confusing love with the distractions of sex. In her initial statements, Ti-Grace Atkinson proposed that lesbianism was primarily an alternative sexual choice and thus represented a distraction rather than a solution to heterosexual sex (Echols, 1989). Later, however, she defined lesbianism as a potent political choice that could help eliminate the power of men over women (Atkinson, 1974). She stated, "Feminism is the theory; lesbianism is the practice" (quoted in Koedt, 1973, p. 246).

A second influential member of The Feminists was Kate Millett, whose book titled *Sexual Politics* (1970) analyzed how sex is a status category with political implications. Millett (1970) argued that male supremacy is not based on biological difference but on a belief system founded on the "needs and values of the dominant group and dictated by what its members cherish in themselves and find convenient in subordinates: aggression, intelligence, force, and efficacy in the male; passivity, ignorance, docility, 'virtue,' and ineffectuality in the female" (p. 26). Millett identified how conditioning, family relations, class differences, economic conditions, violence and force, psychological factors, and religion support and reinforce patriarchal values across generations. She concluded that "patriarchy's greatest psychological weapon is simply its universality and longevity" (p. 58). Although she noted that class is also a powerful force in molding behavior, "patriarchy has a more tenacious hold through its successful habit of passing itself off as nature" (p. 58).

The Radicalesbians

Although some radical feminists viewed lesbianism primarily as a sexual choice and a substitute for working toward equal heterosexual relationships, other radical feminists described the lesbian lifestyle as a profoundly political choice and an egalitarian alternative to the oppressive aspects of heterosexual arrangements. The Radicalesbians were among the first to challenge the heterosexism of heterosexual feminists and to describe lesbian experience in positive terms. In their manifesto, titled "The Woman Identified Woman," the Radicalesbians (1973) stated that the lesbian "is the woman who, often beginning at an extremely early age, acts in accordance with her inner compulsion to be a more complete and freer human being than her society . . . cares to allow her" (p. 240). Based on her ongoing, continuous struggle with heterosexist society, the lesbian is "forced to evolve her own life pattern" and learns earlier than her heterosexual sisters about "the essential aloneness of life (which the myth of marriage obscures)" (p. 240). The manifesto noted that feminists often avoid dealing with lesbianism, and that fear of lesbianism frightens women into assuming a less militant stance, separates women from one another, and reinforces the notion that "male acceptability is primary" (p. 243). The Radicalesbians contended that "only women can give to each other a new sense of self" and that "our energies must flow toward our sisters, not backward toward our oppressors" (p. 245).

The Furies

Although the Radicalesbians worked primarily toward creating a new way of thinking about lesbians, a second lesbian feminist group, the Furies, viewed lesbianism as a way to intensify the struggle for liberation (Echols, 1989; Myron and Bunch, 1975). The Furies advocated lesbian separatism as an opportunity to stop justifying themselves to society and to

> build our own pride, strength, and unity as a people, to develop an analysis of our particular oppression, and to create a political ideology and strategy that would both force the movement's recognition of us and lead to the end of male supremacy. (Bunch, [1976] 1987, p. 185)

Critical of heterosexual women, Rita Mae Brown stated, "Straight women are confused by men, don't put women first" (1975, p. 74). Charlotte Bunch noted that heterosexuality often separates women from one another, and encourages women to compete for and define themselves through men. However, "lesbianism threatens male supremacy at its core. When politically conscious and organized, it is central to destroying our sexist, racist, capitalist, imperialist system" (Bunch, [1972] 1987, p. 161). Lesbianism dismantles beliefs about women's inferiority and erases women's need for men. The independence of the lesbian woman is a "basic threat" (p. 164) to the power of men over women; lesbians are more likely to seek radical solutions and to fight to change society because they have no vested interest in maintaining the various institutions that support heterosexuality (e.g., church, the state, schools, health systems). Bunch ([1972] 1987) concluded, "Lesbianism is the key to liberation and only women who cut their ties to male privilege can be trusted to remain serious in the struggle against male dominance" (p. 166). Charlotte Bunch ([1978] 1987) distinguished between a lesbian and woman-identified woman: a woman-identified woman is a feminist who "adopts a lesbian-feminist ideology and enacts that understanding in her life" (p. 198), whether or not she defines herself as lesbian in a sexual sense. Thus, lesbian feminism could be endorsed by gay or straight men and women.

Male Dominance, Violence, and Sexuality

Although the theoretical assumptions associated with various radical feminist groups were diverse, they shared the view that violence against women is pervasive and damaging. Radical feminists generated a variety of theories about and activist responses to issues regarding violence against women. Barbara Mehrhof and Pamela Kearon (1971) were among the first to describe rape as a political act of oppression, a terrorist act for maintaining women's subordination. In her highly influential book titled *Against Our Will,* Susan Brownmiller (1975, 1999) defined rape as an act of violence rather than sex, as a way in which sexual violence is culturally condoned, and as a method for establishing the power of masculinity. In contrast to Susan Brownmiller's efforts to separate sexuality and violence, Robin Morgan (1980) described rape as "the perfected act of male sexuality in a patriarchal culture—it is the ultimate metaphor for domination, violence, subjugation, and possession" (p. 134). In similar fashion, Andrea Dworkin (1981) described rape as "the defining paradigm of sexuality" (p. 136).

Catherine MacKinnon (1989) declared, "Male dominance is sexual" (p. 127). Sexuality is the medium through which male supremacy defines, eroticizes, and confines men and women, their gender identities, and their sexual pleasure. Thus, male-defined sexuality is forced on women and maintains male dominance as a political system. Catherine MacKinnon ([1982] 1993) argued that violence and coercion are related integrally to sexuality in our society and thus violence and coercion are normative aspects of heterosexual sex. Because of the difficulty separating violence and sexuality in rape, she defined rape as more than the displacement of power into the realm of sexuality but as "an expression of male sexuality, the social imperatives of which define all women" ([1982] 1993, pp. 208-209). Catherine MacKinnon (1989) added that the legal system renders "male dominance both invisible and legitimate by adopting the male point of view" (p. 237). The state defines the social order in the interests of men by "embodying and ensuring male control over women's sexuality at every level, occasionally cushioning, qualifying, or de jure prohibiting its excesses when necessary to its normalization" (MacKinnon, [1982] 1993, p. 207). According to MacKinnon, laws define rape as violent acts perpetrated by deviant rapists; they do not address the conditions that normalize male violence against women.

In general, radical feminists have drawn important connections between sexuality and the full range of ways in which sex, coercion, and violence are used against women. Organizations such as Women Against Violence in Pornography and Media (WAVPM) directed efforts against the pornography industry (Russell and Lederer, 1980). Robin Morgan (1980) argued that rape and pornography are closely intertwined, stating, "Pornography is the theory, and rape the practice" (p. 139). According to many radical feminists, pornography becomes sexual reality because it defines women; men are trained to have sex with an image or object, not a real woman. Through pornography, the inequality of men and women appears natural or sexy, and men become conditioned to experience sexual arousal when themes of dominance, submission, and violence are present (Kappeler, 1986; Russell and Lederer, 1980; Russo, 1987). Women's self-determination and consent are erased.

Some feminists believe that radical feminists have overemphasized and oversimplified women's victimization, relied on confusing and ambiguous definitions of pornography and violence, and inadvertently advocated sexual repression rather than sexual liberation (Berger, Searles, and Cottle, 1991; Russo, 1987; Tong, 1998). Other opponents of radical feminist antipornography efforts point to the importance of supporting free speech rights of individuals. However, Andrea Dworkin (1980) found this position indefensible, arguing that in the name of freedom and the "absolute integrity" (p. 154) of the First Amendment, men have created images of women who are bound, shackled, and mutilated, and have used pornography to rape, torture, and terrorize women into silence. The impact of pornography on women remains an important area of contention within feminist theory in the twenty-first century.

Summary of Radical Feminist Contributions

Radical feminist theories assume that gender distinctions and restrictions encompass virtually all aspects of life; however, these distinctions are rarely questioned by most individuals because they are considered "natural." From a strict radical feminist perspective, women's oppression is the most fundamental and pervasive form of oppression. It is rooted in patriarchy, which is characterized by male dominance, competition, and heterosexism. A central objective of radical feminist change efforts is to illuminate how gender divisions influence basic aspects of living, such as thinking patterns, social/sexual relationships, physical appearance, dress, and work. Radical feminists view male power and male control over women's bodies as dominating every area of life, including work, love, marriage, violence against women, housework, childbearing, and child care. According to this view, culturally defined gender roles and concepts of masculinity and femininity distort personhood and support patriarchy, and these roles should be abolished. Furthermore, institutions such as the family and church are so completely permeated by patriarchy that they must be obliterated and replaced with new structures (Donovan, 2000; Ferree and Hess, 1995; Freedman, 2002; Jaggar, 1983; Tong, 1998).

Because of their belief in the pervasive nature of male domination in society, radical feminists have sometimes advocated separatism as a strategy for change. To counter the "patriarchal imperative that males *must have access* to women" (Frye, 1983, p. 103), some radical women believed that by choosing to participate in alternative institutions they were destroying patriarchal power. By participating in all-female consciousness-raising groups and all-women social events and businesses, women could actively refuse to endorse normative cultural values and destroy long-standing blocks of power. Women's health centers and institutions have also provided ways for women to gain control over their own bodies and destiny within nonhierarchical climates (Ferree and Hess, 1985; Jaggar, 1983). However, radical feminists believe that feminists must not only participate in supportive women's communities but also adopt a mandate for political change. Political change efforts have included collective actions against rape, war, and other forms of violence, as well as creative art and literary contributions that challenge the status quo.

The "classic" radical feminist views described in this section are less salient within twenty-first-century circles than they were in the 1970s. Those who remain influenced by radical feminist positions are less likely to take dualist positions about oppression, are less likely to suggest that a single factor (e.g., patriarchy) is responsible for oppression, and are more likely to acknowledge the complex intersections that influence identity, oppression, and privilege.

Socialist Feminism

To use the following items as a form of self-assessment, respond to each statement with a "yes" or "no." Agreement with these items is indicative of consistency between your beliefs and the basic tenets of socialist feminism.

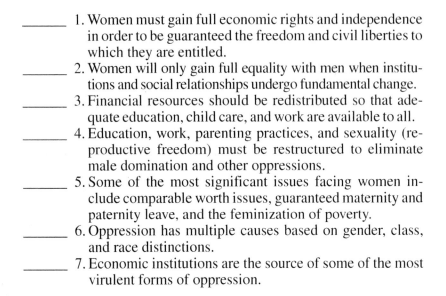

_____ 1. Women must gain full economic rights and independence in order to be guaranteed the freedom and civil liberties to which they are entitled.

_____ 2. Women will only gain full equality with men when institutions and social relationships undergo fundamental change.

_____ 3. Financial resources should be redistributed so that adequate education, child care, and work are available to all.

_____ 4. Education, work, parenting practices, and sexuality (reproductive freedom) must be restructured to eliminate male domination and other oppressions.

_____ 5. Some of the most significant issues facing women include comparable worth issues, guaranteed maternity and paternity leave, and the feminization of poverty.

_____ 6. Oppression has multiple causes based on gender, class, and race distinctions.

_____ 7. Economic institutions are the source of some of the most virulent forms of oppression.

Early Socialist Feminism

Early-nineteenth-century socialist feminists were influenced by utopian socialists who established small experimental, cooperative communities designed to replace systems of economic competition and exploitation. Feminist socialists hoped that within utopian communities men and women would share domestic tasks, household chores, and child care (Banks, 1981; Bartlett, 1988). Charlotte Perkins Gilman viewed women's economic oppression by men as central to their subordinate role in society. In *Women and Economics* (1898) and her utopian novel *Herland* ([1915] 1979), Gilman described communal living arrangements free of male violence, based on class equality and egalitarian work roles, and supportive of communal child rearing. In this context, women would be free to pursue their full potential and attain economic independence.

In contrast to the relatively conservative socialism proposed by Gilman, Emma Goldman's socialist/anarchist feminism of the early twentieth century identified marriage as a major form of women's oppression, arguing that "marriage and love have nothing in common; they are as far apart as the poles; are, in fact, antagonistic to each other" (Goldman, [1917] 1969a, p. 227). She believed that marriage is an economic arrangement which ensures women's dependency: "It incapacitates her for life's struggle, annihilates her social consciousness, paralyzes her imagination, and then imposes its gracious protection, which is in reality a snare, a travesty on human character" (Goldman, [1917] 1969a, p. 235).

Emma Goldman believed that suffrage would do nothing to alter women's realities, society, or a rotten capitalistic system. Instead, the promise of suffrage encouraged women to accept a narrow, artificial, and superficial definition of emancipation, and it blinded woman to "how truly enslaved she is" (Goldman, [1917] 1969c, p. 208). Emma Goldman contended that before true emancipation could occur, the connections between marriage and subordinate status would need to be eliminated and society would need to "do away with the absurd notion of the dualism of the sexes" (Goldman, [1917] 1969b, p. 225). She viewed women's control over their own bodies as especially important to their liberation. Like her contemporary Margaret Sanger, she strongly advocated birth control for women (Douglas, 1970; Solomon, 1987). Although contemporary socialist feminism is viewed primarily as a product of the "new" feminist movement of the 1960s, it is important to note that socialist feminist ideas were expressed throughout the nineteenth and twentieth centuries (Banks, 1981).

Contemporary Socialist Feminism

As with many radical feminist activists, women who chose a feminist socialist orientation during the 1960s felt disenfranchised by the male-dominated new left movements, and they developed manifestos which articulated their demands (Sargent, 1981). Both radical and socialist feminists shared the belief that patriarchy predates capitalism and were critical of the mainstream Marxist belief that capitalism and patriarchy arose alongside each other (Eisenstein, 1979). Socialist feminists also viewed radical feminists as being overly simplistic in conceptualizing oppression, for defining patriarchy as a generalized ahistorical power structure, and for describing gender oppression as similar and universal across classes and cultures (Eisenstein, 1979; Tong, 1998). Second, socialist feminists (e.g., Zillah Eisenstein, 1979) criticized radical feminists for defining sexuality as the central form of oppression and ignoring economic and other complex factors that are oppressive to women. Heidi Hartmann (1981) proposed that although radical feminism provides brilliant insights regarding how sexism operates in the present, its overly psychological analysis can blind feminists to history and the ways in which oppression is modified by era, economics, race, sexual orientation, and culture.

Early manifestos of socialist feminist groups articulated many of the ideals of socialist feminism. The Students for a Democratic Society's (SDS) (1969) National Resolution on Women argued that the struggle for women's freedom must be accompanied by an overthrow of the capitalistic system. Their resolution elaborated three aspects of women's oppression: (1) women serve as "a reserve army of labor" (p. 255) and are forced to work for lower wages than men; (2) women provide free housekeeping services for working men; and (3) women are exploited and oppressed by becoming the target of men's "justified frustration, anger, and shame at their inability to control their natural and social environment" (SDS, 1969, p. 256). Another group, the Charlotte Perkins Gilman Chapter of the New American Movement (1984), focused on creating a synthesis of socialism and feminism. First, they noted that "sexism has a life of its own" (p. 153) which has existed under every economic system; and second, "capitalism determines the particular forms of sexism in a capitalist society" (p. 153). They declared that the goals of feminism, such as day care, reproductive rights, and the elimination of gender roles, cannot be met in a capitalist society but can exist only in a system in which no group is exploited by other groups.

As suggested by the manifestos, socialist feminists have often seen Marxist analyses as useful for articulating the material or economic ways in which women are exploited and alienated under capitalism. Nancy Hartsock (1984) stated,

> Work in a capitalist and patriarchal society means that in our work and in our leisure we do not affirm but deny ourselves; we are not content but unhappy; we do not develop our own capacities, but destroy our bodies and ruin our minds. (p. 270)

Although Marxist concepts provide useful insights about capitalism and class discrimination, a distinctive feminist analysis was also deemed necessary because some aspects of women's oppression are not adequately explained by Marxist analysis, which assumes that women's problems will naturally be eradicated by the overthrow of capitalism or that women's condition is not as important as the oppression of workers (Eisenstein, 1979; Hartmann, 1981; Tong, 1998). Heidi Hartmann (1981) stated, "The 'marriage' of marxism and feminism has been like the marriage of husband and wife depicted in English common law: marxism and feminism are one, and that one is marxism" (p. 2). Hartmann (1981) contended that Marxist analysis provides no insight about why women have lower status than men or why women rather than men are historically assigned to tasks in the home. Ann Oakley (1990) elaborated on this problem, concluding that the housewife role within capitalistic society is

1. exclusively the domain of women,
2. connected to economic dependence,
3. contrasted with primary or "real" work, and
4. seen as having priority over all other roles held by women.

The Integration of Socialist and Psychoanalytic Analysis

Juliet Mitchell's (1969) early essay titled "Women: The Longest Revolution" proposed that four separate systems must be dramatically reconstructed in order for women to achieve liberation:

1. Production, work, and earnings
2. Reproduction
3. Sexuality
4. The responsibility for nurturing and socializing women

Mitchell (1969) stated, "The liberation of women can only be achieved if *all four* structures in which they are integrated are transformed" (p. 166). Mitchell developed an approach that combined psychoanalytic and Marxist analyses, and she proposed that whereas Marxist methods are necessary for overcoming capitalism, feminist applications of psychoanalysis are crucial for overcoming patriarchy (Mitchell, 1974). Mitchell suggested that if Freud's description of psychosexual development is viewed as a social and descriptive analysis rather than as a biologically deterministic account of childhood, the castration and oedipal complexes can be used to explain how early development and oppression operate in a patriarchal society; they explain how people internalize and act out oppressive ideologies. According to Mitchell (1974), psychoanalysis provides a more complete account of socialization than other psychological models because its analysis of the unconscious reveals the invisibility, tenacity, and extent of sexism and explains why traditional ideology is so resistant to change. Because women's oppression is internalized and buried deep within the unconscious, a revolution of the human psyche is necessary for unlocking and undoing women's oppression in private, family domains.

Gayle Rubin's ([1975] 1984) feminist socialist account also used psychoanalysis to explain women's subordinate roles. She stated, "Psychoanalysis provides a description of the mechanisms by which the sexes are divided and deformed, of how bisexual, androgynous infants are transformed into boys and girls" (p. 166). Nancy Chodorow's (1978) analysis of family structure noted that women become the designated and almost exclusive nurturers and caregivers of children. During the pre-oedipal stage of development, girls come to view themselves as similar to their mothers and learn to define themselves in relational and connected terms; boys become aware of their differences from their mothers and learn to define themselves as separate from others. The restructuring of capitalistic society and the participation of fathers in caregiving would eliminate this pattern and allow for greater diversity of human personality. Many cultural feminists also incorporated Chodorow's observations about relational and separate styles of women and men, but have generally ignored Chodorow's early views about capitalism and the need for structural changes in society. A discussion of the limitations of Chodorow's theory from a multicultural perspective appears in the chapter on women of color and feminist therapy (see Chapter 5).

More recently, feminist therapist Ellyn Kaschak (1992) used psychoanalytic theory to identify how the oedipal drama can be used to understand the socially constructed roles of women and men. As an outcome of the oedipal drama, men reject women and identify with powerful men. Men see women as extensions of themselves and feel entitled to women's attentions and seek power and sex in self-serving ways. As part of the oedipal legend, Antigone, the daughter of Oedipus, becomes her father's caretaker after he blinds himself in the wake of his inadvertent incestuous relationship with his wife Jocasta (who is also his mother). Oedipus feels entitled to Antigone's devotion, and she gives up her independence to care for and please her father. Kaschak suggested this scenario exemplifies how women are trained to relate to men in a subservient manner. The basic themes associated with these "complexes" are experienced in myriad ways that are modified by race, class, sexual orientation, and age.

The use of psychoanalytic concepts by some socialist feminists has not been received without criticism by those who believe that elaborate psychoanalytic explanations provide intricate theoretical explanations with no corresponding ideas about how to enact significant change. Ann Foreman (1977) argued that a synthesis of Marxism and psychoanalysis is an "impossible task." Elizabeth Wilson (1990) elaborated, "The last thing feminists need is a theory that teaches them only to marvel anew at the constant recreation of the subjective reality of subordination and which reasserts male domination more securely than ever within theoretical discourse" (p. 224). Wilson suggested that bringing about external and visible change in family and work structures "might do more for our psyches as well as for our pockets than an endless contemplation of how we came to be chained" (p. 224).

Toward Integrative Pluralistic Socialist Feminist Theories

As socialist feminist thinking matured, authors noted that a comprehensive analysis must move beyond traditional considerations of class and gender systems and focus on oppressions that are associated with racism and heterosexism (e.g., Joseph, 1981; Riddiough, 1981). This emphasis on the intersection and interaction of multiple and complex factors led some authors to view socialist feminism as a potentially unifying force for feminism. Floya Anthias and Nira Yuval-Davis (1990) stated that gender, class, and ethnicity "are intermeshed in such a way that we cannot see them as additive or prioritize abstractly any one of them" (p. 110). They added that there is no unitary category of women; each category modifies another and may be experienced differently based on the contexts in which they come together. Theorists, researchers, and activists must be aware of the multiple ways in which gender influences women's lives and must consistently recognize the plurality of experience. Gender is experienced differently by various groups of women; furthermore, some women view gender oppression as less salient than issues such as racism and classism. Socialist feminists have been influential in identifying the importance of developing complex and pluralistic feminisms (Jaggar, 1983; Tong, 1998). Because of its simultaneous attention to multiple factors, Nellie Wong (1991) indicated that no woman is left out of socialist feminist analysis:

> Socialist feminism is a radical, disciplined, and all-encompassing solution to the problems of race, sex, sexuality, and class struggle. Socialist feminism lives in the battles of all people of color, in the lesbian and gay movement, and in the class struggle. (p. 290)

Summary of Socialist Feminist Themes

Whereas radical feminism identifies gender oppression as the fundamental source of women's oppression, socialist feminism is linked to the belief that oppression is influenced by gender but is also shaped by race, nationality, and class. Socialist feminism is based on the assumption that gender status is imposed and defined by social relationships, embedded in historical factors, and situated in systems that organize social production. Early gender learning is reinforced through a variety of social mechanisms, such as work and child-rearing practices, and modified by class and race (Jaggar, 1983; Tong, 1998).

Contemporary socialist feminist thought attempts to respond to the intersections of oppressions that are discussed by other feminist philosophies: the structures of production, class, and capitalism stressed by strict Marxist feminists; the control of reproduction and sexuality emphasized by radical feminists; and the impact of socialization discussed by liberal feminists (Tong, 1998). In general, socialist feminists have proposed that the realization of human potential will not be made possible through the legislation of individual rights alone but must involve the restructuring of life in both personal and public spheres. The restructuring of family life and decrease in alienation and oppression will be made possible in part through universal access to adequate child care, education, housing, birth control, and maternity/paternity leave. The gendered structure of paid and unpaid labor forces is a key issue, and socialist feminists have emphasized the importance of increasing women's options, modeling new social relationships, and valuing all forms of work, both public and private. The development of women's alternative work and social organizations is also important because such involvement allows women to model new social relationships, overcome a sense of alienation from creative work and activity, and realize their goals in a supportive atmosphere (Hartsock, 1984). In summary, socialist feminists have focused on removing structural and psychological barriers to equality as well as responding to the intersections of oppression (Ferree and Hess, 1985; Tong, 1998).

SOCIAL CHANGE THEMES IN FEMINIST THERAPY

Radical and socialist feminisms were among the first approaches to emphasize the centrality of social change and societal transformation, and they became the foundation for early definitions of feminist therapy that emphasized social activism. Feminist therapists with radical social change orientations often defined feminist therapy in ways that combined an analysis of the subjugation of women as a fundamental form of oppression (radical feminism) with the class, political, and economic systems that victimize women (socialist feminism). For example, Kirk (1983) defined feminist therapy as

> action-oriented and predicated on an analysis, not only of the plight of women in society, but of the generally oppressive nature of patriarchy, the corporate capitalist system, and the political and social institutions which they have created. It is also predicated on an understanding of how these systems oppress women in particular as well as other groups. (p. 179)

Radical and socialist feminist approaches have been the target of criticism during recent years for being based primarily on the lives and concerns of white middle-class women as well as for emphasizing gender as a primary or the most critical focus of oppression in women's lives. Despite their limitations, these feminist approaches became a catalyst for social change and classic definitions of feminist therapy, and formed an initial foundation or orienting focus for more inclusive recent feminisms that emphasize social change themes (e.g., women-of-color feminisms). The following sections begin with a discussion of important structures and themes in the early practice of social change feminist therapies and briefly trace changes and modifications over time. Later sections then summarize the contributions of specific feminist therapists whose approaches, which represent a rich mosaic of diverse viewpoints, can be categorized at least roughly within a social change tradition. The chapter concludes with an overview of the legacy of radical social change feminisms in feminist therapy. Some of the more recent approaches discussed in later sections of this chapter (e.g., Brown, 1994; Herman, 1992; Walker, 1994) incorporate aspects of feminist thought described in subsequent chapters (e.g., women-of-color feminisms, postmodern feminism). However, because of their affinity with many of the social change roots of feminisms, they are included in this chapter.

As noted in Chapter 2, the early years of feminist therapy were characterized by a questioning approach (which included reformist efforts that were lodged primarily within established mental health professions) and a radical approach (which was associated with elements of the feminist movement that sought to change the very nature and focus of mental health practices) (Ballou and Gabalac, 1985). This chapter explores contributions relevant to a radical focus. It is important to clarify that Mary Ballou and Nancy Gabalac's use of the term *radical* was not limited to radical feminist theory. Their use of *radical* refers to dictionary definitions such as "fundamental," "thorough," or "change at the very roots of a society." The word *radical* refers to forms of feminist psychotherapy that have been influenced by a variety of social change feminist perspectives, including radical feminist theory, socialist feminist theory, and a variety of other feminisms that highlight the importance of liberation and social change.

Consciousness Raising: Radical Alternative to Androcentric Approaches

To understand the earliest forms of radical feminist therapy, it is necessary to summarize the evolving role of consciousness raising during the early years of the "new" feminist movement. Radical feminist women believed that most theories of women's experiences were steeped in androcentric assumptions and reflected the male-dominated disciplines and institutions which inspired them, and CR became a method for arriving at new theories and methods based on women's lives. Kathie Sarachild (1975) stated, "You might say we wanted to pull up weeds in the garden by their roots, not just pick off the leaves at the top to make things look good momentarily" (p. 144). Feminist groups explored the origins of women's problems by studying topics such as work, motherhood, and childhood as they were experienced personally by women. All generalizations about women were tested against the "living practice and action" (p. 145), and CR was defined as the "scientific method of research" (p. 145).

Consciousness-raising groups functioned in a spontaneous manner with a minimum amount of structure and a commitment to nonhierarchical norms which endorsed decision making by consensus and specified that each person shared equal responsibility for group content and process. Groups generally consisted of five to fifteen members who came together to share their perceptions and concerns and use their findings to develop a program of liberation (Redstockings, 1969). One of the first descriptions of CR groups identified the following components:

1. Expanding consciousness through personal testimony and generalization from personal experience
2. Discussing how women can overcome denial and delusions and "dare to see" oppression for what it is
3. Developing radical feminist theory that conceptualizes how oppression occurs in everyday life and how personal privilege, such as white skin and education privilege, may perpetuate oppression (Sarachild, 1970)

Pamela Allen (1971) described the CR group process as consisting of four phases of:

1. *opening up*, a time when women express their individual needs in a nonjudgmental atmosphere;
2. *sharing*, the revelation of personal material for the purpose of identifying the commonalities of women's experiences;
3. *analyzing*, or going beyond personal experience to objectively consider women's predicament; and
4. *abstracting*, or building a vision for action.

The purpose of CR was "to get closer to the truth" (Sarachild, 1975, p. 148). Carol Hanisch's (1971) paper titled "The Personal Is Political" declared that through participation in CR, women discover that personal problems can only be understood as political problems. As an extension of the CR process, group members became engaged in actions designed to increase public awareness about sexism. These public actions, which consisted of "zap" actions, speak-outs, protests, writings, and media events, "would waken more and more women to an understanding of what their problems were" (Sarachild, 1975, p. 149). Consciousness raising provided a method for gaining new information, analyzing obstacles, and setting new priorities for activism.

Although the primary intent of the original CR groups was to articulate social problems, the discussion of personal dilemmas was experienced as therapeutic by many members. Marilyn Zweig (1971) noted, "Although we are not a therapeutic group and do not try to solve personal problems of individual women, we want to study ways to make the condition of all women better so that individual women have fewer problems" (p. 163). Thus, the CR group often helped individual women "make a better life" (p. 163) and provided a "haven from hassles" (Payne, 1973).

By the mid-1970s, the political awareness or radicalizing function of CR groups became less salient, and women increasingly joined CR groups to achieve personal growth (Kirsch, 1987; Kravetz, 1978, 1980; Lieberman and Bond, 1976). Although CR groups continued to serve a political and ideological function, the self-reports of group members suggested that personal change, rather than political or ideological change, was the primary benefit derived from these groups (Lieberman et al., 1979; Warren, 1976). Diane Kravetz's (1978, 1987) reviews of the research literature identified the following personal benefits of CR groups:

- Increased feelings of self-esteem and decreased feelings of personal inadequacy
- Increased personal and intellectual autonomy
- Awareness of similarities among women and improved relationships with women
- A new ability to express feelings such as anger

- Change in interpersonal roles and relationships
- The development of a sociopolitical analysis of the female experience and women's oppression

Consciousness Raising: Foundation for Feminist Therapy

Women psychotherapists who participated as members of CR groups were changed and radicalized through their interactions with other women. They began to integrate CR with therapeutic skills to combat oppression in their professional work, and the possibility of feminist therapy emerged (Lerman, 1987). Some feminists questioned whether feminist therapy was possible because it borrowed concepts from an institution that contributed to the oppression of women. For example, Phyllis Chesler (1971) noted that the majority of psychotherapists were male, that they acted as extensions and enforcers of the political institution of psychotherapy and promoted the "covertly or overtly patriarchal, autocratic, and coercive values and techniques of psychotherapy" (p. 375). She also described psychotherapy as mirroring the inequality of marital relationships:

> Both psychotherapy and marriage isolate women from each other; both emphasize individual rather than collective solutions to woman's unhappiness; both are based on a woman's helplessness and dependence on a stronger male authority figure; both may, in fact, be viewed as reenactments of a little girl's relation to her father in a patriarchal society; both control and oppress women similarly. (p. 373)

Although psychotherapy "psychologizes, personalizes, and depoliticalizes social issues" (Hurvitz, 1973, p. 235), many feminists believed that to "abandon therapy out of hand is at once to refuse to satisfy an obvious personal need and to sacrifice a tool of potentially enormous importance to the movement" (Chase, 1977, p. 20). Karen Chase argued that feminists would need to "dismantle the professional/patient hierarchy, to discount formal accreditation, and to reconstruct the therapeutic situation on a basis of mutuality" (p. 20). In addition to removing the therapist from the role of "high priest" (p. 20), symptoms would need to be redefined as appropriate reactions to inappropriate situations. New forms of therapy for women would need to be constructed according to radically different models and norms rather than traditional therapy. This new model was described as

> a radical therapy of equals (in which) . . . the process would be democratized, the perspective would be on the "pathological" forces in the culture that uniquely damage women, and the therapeutic goals would go beyond internal psychic changes to creating new sensibilities, ambiances, and social contexts. (Walstedt, quoted in Sturdivant, 1980, p. 10)

Karen Lindsey (1974) added,

> The women's movement needs to form counter structures, therapy forms which incorporate some of the skills and knowledge of the existing structures (of therapy), but which gear them toward helping women find their own values and needs, rather than molding them into prefabricated roles. (p. 2)

Although some radically oriented feminists viewed self-help as the only appropriate structure for integrating the political and personal, others formed therapy groups that retained many of the characteristics of CR. As the therapeutic benefits of CR became increasingly apparent, CR groups were promoted as an alternative or adjunct to therapy (Barrett et al., 1974; Brodsky, 1977; Glaser, 1976; Kirsch, 1974, 1987; Kravetz, 1976, 1980; Lieberman and Bond, 1976; Rice and Rice, 1973; Warren, 1976). In addition to its personal benefits, CR offered a structure that was radically different from traditional psychotherapy. In one of the earliest statements on the mental health benefits of CR, Annette Brodsky (1976) indicated that CR groups help women become aware of how the "problem with no name" is exhibited in their personal lives, and encourage women to fight the stagnation of role confinement. By adopting CR as a model of therapy, therapists can "confirm the reality" of women's experiences; women no longer need to deny experiences of discrimination or "pass them off as projections" (Brodsky, 1976, p. 376). The therapist serves as a "supporter and believer" (p. 375) of women's competence, helps women become aware of the range of goals and options available to them, and acts as an effective coping role model. Barbara Kirsch (1974) added that CR as psychotherapy affirms women's views of reality, transforms consciousness, provides a release from conditioning, and highlights "the need to change society by showing individuals that their 'personal' problems are rooted in sociocultural phenomena" (p. 337).

Many of the norms of consciousness raising were incorporated within early forms of radical feminist group therapy, including

- an emphasis on egalitarianism,
- an understanding that oppression and social conditioning are central to understanding women's distress,
- the assumption that the sharing of personal issues contributes to a more complete understanding of social and political issues, and
- the belief that awareness should be matched with action.

In keeping with CR principles, feminist therapy groups emphasized the importance of "collective rather than hierarchical structures, and [the] equal sharing of resources, power, and responsibility" (Marecek and Kravetz, 1977, p. 326). Therapy groups provided an effective antidote to negative gender socialization because women could gain power by practicing new skills in a safe environment. Women could facilitate change in their lives by making the following transitions in thinking:

> "There is something wrong with me as a woman or as a person" to "There's something wrong in society." Anger could be rechanneled into active, open confrontation with the oppressing agent, increasing the potential for a sense of mastery and for more reciprocal human relationships. (Barrett et al., 1974, p. 14)

In contrast to traditional leaderless CR groups, feminist therapy groups were led by one or more trained leaders who helped members redefine issues of women, separate internal from external causes of problems, identify "corrective" actions, and develop productive personal responses (Brodsky, 1976; Johnson, 1976; Kaschak, 1981; Kravetz, 1978; Leidig, 1977). The group process diluted the power of the therapist and decreased power imbalances between therapist and clients because all members not only received assistance but also provided emotional support to one another (Burden and Gottlieb, 1987; Kaschak, 1981; Rawlings and Carter, 1977). In contrast to individual therapy, which confines growth by limiting the number who receive assistance to a privileged few, groups provided a mechanism for reaching many women and energizing them to engage in active resistance (Wyckoff, 1977b).

Feminist therapy collectives emerged in many parts of the United States during the early 1970s and were often associated with feminist health clinics or women's centers. Some of these collectives were founded by professionally trained mental health professionals who had become radicalized through their experiences in CR groups and, as a consequence, preferred to work outside of hierarchical organizations that resembled or replicated oppressive patriarchal structures. Other collectives included both paraprofessional and professional therapists and provided ongoing training programs for members of the community who desired to lead therapy groups. A typical experience of feminist therapy within one of the early collectives included attending an initial exploratory group in which each woman could ask questions, consider her level of interest in therapy, and identify aspects of her life that she would like to explore. If she decided to continue in group therapy, she signed a twelve-week contract that identified what problems she would address in therapy. During the twelve-week therapy contract, she examined these issues and practiced new behaviors in the presence of group members who offered support and confrontation. At the conclusion of twelve weeks, she evaluated her progress and renewed her contract if she desired to work on additional issues.

One of the few research studies of feminist therapy compared the experiences of twenty-four women who received group therapy in a feminist therapy collective with similar clients who participated in individual therapy with male therapists (Johnson, 1976). Although the mean length of therapy was four months for collective clients and ten months for the comparison sample, both groups showed similar levels of improvement and satisfaction. The top three factors that collective clients saw as central to their improvement included experiencing a sense of belongingness and acceptance by the group, learning how to relate effectively in an interpersonal environment, and working with therapists who viewed them as competent.

A second research study (Marecek, Kravetz, and Finn, 1979) compared the responses of approximately 400 CR group members who had participated in either feminist therapy (not necessarily group feminist therapy) or traditional therapy. Women who experienced feminist therapy reported a greater number of positive evaluations than did women who were clients in traditional therapy. Sixty-seven percent of women in feminist therapy and 38 percent of women in traditional therapy reported that their experiences were very helpful. Both early studies of feminist therapy (Johnson, 1976; Marecek, Kravetz, and Finn, 1979) demonstrated that feminist therapy facilitates empowerment, affirmation, and validation in an environment which relies on interactions among women as important therapeutic components.

One of the most influential descriptions of feminist therapy, which was authored by Edna Rawlings and Diane Carter (1977), reflected many of the values of social change feminisms. Their definition stated that

1. the goal of feminist therapy is social and political change;
2. oppression and environmental stress are major causes of "pathology" but should not be used as excuses to avoid personal responsibility;
3. diagnostic labels should be rejected because they have been used as instruments of oppression and focus on deficits rather than strengths;
4. feminist therapy can be accomplished most effectively in groups;
5. egalitarianism and efforts to equalize power in the therapy relationship are central to empowerment;
6. biologically based theories of male-female differences must be rejected;
7. traditional role differences between men and women must be erased in order to break down the legacy of sex-role stereotypes; and
8. therapists' participation in social change activities on behalf of women is an important extension of their therapeutic role.

These principles, which were applied to group feminist therapy, also became the foundation for individual feminist therapy practice.

During the early years of feminist therapy, feminist counseling groups emphasized the shared oppression of women and the external sources of their problems. Women were typically assigned to groups on the basis of convenience rather than type of presenting problem, and individual differences between women were minimized to heighten awareness of similarities among women. By the mid-1980s, group members were less likely to come together by virtue of their feminist views; more often they assembled because they shared a specific problem. A survey of feminist therapists during the mid-1980s revealed that although approximately three-fourths of feminist therapists conducted groups, these groups tended to focus on specific issues (e.g., eating disorders) rather than on the general themes that received greater attention during the 1970s. A majority of therapists indicated that the demand for feminist groups had decreased, and only one-fourth of the therapists facilitated groups that resembled feminist therapy collective groups (Johnson, 1987).

As feminist groups became more diverse and complex, group approaches were recommended for specific problems such as sexual abuse and other forms of sexual violence, body image issues, battering, and eating disorders (Enns, 1993). Greater emphasis was placed on the successful individual resolution of issues and less emphasis was placed on the political ramifications of personal issues. By the early 1980s, individual feminist therapy was the most typical form of feminist practice (Kaschak, 1981). Although noting the significant benefits of individual work, Longres and McLeod (1980) also saw disadvantages, indicating that "the unique capacities of people are made so evident that it is next to impossible not to treat those incapacities as *the* problems" (p. 275). In contrast, "feminist groupwork delabels, deconstructs boundaries, expands a sense of personal vision and makes the connections between these and wider socio-economic forces. Feminist groupwork breaks down the destructiveness of individualism" (Butler and Wintram, 1991, p. 188). The connections between the personal and political are often less obvious in individual therapy than in group therapy. The appropriate balance of feminist individual and group work remains an important issue in the twenty-first century.

The Radical Antitherapy Position and Self-Help

Although feminist therapy based on CR processes was endorsed by many radical therapists, some found it impossible to imagine that the institutionalized sexism of psychotherapy could be altered. Carol Hanisch (1971) stated,

> [T]he very word "therapy" is obviously a misnomer if carried to its logical conclusion. Therapy assumes that someone is sick and that there is a cure, e.g., a personal solution. I am greatly of-

fended that I or any other woman is thought to *need* therapy in the first place. Women are messed over, not messed up! We need to change the objective conditions, not adjust to them. Therapy is adjusting to your bad personal alternative. (p. 153)

Dorothy Tennov (1973) also viewed the terms *feminist* and *therapy* as mutually contradictory, noting that although "some psychotherapists have become activists in the women's movement, and have tried of late to 'liberate' women instead of 'adjusting' them, does not remove the problem. . . . Feminists do not practice *therapy* on their sisters" (p. 110).

Dorothy Tennov (1973) prioritized changing social structures over changing individuals and viewed self-help as the only legitimate alternative for women who were seeking help with personal issues. This point of view has remained an important dissenting voice within radical feminism. For example, Celia Kitzinger and Rachel Perkins (1993, p. 3) drew attention "to the political problems inherent in *the very idea* of 'feminist therapy' or 'feminist psychology.'" They argued, "Feminism tells us our problems are caused by oppression; psychology tells us they're all in the mind—at least, the important ones are, the ones we can do something about in therapy" (p. 7). They added, "Whatever it pretends, psychology is never 'apolitical.' It always serves to obscure larger social and political issues (sexism, heterosexism, racism, classism), converting them into individual pathologies by an insistent focus on the personal" (p. 6).

Although some radical feminists have believed that feminism and therapy are incompatible (e.g., Tennov, 1973; Kitzinger and Perkins, 1993), they have typically viewed self-help and feminism as highly compatible. Ann Withorn (1980) noted the widely divergent characteristics of self-help groups. One end of the self-help continuum is represented by politically focused feminist groups that are characterized by "self-conscious, empowering democratic effort where women help each other and often provide an analysis and an example from which to criticize and make feminist demands on the system" (Withorn, 1980, p. 26). Groups that connect individual solutions with political actions include women's health collectives, abortion referral services, and rape crisis centers (see next section on crisis centers). These feminist self-help systems typically focus on health, prevention, and personal growth rather than on recovery from illness. Members rely on mutual sharing, advice, support, and the pooling of member resources (Marecek and Kravetz, 1977; Withorn, 1980).

Participation in self-help does not ensure that connections between personal and political issues are addressed. One end of the self-help spectrum consists of groups that focus on specific personal problems, such as twelve-step recovery groups and codependency groups (Withorn, 1980). In contrast to activist self-help groups, codependency groups typically define the victim of abuse or the partner of an addicted person as coculpable with the addicted person or perpetrator of abuse. As a result, they may neglect power differentials between partners or between the perpetrator and the abused person (van Wormer, 1989). The political implications of codependent behavior, such as its similarity to women's prescribed cultural role and its role as a survival skill in a patriarchal environment in which issues of unequal power and dominance exist, are infrequently addressed.

Although many codependency self-help groups adopted the model of the CR group, the ideology and emphases of these two types of groups are markedly different. CR groups emphasize competency and an analysis of the social origins of problems, challenge power relations in the larger society, and focus efforts on empowering the group *and* individuals. In contrast, codependency and "process addition" groups have often relied on a deficit or "disease" model of personality, examine personal and family roots of problems, encourage surrender to a "higher power" rather than involvement in social activism, and emphasize individual healing and empowerment over social change (Kasl, 1992).

Violence Against Women and the Crisis Center Movement

While feminist therapy collectives and self-help alternatives were being established, grassroots rape crisis and domestic violence centers were emerging throughout the United States, Canada, and Europe. The first rape crisis centers were founded in 1970 by grassroots, community-based feminist organizations, and the antirape movement was influenced in a significant way by radical feminist perspectives, which identified "sexual violence against women as the embodiment of patriarchy" (Koss and Harvey, 1991, p. 123) and a threat to all women. This feminist analysis conceptualized rape and the fear of rape as supporting and reinforcing male power and the social control of women. In response to their fear of rape, women lead more constricted lives, search for male protection, and limit their efforts toward becoming autonomous and independent. Furthermore, society often sees women as responsible for their own victimization, and traditional legal and medical procedures for survivors support victim blaming. In order to counteract the social control of women through patriarchy, "a feminist response must do just the opposite: encourage choice, affirm independence, and aid women's cultivation of personal and social power" (Koss and Harvey, 1991, p. 126). The rape crisis center is a context in which women are believed, supported, and receive direct help for working through the aftermath of sexual violence.

During the mid-1970s, feminist crisis workers described the aftermath of rape as rape trauma syndrome (Burgess and Holmstrom, 1974) and created a variety of services for rape survivors including crisis hotlines, single session debriefing and crisis management, peer support groups, self-defense training, individual and group counseling, medical assistance, rape exams, and legal assistance (Koss and Harvey, 1991; O'Sullivan, 1976). Services for rape survivors focused primarily on helping women work through their shattered beliefs and restoring mastery and choice.

Rape crisis centers have offered a range of group services that include self-help groups, education groups, crisis intervention groups, and formal psychotherapy groups. The basic goals of these groups are to communicate that the victim's actions and responses to violence were based on her need to survive, establish and reinforce her status as a survivor, decrease her isolation and self-blame, validate feelings, facilitate grief and mourning about psychological losses, and identify new forms of meaning. Consistent with feminist therapy principles, group members are encouraged to participate in both personal recovery and social change. When sufficient personal healing is accomplished, survivors often provide training about the dynamics of sexual assault, become volunteer crisis workers, or participate in community speakers' bureaus, antirape task forces, or "Take Back the Night" rallies (Koss and Harvey, 1991).

Rape crisis centers have usually considered social change activities as an essential extension of their services to individual assault survivors. These social change activities emphasize the importance of community education, risk awareness, and self-defense training for women. They also foster training programs designed to sensitize legal, medical, and mental health personnel to the needs of victims. Many efforts have focused on correcting myths about rape and informing the public about date and acquaintance rape. Rape crisis personnel also engage in political activism and lobbying activities directed toward the passage of legislation designed to protect women's rights, define sexual assault in more accurate and less restrictive ways (e.g., not just forceful penetration), establish consequences for those who act violently toward others, and reform the legal system so that women who bring charges against perpetrators are not revictimized (Koss and Harvey, 1991). After reviewing the programs and efforts of rape crisis centers from 1970 to 1990, Mary Koss and Mary Harvey (1991) concluded that crisis centers have had a "profound impact on virtually all aspects of the larger society's response to rape" (p. 120).

The emergence of the battered women's movement owes much to the inspiration of feminist antirape programs. Like the rape crisis movement, the battered women's movement was founded on the belief that violence against women is rooted in male domination, and women's situations can be changed only through the pairing of services to women with political change efforts (Whalen, 1996). Battering was defined as a consequence of "male domination within and outside the family" (Schechter, 1982, p. 216). In contrast to the mythology of battered women as passive or helpless, the battered women's movement conceptualized battered women's behaviors as active efforts to struggle and cope effectively with limited options.

Battered women have often become radicalized through their experience with shelters and at some point often become involved in political activism and volunteer work. As a first step, the shelter provides a safe space for women, which represents a first gigantic step in building strength in women and offering hope. As battered women share pain with one another, they overcome their isolation and feel released from personal blame. Responsibility for violent abuse is "placed squarely in the hands of a violent man" (Schechter, 1982, p. 315). Susan Schechter stated, "In literally six to eight weeks, shelters not only change women's self-perceptions but also their thoughts about male-female relationships, sex roles, and the meanings of violence" (p. 316). Through interaction with one another, women often develop a new pride in themselves as a group and gain a new political analysis of violence against women, which can eventually lead to their own involvement in activism. Through the collective efforts of battered women and activists, the battered women's movement "created the first public spaces in history through which women were offered visible alternatives to violent men. It is not grandiose to suggest that . . . the battered women's movement has transformed the world for many" (Schechter, 1982, p. 321).

In keeping with the radical feminist perspective that services for women need to be defined in dramatically different ways than traditional institutions, many feminist service organizations, including women's health centers, rape crisis centers, and domestic violence programs, have experimented with models which revolutionize women's experience with service institutions. These feminist agencies seek to eliminate hierarchical structures that foster social inequality, dependency, and powerlessness; and establish shared decision-making models designed to contribute to the empowerment of volunteers, professional staff members, and clients. These organizational structures are based on the assumption that women must have control over their own bodies and personal choices, and that an egalitarian structure facilitates women's abilities to choose (Whalen, 1996). The use of self-help groups, consciousness raising, and collective action also highlight the competency of women. In other words, "the process and the product must both adhere to basic feminist principles" (Kravetz and Jones, 1991, p. 237). These organizations have also sought to link services with political change, with the hope that women would become radicalized by experiencing these services.

As services for women evolved, the structure and services of rape crisis centers and domestic violence projects became more diverse. Whereas some centers emphasized victim services over social change activities, others have maintained their commitment to both personal service and social change. It has been difficult for many feminist agencies to sustain a high level of energy over an extended period of time, and some volunteers eventually become exhausted from dealing with the struggles of maintaining services despite poor funding or lack of strong community support (Matthews, 1994). Many original grants to rape crisis centers, shelters, and health centers represented "seed money" that was only guaranteed for several years, and many feminist organizations have concluded that they need to seek government funding to continue. Government funding provides increased resources and opportunities for expansion but also leads to greater complexity of organizational structure and staffing patterns, and results in more agency regulations. Although many organizations started with deeply committed volunteers who participated in all aspects of decision making, increased funding also led to more specialization, hierarchical structures, and the hiring of professional administrators or staff to provide many services to women. Despite the presence of complex issues, the services of women's crisis centers, shelters, and health centers endure as radical alternatives to traditional mental health services (Koss and Harvey, 1991; Matthews, 1994; Whalen, 1996).

In her 1981 discussion of feminist therapy, which was then at the end of its first decade, Ellyn Kaschak distinguished between radical grassroots feminist therapy and radical professional therapy. Whereas grassroots radical feminist counselors were most typically trained in alternative women's settings and often worked within feminist crisis centers and collectives, professional radical feminist therapists typically received their training in academic institutions and tended to work in more formal agencies. Professionally trained therapists tended to rely primarily on individual and group interventions; grassroots therapists more frequently emphasized the importance of societal issues and group interventions designed to influence social change. Susan Schechter (1982) argued that too often, as professional services increased, "political analysis disappeared, was changed, or was considered beyond the scope of professional concern" (p. 107). Thus, grassroots activists have often feared that "professionalization" will result in a loss of political and social vision (Cooper-White, 1989; Whalen, 1996).

Professionalization is also associated with more formal organizational structures. Rape crisis centers, battered women's shelters, and feminist therapy collectives of the early 1970s were committed to antihierarchical, egalitarian structures, which minimized differences between personnel based on status or specialized knowledge (Whalen, 1996). Employees and volunteers often refused to become aligned with formal mental health organizations for fear of being subtly coopted by such organizations. However, most feminist organizations gradually adopted more formal structures and policies in order to secure the financial support necessary to serve their clientele, develop a structure that would sustain services over time, ensure the accountability of workers, and resolve conflicts among service providers (Reinelt, 1995). Jo Freeman (1995) noted that "movements are not institutions, but to survive beyond the initial burst of spontaneity they must take on many of the characteristics of institutions" (p. 404).

The work of crisis centers inspired by radical feminists continues to be highly influential, but sustaining funding for these organizations and retaining their original mission is often challenging. Many antiviolence agencies are dependent on state and national antiviolence budgets, and they must reapply regularly for this funding. The need to maintain funding that is dependent on the goodwill of politicians may limit the range of political activities that feminist institutions might otherwise support (Mardorossian, 2002).

THE VARIETIES OF SOCIAL CHANGE FEMINIST THERAPIES

Whereas the previous sections have described general themes, issues, and institutions associated with radical feminist therapies and self-help, this section summarizes the unique contributions of specific individuals who have proposed feminist therapy approaches that are consistent with many of the principles of radical social change feminisms. It is organized chronologically and describes a variety of perspectives that were published between 1971 and 1994.

The Radical Therapy Movement and Radical Feminist Therapy

During the early years of radical feminist therapy, some therapists were closely aligned to the goals and origins of the radical therapy movement, which was organized by men and women who sought to raise awareness of the oppressive nature of psychiatry and psychotherapy. The aim of radical therapy is captured by the inscription inside the cover of *The Radical Therapist* (Agel, 1971): "Therapy is political change, not peanut butter." Michael Glenn (1971) declared,

> Therapy is change, not adjustment. This *means* change—social, personal, and political. . . . A "struggle for mental health" is bullshit unless it involves changing this society which turns us

into machines, alienates us from one another and our work, and binds us into racist, sexist, and imperialist practices. (p. xi)

The radical therapy Manifesto (Anonymous, 1971) identified the following major goals:

1. The liberation of therapists and the systems they work in, which are "unresponsive, bulky, privileged, and stiff" and which reinforce a "tangle of midwife myths, fantasy, and outright bias" (p. xvii)
2. The development of new training programs that are nonhierarchal, remove artificial boundaries between "professionals" and laypeople, and use more open, responsive, and creative methods
3. The elaboration of a new psychology of women and liberating theories of family and social life
4. The development of therapy programs that can be monitored and controlled by clients
5. The creation of new techniques of therapy that are readily accessible to all people (not just the middle-class elite)
6. The confrontation of social injustice ranging from the violation of natural resources to the "encroachment of our minds" (p. xxii) through the means of advertising, biased education, and gender role stereotyping

Hogie Wyckoff (1971, 1977a,b) developed a form of radical feminist therapy that combined feminism and principles of radical therapy. According to her definition of feminist therapy, psychotherapy *is* a political activity; therapists are community organizers who teach problem-solving skills and political awareness (Wyckoff, 1977a). In addition, radical therapists used the term *psychiatry* to communicate that radical therapists are "soul healers" as defined by the original Greek meaning of the word psychiatry, and to emphasize "the competency of our work and the coopting of power from the medical establishment" (Wyckoff, 1977a, p. 371). Radical psychiatry was founded on several basic principles. First, in the absence of oppression, people are "okay" and live productive lives in harmony with one another. However, coercion and discrimination lead to alienation, which represents a central component of all psychiatric problems and involves "a sense of not being right with oneself, the world, or humankind" (Wyckoff, 1977a, pp. 371-372). Wyckoff (1977a) indicated that the most typical ways in which women feel alienation include coercive or unsatisfactory experiences of sexuality, lack of recognition or minimization of their work, and self-contempt for themselves and their bodies.

For liberation to occur, individuals must negotiate the steps of awareness and contact. Awareness occurs when women explore how they were "deceived or mystified into colluding with their oppression" (Wyckoff, 1977a, p. 372) and how they learned to believe that something is wrong with them rather than with a corrupt society. When consciousness is raised, awareness leads to anger, which becomes a useful force for fighting the "real culprit" (p. 373) and reclaiming humanity. Anger is a first step toward contact, which involves working with and gaining support from others who are working toward liberation. Contact with other humans counteracts alienation and isolation. Through connection with a supportive group, people experience permission to engage oppressive agents and gain protection from the potential retaliation of oppressive people.

Hogie Wyckoff (1971) also believed that group work reinforces the principle that "there are no individual solutions for oppressed people" (p. 182). The group experience does not detract from political action but helps women enact changes in their own lives so they can "carry on their struggle in a more vital way" (p. 187). Groups also encourage women to develop a sense of sisterhood and to test their problem-solving skills in a ready-made social situation (Wyckoff, 1971). Each group member develops a contract with the group; the contract both guides problem-solving efforts and guards against the facilitator imposing personal values on the client (1977b).

According to Hogie Wyckoff (1977a) this form of radical feminist therapy

- explains how freedom and spontaneity are repressed and can be regained;
- describes in clear terms how gender roles are conditioned, and how oppression is internalized and maintained;
- ties the identification of personal issues to concrete, straightforward problem-solving skills;

- provides practice in helping women act on their own behalf and try out new skills rather than being victims; and
- suggests language and techniques for implementing self-nurturing activities.

Although radical psychiatry received relatively brief visibility within radical feminist therapy, its critique and alternative approaches remain important reminders to feminist therapists about the power of "mainstream" mental health professions to co-opt the work of practitioners who work for social justice.

Miriam Greenspan's Radical Socialist Perspective

Miriam Greenspan's (1993) book, *A New Approach to Women and Therapy,* made important contributions to feminist therapy by integrating radical feminist theoretical perspectives regarding the body as a focus of oppression, liberal feminist perspectives on how women are trained to behave as victims, and a socialist feminist view of how economic factors and traditional labor divisions oppress women. Consistent with a radical perspective, Greenspan (1993) stated that "under a system of male rule, a woman's body is the source of her power" and "woman must develop herself as a body for men" (p. 163). Greenspan also described how women develop victim traits, such as indirect communication, internalized anger, dependency, depression, and indirect expressions of power, as methods of coping with an oppressive social system. Because psychiatric labels place blame on women and not on the circumstances that create their problems, Greenspan (1993) argued that these labels should be abandoned and replaced with descriptive terminology; symptoms are a "response to an untenable psychopolitical situation" (p. 264) and within each symptom is a "seed of strength which lies dormant" (p. 265). Female "craziness" is a form of wisdom, and symptoms such as being overweight represent a "great refusal" (p. 268) to be controlled or to fulfill narrow expectations of what women's bodies should be.

In keeping with a socialist feminist orientation, Greenspan indicated that gaining insight about the socioeconomic subordination of women is central to understanding their experiences. Patriarchy and capitalism cooperate to define women and assign women to perform the work of the private and family spheres. It is in this context that women's work is most devalued, which encourages women to develop relational skills in order to cope and survive. Women's wage-less work involves meeting the needs of others; through this activity, women's identity is constructed. Children and men are the beneficiaries of women's work; women's work makes it possible for them to enter and maintain a capitalist system. To halt women's loss of identity in their relationships and families, Greenspan believes that radical economic and ideological notions about motherhood will need to change. In contrast to cultural feminist theories that tend to see women's relational capacity through interpersonal and intrapsychic lenses, Greenspan concluded that it is dangerous to separate women's relational strengths from the economic and material sources that support them.

In a 1995 autobiographical statement, Greenspan noted that she wrote *A New Approach to Women and Therapy* in order to "consolidate the best of grassroots feminist therapy in the form of a book that women could use as both providers and consumers of therapy" (p. 235). Her thoughts about conducting therapy are embedded in a series of case studies designed to inform potential clients about what they can expect in feminist and traditional therapy. Thus it fulfilled important goals of feminist therapy: it demystified therapy and empowered clients by providing information.

Bonnie Burstow's Radical Feminist Therapy

Bonnie Burstow (1992) charged that many of the books on feminist therapy are "not very feminist" and "none take a radical feminist line" (p. xiii). She criticized feminist therapy for treating psychiatry as "simply like any other field that needs to be tidied up" (p. xiii) and devoting only limited attention to "isms" such as racism, homophobia, and anti-Semitism. She also argued that feminist therapists have operated under the unspoken assumption that feminist therapy clients will be white, able-bodied, gentile women, and that they have avoided working with pathologized populations such as prostitutes, ex-inmates, psychiatrized women, drug-dependent women, and women who engage in self-mutilation. A major goal of Burstow's book was to provide practical suggestions to feminist therapists for working with diverse groups of women (e.g., women of color, women with disabilities) and issues that are often ignored (e.g., problems related to violence).

Bonnie Burstow (1992) sought to "radicalize feminist therapy further" (p. xiv) by working from a feminist foundation that sees gender and sex as central to the ways in which women are oppressed, especially through the physical violation of women's bodies. Violence is a crucial focus for feminist therapy because "women's bodies are arranged, maimed, jeopardized, and tailored for the purposes of men-defined eroticism" (p. 4). According to Burstow, all women are either subject to violence or must deal with the threat of violence throughout their lives; conceptualizing issues through the lens of violence against women gives meaning and perspective to other issues that women experience. The existential feminist position of Simone de Beauvior (1952) is another cornerstone of Burstow's approach; it views freedom as "severely and often brutally conditioned but not totally 'determined' by our social and human situation" (Burstow, 1992, p. xvi). Women remain agents capable of choice despite facing limited options and enormous pressures.

A final assumption of Burstow's approach is the belief that psychiatry is a "fundamentally oppressive institution" (p. xvi). Despite feminist efforts to reform psychiatry, it remains fundamentally oppressive because psychiatry

1. limits individual freedom through mandated hospitalization and drug treatment,
2. represents a massive growth industry designed to serve its own interests and those of large pharmaceutical companies,
3. pathologizes different lifestyles by labeling them as personality disorders, and
4. relies on drugs to manage people rather than facilitate their growth.

Despite so-called changes in psychiatry, "defiant women are blamed, are punished, and are threatened with perpetual sickness and perpetual 'treatment' if they do not cooperate with narrowly defined treatment" (Burstow, 1992, p. 35).

An important principle of therapy involves expressing solidarity and "honest outrage" (Burstow, 1992, p. 151) about the injuries and injustices a person has faced. The therapist's use of solidarity is critical for empowerment because it involves identifying commonalities and bonds between women, communicates empathy, and views the analysis of sexism and oppression as inextricably connected to understanding women's issues. Body work also represents "powerful stuff" (p. 62) for unearthing issues, engaging anger, gaining energy, exploring sexuality on women's terms, and developing a new body image. Burstow proposed that a focus on the physical self is especially healing for women who have been violated through their bodies. Finally, she views systemic oppression as a fundamental contributor to women's concerns and believes that political advocacy is an important commitment for therapists who desire to effect real change in society (Burstow, 1992, 2003).

One of Burstow's (1992) positions is an antipsychiatry perspective, which includes the rejection of drug treatment and psychiatric hospitalization. She refers to individuals who have been hospitalized for mental health reasons as "psychiatric survivors" (p. 235) and believes that feminist therapists should help these clients explore how they have been oppressed by the psychiatric system, offer concrete and practical assistance, and protect them from further psychiatrization (Burstow, 2002). According to Burstow (1992), the following important messages should be communicated to the client:

- Psychiatric treatment is "without basis."
- Drugs and electroconvulsive therapy do enormous damage.
- Violation of women by the psychiatric profession is an extension of their violation as women by other institutions and people.
- "Going mad" is a way of "getting in touch with feelings and realities that were suppressed" (p. 245).
- Drugs prevent women from working through their problems.

Burstow recommends assisting clients by helping them secure advocacy and legal assistance to prevent "future psychiatric intrusion" (p. 252), as well as become involved in support groups and community protests of psychiatrization.

Bonnie Burstow's (1992) position diverges from the radical feminist views of Celia Kitzinger and Rachel Perkins (1993), who stated that although medication has often been used with female clients in abusive ways, there are appropriate uses of medication with highly disabled clients. More specifically, "drugs are quite literally a lifesaver when distress becomes too great to tolerate" (Kitzinger and Perkins, 1993, p. 179). Like Bonnie Burstow, however, Rachel Perkins (1991b) criticized feminist therapists for neglecting women with long-term mental health problems. Perkins (1991b) contended that services for long-term mental health clients should parallel treatment of physically disabled clients, for whom support systems are adapted to the needs of individuals. Similarly, the radical feminist therapist should help "socially disabled" women find shelters and safe havens as alternatives to hospitalization, and help structure their gradual withdrawal from medication, which is "one of the most liberatory acts that survivors can perform" (Burstow, 1992, p. 259). Feminists should abandon the notion that psychotherapy offers the full range of coping skills necessary for survival, and instead

1. refuse to withdraw from socially disabled women and engage in genuine friendship,
2. offer practical assistance designed to help women cope with essential day-to-day tasks,
3. create asylums where socially disabled women can gain relief from the stresses of the social world in a safe and supportive environment, and, when appropriate,
4. help socially disabled women gain access to medications that reduce the incapacitating effects of their problems (Kitzinger and Perkins, 1993).

Lenore Walker: Battered Woman Syndrome and Survivor Therapy

Lenore Walker's contributions have spanned several decades, beginning with the publication of *The Battered Woman* (1979) and eventually leading to the formulation of survivor therapy, a form of feminist therapy for survivors of interpersonal violence (Walker, 1994). According to Walker, battered women become psychological hostages after experiencing repeated episodes of violence that cycle through phases of tension building, intense battering incidents, and periods of loving contrition. Battering relationships often result in women's learned helplessness, which minimizes pain and ensures immediate survival. Learned helplessness also explains, at least in part, why leaving battering relationships is difficult (Walker, 1979, 1984, 1989). Walker clarified that although battered women's behaviors are sometimes interpreted as passivity or as "self-defeating," these behaviors represent a series of coping skills that increase the likelihood of their own and their children's survival. Consistent with radical feminist views, Walker placed responsibility for battering on the "androcentric need for power" (1989, p. 695) and men's desire to control others. Although Lenore Walker's has focused primarily on the reempowerment of individual women through therapy and forensic practice, she has also been supportive of the shelter movement, advocated changes in police and legal practices, and viewed the role of community support and advocacy as central to overcoming violence (Walker, 1979, 1989).

Battered woman syndrome resembles rape trauma syndrome (Burgess and Holmstrom, 1974) in that both conditions connect the personal and political by conceptualizing symptoms as appropriate and understandable responses to extreme crisis and trauma, and by avoiding the victim blaming associated with many diagnostic categories. According to Walker (1989, 1991), both rape trauma and battered woman syndromes can be seen as subtypes of post-traumatic stress disorder, a diagnostic category that first appeared in the DSM-III (American Psychiatric Association, 1980). Many feminist therapists who had earlier eschewed all diagnostic labeling have viewed PTSD a potentially nonstigmatizing method for conceptualizing women's distress. Walker (1991) stated that "PTSD stresses the abnormal nature of the stressor which causes the mental health symptoms, not individual pathology" (p. 22). In addition, it "takes the onus of blame away from the individual woman, yet still lets psychotherapists work with her in finding her own way to heal and move on with her life" (p. 22). Finally, it integrates multiple symptoms within a straightforward framework and thus supports the development of more comprehensive models for understanding women's reactions to trauma (Goodman, Koss, and Russo, 1993).

Lenore Walker has also been a tireless activist who, with other feminist psychologists, protested the creation and inclusion of masochistic personality disorder (later renamed self-defeating personality disorder) in the DSM-III-R (American Psychiatric Association, 1987) and DSM-IV (American Psychiatric Association, 1994). Lenore Walker and Marianne Dutton-Douglas (1988) proposed that up to 85 percent of normally socialized women exhibit many of the criteria of self-defeating personality disorder (SDPD), which describes the behaviors of persons who remain passive and immobilized in exploitive relationships. Feminist psychologists noted that such a label could be used to blame women for being the target of violence rather than placing responsibility on society and abusive partners. Furthermore, SDPD did not acknowledge the survival value of learned sacrificial or pacifying behaviors for reducing the emotional or physical violence that accompanies abusive relationships. To raise consciousness and further point out the oppressiveness of this label, Paula Caplan (1991, 1995) proposed a new diagnostic category: delusional dominating personality disorder, which represents SDPD's counterpart and conceptualizes dominating behaviors as overconformity to a traditional "real man" image. The activism of feminist psychologists such as Lenore Walker and Paula Caplan was crucial in eliminating further consideration of this disorder; no mention of the category appeared in DSM-IV (American Psychiatric Association, 1994).

Survivor therapy (Walker, 1994) integrates principles of feminist and trauma theory and emphasizes safety and reempowerment. The safety phase, or feminist crisis intervention, involves assessing the potential for violence as well as creating safety and escape plans. Reempowerment emphasizes

- helping a woman regain a sense of control and power over her life, including gaining financial independence;
- validating her experience, bearing witness to her story, and supporting her healing from trauma;
- focusing on strengths that build self-esteem, and decision-making skills; and
- decreasing isolation by establishing supportive connections with others.

Some feminists view Walker's contributions as more reformist than radical, and others conceptualize her model of learned helplessness as potentially victim blaming because it places greater emphasis on a woman's weaknesses rather than her resourcefulness and coping skills and does little to address structural inequities that support abuse (Gondolf, 1988; Rothenberg, 2003; Whalen, 1996). However, her assertion that pathology is lodged in male violence rather than in women's personality traits, her emphasis on treating battered women as their own best experts, and her activism against potentially oppressive diagnoses reflect important components of a radical social change emphasis. Bess Rothenberg (2003) concluded that Walker's work has garnered support for the battered women's movement while also taking attention away from the collective plight of abused women. As such, the battered woman syndrome and related efforts to work with abuse victims can be viewed as a "cultural compromise" (p. 771).

Judith Herman on Trauma and Recovery

Like many other feminist therapists, Judith Herman participated in a consciousness-raising group, which then became a catalyst for her participation as a feminist therapist in the Women's Mental Health Collective. She gained additional awareness of the extensive impact of sexual and domestic violence on women through work with her patients, which also contributed to her goal of transforming psychology of women (Herman and Ojerholm, 1995). In addition to conducting groundbreaking research on sexual abuse (Herman, 1981), she raised concerns about the ways in which the conceptualization of many personality disorders contribute to the blaming of victims. She also reframed borderline personality disorder as a posttraumatic condition.

To expand therapists' thinking about the nature of posttraumatic conditions, Herman proposed a new category of disorders termed "complex post-traumatic stress disorder." In contrast to simple PTSD, which describes the typical reactions to single traumatic events, complex post-traumatic stress disorder describes a complicated set of reactions to "a history of subjection to totalitarian control over a prolonged period (months to years)" (Herman, 1992, p. 121). Concentration camp survivors and survivors of sexual trauma or battering are examples of individuals who may experience this disorder, which typically involves alterations in affect regulation, consciousness, self-perception, and meaning systems. Alterations of victims' perceptions of perpetrators and disruptions in relationships with others may also be a part of this constellation of symptoms (Herman, 1992). This conceptualization offers a new and nonpejorative way of organizing symptom patterns that are often labeled as borderline, dissociative, or somatization problems.

Bonnie Burstow (2003), whose model of radical feminist therapy was described earlier in this chapter, believes that despite Judith Herman's significant contribution to trauma theory, her conceptualization of complex PTSD relies on "largely accepted psychiatric underpinnings" (p. 1293), which may reinforce victim identities of clients and allow feminist therapists to be "co-opted by organs of the state that traditionally traumatize our clients" (p. 1316). Ongoing controversies about the degree to which feminist therapists can use traditional diagnosis as a tool to empower their clients are revisited in the final chapter of this book.

Judith Herman (1992) also identified three primary phases of healing from interpersonal trauma: safety, remembrance and mourning, and reconnection. During the initial phase, the feminist therapist works toward helping clients (1) feel a sense of psychological safety, stability, and control; (2) develop skills for daily living and self-care; and (3) cope effectively with intrusive and immediate trauma symptoms. During the phase of remembrance and mourning, clients face the task of coming to terms with long-term trauma by grieving losses associated with abuse and violence, and re-creating a sense of meaning. Through a series of carefully timed and paced emotionally corrective experiences, memories of abuse are no longer associated with shame but with dignity and new beliefs about the capacity to thrive. A final phase of reconnection involves dealing with unresolved issues such as sexual, relational, family, and social concerns. Herman's model also speaks to the importance of matching individual healing with social change.

Laura Brown: Feminist Therapy As Subversive Dialogue

Laura Brown (1997) identified three social movements that influenced her approach: the feminist movement, the civil rights movement for gay and lesbian rights, and the social activism of adult survivors of interpersonal violence. She refers to her work as the practice of social justice and the "private practice of subversion" (p. 449), and has made contributions to multiple areas relevant to feminist therapy including feminist ethics (e.g., Brown, 1991b, 1995), feminist multiculturalism and antiracism (e.g., Brown, 1990a, 1995), feminist conceptualizations of distress (e.g., Brown 1994, 2000b), feminist gender-role analysis (Brown, 1986, 1990b), feminist forensic practice (Brown, 2000a), and lesbian feminist psychotherapy (Brown, 1992b).

Laura Brown's contributions to conceptualizing distress have been especially noteworthy and diverge from the views of radical feminist therapists such as Rachel Perkins, Bonnie Burstow, and Celia Kitzinger. Brown (1994) noted that although some radical feminist therapists have concluded that diagnosis is "irrelevant" or "no more than negative labeling" (p. 125), this position may be considered naive. If all of the complex problems that clients bring to therapy are reduced to "feeling bad," the therapist has an inadequate framework for guiding the client toward wholeness. On the other hand, distress cannot be adequately understood by using formal diagnostic categories alone.

According to Laura Brown (1994), feminist constructions of distress must take into account the unique context and experiences of the client, avoid conceptualizing "disorder" as lodged in the individual, and consider the functional or usefulness of behaviors for meeting the client's goals. In addition, considerations related to distress are secondary to the identifications of the client's skills and resources. Finally, distress "is conceived of as a potential outcome of behaviors that are empowering and affirming to the person and/or the social network . . . rather than as evidence of the presence of a disorder" (p. 377). It is essential for feminist therapists and their clients to "work jointly to develop organized hypotheses about the nature, origins, and meanings of the client's distress" (1994, p. 128). Such a process helps the client and therapist name the distress accurately; identify the complex individual, biological, interpersonal, and social/contextual factors that contribute to the client's issues; and clarify the course and goals of therapy.

In keeping with this position, Laura Brown (1994) recommended the use of an integrative biopsychosocial perspective for understanding the client's experience and proposed that biological treatments can be integrated with methods which focus on interpersonal and sociopolitical factors. All options for healing, however, must be presented to clients in an open and noncoercive manner that articulates the potentially positive contributions of the option as well as limitations.

In contrast to radical social change therapists who rejected most tools of traditional psychology, Laura Brown (1994) has adopted a flexible position, suggesting that although traditional psychological tools have often been used to oppress women, feminist therapists can also use traditional tools to sabotage and transform patriarchal systems. However, she has been more critical than Lenore Walker of diagnostic categories like PTSD, arguing that PTSD is inadequate for conceptualizing the diverse and often insidious traumas that clients experience.

Laura Brown (1994) recommended the use of "subversive practices" that allow one to use conventional tools while maintaining a cautious and skeptical attitude. According to Brown, the assumption that the master's tools cannot be used to dismantle the master's house (Lorde, 1984) limits the flexibility of feminists. She argued that the master's tools "can be a chainsaw, cutting down a person's sense of worth or value; or they can be turned on the structures of patriarchy, cutting the latter down to size or nicely remodeling them to be a better fit" (Brown, 1994, p. 192). In order to provide alternative models of conceptualization, feminist therapists seek to understand the social meanings of traditional diagnosis, consider how they can be used to oppress individuals, and reshape these tools for feminist change. A feminist therapist can also translate the information derived from diagnosis, psychological tests, and other traditional tools in order to realize feminist goals. Although the "master's tools" cannot be the only tools for transforming psychotherapy, they can be used to "reforge, reshape, and transform each possibility for oppression into one of liberation and social change" (Brown, 1994, p. 199). This approach is consistent with a radical postmodern position, which recognizes the limitations of all conceptual frameworks but uses these incomplete road maps to provide useful but imperfect models for practice.

Similarity and Difference Among Social Change Feminist Therapy Approaches

This section has summarized six approaches to social change in feminist therapy. Common to all descriptions of social change feminist therapy is the goal of transforming assessment and practice. Contributors to these approaches hold varied views, however, with regard to the contexts in and strategies with which social change can be best implemented. In general, those from the radical therapy tradition (e.g., Miriam Greenspan and Bonnie Burstow) have chosen to work outside of "professional" circles of psychology, believing that it is difficult to transform help-giving traditions from within. Laura Walker, Laura Brown, and Judith Herman have also viewed social transformation as a central component of their approaches but have not rejected the potential contributions of professional psychology or psychiatry as tools for supporting some aspects of transformation. It is also important to note that these contributors have proposed models which are more inclusive than those set forth by many early radical feminist theorists. Most authors who have contributed to radical social change thought since 1990 have addressed factors such as class, culture, ethnicity, and sexual orientation and the way in which they may profoundly influence women's gendered experiences. Many of these approaches are compatible with a wide array of feminist theories such as women-of-color feminisms, lesbian feminism, and postmodern feminism.

Ongoing Issues: Diagnosis and Feminist Ethics

Feminist therapy owes a significant debt to the basic tenets and ideals of radical social change feminisms. The final section of this chapter briefly addresses two ongoing issues related to the legacy of social change feminisms in feminist therapy: diagnosis and feminist ethics.

The Politics of Diagnosis in Feminist Therapy

Edna Rawlings and Diane Carter (1977) stated that feminist therapists do not use diagnostic labels because they reflect the inappropriate application of social power, ignore environmental influences on symptom formation, represent a major instrument of oppression, and reduce the therapist's respect for clients. Consistent with this view, radical feminist efforts have directed less attention to diagnosing and controlling symptoms and more on exploring the role of symptoms in clients' lives (Gilbert, 1980; Marecek and Kravetz, 1977; Rawlings and Carter, 1977).

Although liberal feminist therapists have focused primarily on eliminating sex bias in diagnosis and calling for diagnostic categories that are equally valid for women and men, radical feminists have often rejected traditional systems, avoided diagnostic labels, and utilized descriptive narratives and gender-role analysis (Brown, 1986, 1990b) to assess the meaning of clients' problems. Each of the specific contributors whose work was discussed in this chapter have been critical of traditional diagnosis and have proposed divergent ways of coping with these limitations by (1) rejecting all forms of formal diagnosis, (2) proposing new categories for conceptualizing women's concerns, or (3) reframing traditional diagnostic categories in feminist terms.

In the twenty-first century, radical feminist therapists are less likely than radical feminist therapists of the 1970s to reject the use of conventional diagnostic labels altogether, but have focused on developing categories that place symptoms in context and provide a respectful foundation for working with clients. Given increased knowledge about biological contributions to some disorders, contemporary feminist therapists are less likely than early feminist therapists to reject the use of labels such as schizophrenia, bipolar disorder, or depression. However, they typically remain opposed to the use of such a term as borderline personality disorder, which is associated with pejorative and pessimistic views of clients. Categories such as complex post-traumatic stress disorder, which help organize the complex and multifaceted symptoms of clients and draw connections between distress and oppression or abuse, are more likely to be acceptable to radically oriented therapists than labels such as BPD. Many social change feminist therapists view themselves as engaging in "subversive practices," which involves using diagnostic categories to meet clients' needs to access health insurance coverage but avoiding the use of diagnosis whenever possible.

Although radical feminist therapists hold varied perspectives about the utility of diagnostic labels, they agree that assessment of a client's problems must be based on a shared dialogue between the therapist and client. Through such discussion, clients achieve greater understanding of the personal, cultural, and social aspects of their problems. Feminist therapists inform clients about their hypotheses, how these were developed, and what theories and beliefs influenced their thinking (Brown and Walker, 1990). Conceptualizations are tested with clients, who are encouraged to ask questions or propose alternatives. Therapists also explain why they do or do not reject the use of traditional diagnoses. Given the importance of these issues to the future of feminist therapy, they will be revisited in the final chapter of this book.

Social Change Feminisms and Feminist Ethics

During the earliest years of feminist therapy, some feminist therapists naively assumed that when both the therapist and client were women, the type of power issues associated with hierarchical, patriarchal structures and relationships would not be evident in feminist therapy (Lerman and Rigby, 1990). The early radical feminist position of "undifferentiated egalitarianism" (Adleman and Barrett, 1990) represented a false sense of equality and a simplistic view of the actual power differentials that exist between therapists and clients. Although calling oneself a feminist therapist involves making a commitment to equality, the title *feminist therapist* does not insulate one from engaging in ethically problematic behaviors, including the inappropriate use of power, boundary violations, and sexual victimization of clients (Brown, 1991b).

As feminist therapy has matured, feminist therapists have recognized the importance of examining feminist ethical practices, and these themes are reflected in the FTI's (2000) *Feminist Therapy Institute Code of Ethics* and other influential publications on feminist ethics on feminist practice (e.g., Brabeck, 2000; Rave and Larsen, 1995). Although feminist social change ethics address many of the same issues as traditional ethics, such as the nature, consequences, and motives associated with ethical and unethical actions (Tong, 1993), sterile rules and regulations such as those presented in many traditional codes of ethics are inadequate for supporting feminist practice. The FTI code of ethics (1990, 2000) consists of aspirational guidelines that articulate the implications of social change feminisms for the practice of psychotherapy, training, and research (Rave and Larsen, 1990). First, the code clearly exemplifies the perspective that the personal is political and reflects a proactive stance designed to eliminate oppression and empower women as a group. Second, it pays particular attention to the specific concerns of women as therapists and as clients. Third, it proposes guidelines for dealing with potentially risky situations associated with overlapping relationships. Fourth, it acknowledges that power differences between clients and therapists do exist and proposes ways in which the power of therapists can be used in their clients' best interests. Fifth, it attends to diversities of race, class, age, and ability and calls on therapists to engage in constant monitoring of their attitudes, behaviors, and knowledge. It also highlights the importance of self-care as a tool for ensuring the personal health of the therapist. Sixth, it articulates the responsibility of feminist therapists to address social change as well as personal issues (FTI, 1990, 2000; Rave and Larsen, 1990).

In general, feminist social change ethical principles are characterized by several overarching themes (Brabeck and Ting, 2000). First, the experiences of women and the subjective knowledge of women, which have often been ignored in traditional ethical treatises, hold significance for ethical codes and behaviors and provide illumination about ethical issues. In addition, feminist critiques of distortions and bias in knowledge and practice must also address multiple "discriminatory distortions" (Brabeck and Ting, 2000, p. 26) related to social statuses such as race, age, class, ethnicity, and homophobia. Finally, feminist values and ethics incorporate the analysis of power dynamics, and are designed to lead to actions that seek to achieve social justice (Brabeck and Ting, 2000). Radical social change feminist therapy is about transformation. Preparing to participate effectively in an ethics of social change requires that the feminist therapist adopt self-reflective attitudes which help them identify and correct ethnocentrism, inadvertent biases, and unexamined assumptions in their theory and practice.

CONCLUDING COMMENTS

Feminists who are influenced by radical and socialist feminist perspectives assume a wide range of positions regarding the degree to which mainstream psychotherapy can be integrated with psychotherapy principles. Kitzinger and Perkins (1993) reject psychotherapy as a viable method for solving women's problems, and Burstow (1992) rejects many of the tools and ethical stances of mainstream psychology. Laura Brown (1994), however, views radical postmodern feminist psychotherapy as a crucial tool for empowering individuals to become involved in social change. While highly critical of the sexism, racism, and heterosexism that permeate much traditional psychological thinking, she believes that feminist therapists can use many mainstream psychological tools to achieve radical feminist goals.

Despite differences regarding how radical feminist goals are interpreted, "the personal is political" remains a central theme of radical social change feminist therapy. Within therapy, "a client comes to perceive her problem as just one knot in a power network that ties up many peers with seemingly equal tightness" (Elias, 1975, p. 58). She then recognizes the intricate connections between personal issues and the social context in which she lives. A salient emphasis of radical forms of feminist therapy is that women's problems are not only the result of unequal opportunity (a liberal feminist position) but are also the consequence of the devaluation of women that permeates the very structure of institutions such as the church, legislative bodies, the justice system, education, and the family.

At the beginning of the twenty-first century, feminist social change practice has moved beyond the original positions of radical feminism, which has sometimes been characterized as white women's feminism, placing exclusive emphasis on gender oppression, and ignoring the many other complex social identities, oppressions, and privileges that shape women's lives. Recent radical social change feminisms reflect the early values of radical feminism but also attend to diversities and power differences among women. The transformation of social systems remains a salient goal of feminist psychotherapy, and radical feminist therapy offers a "disruptive force" (Brown, 1994, p. 29) and a "subversive dialogue" designed to resist and "subvert patriarchal dominance at the most subtle and powerful levels, as it is internalized and personified in the lives of therapists and their clients, colleagues, and communities" (Brown, 1994, p. 17).

Chapter 4

Cultural Feminist Theory and Feminist Therapy

Cultural feminism has historically emphasized the unique or special qualities of women's lives. Cultural feminists have tended to define women's experiences as distinctly different from men's experiences, and have sought to change society's priorities through the introduction of "feminine" strengths and priorities, such as cooperation, relational qualities, and nurturing activities. Cultural feminism has inspired a diverse array of theories relevant to women's personality and priorities, ethics, and ecological concerns. It has also been the focus of criticism by those who see this tradition as based primarily on white, middle-class women's experience and as contributing to overgeneralizations about women's experience. This chapter summarizes the evolution of cultural feminist theory, discusses its strengths and limitations, describes its major influences on feminist personality theories and psychotherapies, and notes ways in which psychological theories embedded in cultural feminist thought have been revised in order to address the diversity among women.

AN OVERVIEW OF CULTURAL FEMINIST THEORY

To use the following items as a form of self-assessment, respond to each statement with a "yes" or "no."

_____ 1. A major cause of sexism and oppression is the devaluation of traditional feminine qualities and the overvaluation of masculine values and patriarchy.

_____ 2. The goal of feminism should be to revalue women's traditional strengths so that women can infuse the society with values based on cooperation.

_____ 3. Solutions to sexism will come through women's discovery of internal truths, relationships with other women, and the "feminization" of the culture.

_____ 4. Key issues for women involve developing a sense of ethics based on caring and relationship values, and organizing around issues of nonviolence.

_____ 5. Women's cooperation with other women and involvement in organized peace efforts of all kinds will give them the necessary power to influence and change society.

Agreement with these statements suggests that your views are consistent with the basic themes of cultural feminism.

Early Cultural Feminism

Cultural feminism shares a rich nineteenth-century heritage with liberal feminism. Cultural and liberal feminists of the nineteenth century often proposed conflicting beliefs about women's liberation: Liberal enlightenment feminists tended to emphasize the importance of rationality and the similarity between men and women, and cultural feminists focused on nonrational, intuitive aspects of life and the special qualities of women that were presumed to make them different from or superior to men. Early cultural feminists such as Margaret Fuller ([1945] 1976), Jane Addams ([1913] 1960), and Charlotte Perkins Gilman ([1915] 1979, 1923) envisioned cultural transformations based on matriarchal visions. They typically defined women's experiences as distinctly different from men's experiences and sought to revere and valorize traditional feminine and maternal strengths.

Margaret Fuller's ([1845] 1976) early cultural feminist perspective emphasized the special strengths of women and women's differences from men. She stated, "The especial genius of Woman I believe to be electrical in movement, intuitive in function, spiritual in tendency" (Fuller [1845] 1976, p. 263). She associated female strengths with harmony, beauty, and love, and male attributes with energy, power, and intellect. She noted that although "there is no wholly masculine man, no purely feminine woman . . . male and female represent the two sides of the great radical dualism" (p. 263). Margaret Fuller ([1845] 1976) believed that women would transform culture by exhibiting a gentle heroism and bringing the world "more thoroughly and deeply into harmony with her nature" (p. 262); she stated: "Should these faculties have free play, I believe they will open new, deeper and purer sources of joyous inspiration than have as yet refreshed the earth" (p. 264).

Although Elizabeth Cady Stanton and Sarah Grimké contributed to a liberal feminist tradition by emphasizing the similarity of men's and women's natures, their later writings proposed that women exhibited moral superiority and power which offered the keys to enlightened motherhood and society's future progress (Banner, 1980; Bartlett, 1988). Stanton ([1891] 1968) argued that the first civilizations were maternal: "The period of woman's supremacy lasted through many centuries, undisputed, accepted as natural and proper wherever it existed, and was called the matriarchate, or mother-age" (p. 143). She contended that although men's early contributions were limited to inventing tools of warfare, women's roles were varied and ranged from mothering to protector, inventor, and breadwinner. Matilda Gage ([1884] 1968) expressed similar sentiments by indicating that the "feminine" principle appeared first and everywhere in science: in chemistry, geology, botany, philology, and biology. She concluded, "When biology becomes more fully understood it will also be universally acknowledged that the primal creative power, like the first manifestation of life, is feminine" (p. 140).

Jane Addams is known for her efforts in the field of social work and her involvement in international peace efforts. She suggested that during earlier centuries women had demonstrated a much wider and more significant role in society as they "dragged home the game and transformed the pelts into shelter and clothing" (Addams, [1913] 1960, p. 109). However, functions such as health and education had been wrested from women and incorporated into institutional departments that were no longer under women's control. She argued that if the tables were turned and women held the more powerful roles granted to men, women would oppose men's suffrage and greater involvement in society for the following reasons:

1. Men's fondness of fighting
2. Their carelessness about health, cleanliness, work conditions, and the well-being of both children and workers
3. Men's emphasis on profit and indifference to human life

4. Their reliance on "savage instincts of punishment and revenge" (p. 111) in their administration of the criminal justice system
5. Men's lack of concern for victims, such as their absence of concern for homeless girls forced into prostitution (Addams, [1913] 1960)

She did not believe that women's suffrage was a guarantee of individual rights or an end in and of itself, but was a means to facilitate women's entry into the social/public sphere so that they could influence the society with new values. Jane Addams's commitment to social reform and pacifism emerged from her belief that women's distinctive values should permeate the family but should also humanize the world and change society.

Charlotte Perkins Gilman identified herself primarily as a humanist and a socialist (Hill, 1980), but many aspects of her thinking are consistent with cultural feminist ideas. She believed that although male traits such as combativeness and assertion had been necessary for the growth and evolution of some aspects of society, the original balance of society needed to be restored through the infusion of values associated with nurturance and cooperation (Donovan, 2000; Hill, 1980). Gilman (1923) viewed feminine traits as superior to masculine traits:

> The innate, underlying difference [between the sexes] is one of principle. On the one hand, the principle of struggle, conflict and competition, the results of which make our "economic problems." On the other, the principle of growth, of culture, of applying services and nourishment in order to produce improvement. (p. 271)

In 1923, women earned the right to vote, and much of the attention of feminist activists was redirected from suffrage to social reform. The cultural feminists of the mid-1900s were often referred to as "social feminists" because they believed the maternal virtues that were typically enacted in the home could provide necessary correctives for social life in general (Black, 1989). As participants in the League of Women Voters, peace movements, and a variety of areas of social reform, these cultural feminist activists believed that maternal and reproductive roles had taught women how to show unselfish commitment to their children, and that this commitment could also benefit disenfranchised children and future children. Social feminists often assumed that because of their connection to children, they could also comprehend more fully the necessity for peace than men; they believe that women, who give birth and nurture life, were less likely to waste time destroying life through war (Black, 1989).

Emergence of Contemporary Cultural Feminism

Liberal, radical, and socialist feminisms dominated the landscape during the early years of the "new" feminist movement. However, cultural feminism reemerged during the mid-1970s as some radical feminists focused less on eradicating sex roles and more on identifying the strengths associated with traditional women's roles. "The Fourth World Manifesto" (Burris, 1973) reiterated the radical feminist principle that female and male cultures are artificial categories defined by male-dominated society and thus represent caricatures of humanity. However, the manifesto also suggested that devalued female traits should not be repudiated but embraced by women:

> We are proud of the female culture of emotion, intuition, love personal relationships, etc., as the most essential human characteristics. It is our male colonizers—it is the male culture—who have defined essential humanity out of their identity and who are "culturally deprived." (1973, p. 355)

The revaluing of motherhood was an important cultural feminist theme. Jane Alpert (1973) asserted that women's biology and capacity to bear and nurture children were the foundation for women's power, and argued that women should claim the "mother right" principle, which called for restructuring the family and society according to the characteristics of an ideal nurturing relationship between a mother and child. These qualities include "empathy, intuitiveness, adaptability, awareness of growth as a process rather than as goal-ended, inventiveness, protective feelings toward others, and a capacity to respond emotionally as well as rationally" (1973, p. 92). When a society embodies these qualities, "[m]atriarchy means nothing less than the end of oppression" (p. 92).

In an elaboration of this theme, Adrienne Rich (1976) stated that women have the unique power to create life, a power of which men are both fearful and jealous. In their attempt to restrict the power of mothers, men have created rules, procedures, and medical practices that control women and alienate them from their own bodies and experiences. Women could regain power by reclaiming the circumstances of childbirth and mothering on their own terms. Some radical feminists were highly critical of these efforts to revalue mothering, stating that it promised women a nonexistent utopia and encouraged women to avoid fighting patriarchy in order to establish separate women's communities designed to "prove to men the error of their ways by shaming them with women's superior morality" (Brooke, 1975, p. 81); they argued that visions of a matriarchal fantasy can offer a retreat from activism and "transform feminism from a political movement to a lifestyle movement" (p. 83).

Cultural feminism was also influenced by those who became disappointed with the limited gains achieved by liberal feminism. Sylvia Hewlett (1986) argued that women had traded their previous protections of traditional marriage for a "lesser life" that included limited financial gain, lower well-being, and pressures to live a superwoman existence. She noted that liberation meant little because it was defined under men's terms, and that women remained "conditioned by and constrained by child-related responsibilities" (p. 401). In similar fashion, Suzanne Gordon (1991) stated that women had been pressured to replace the "feminine mystique" with the "masculine mystique," which is "founded on the assumption that women can find happiness, self-esteem, and self-fulfillment by emulating and ultimately internalizing the ideology of market place society; in other words, by becoming the female equivalent of economic, acquisitive man" (p. 27). Gordon (1991) argued that to help women and society resolve the "crisis of caring" (p. 13), networks of collaboration and community should be integrated within the workplace, which would allow women to revalue and balance care in both work and home settings.

Cultural feminism has influenced a number of contemporary theories and approaches related to feminist ethics, ecofeminism, and feminist standpoint approaches. The following sections summarize influential themes related to these traditions.

Cultural Feminist Contributions to Feminist Ethics

Cultural feminist perspectives on ethics emerged from the recognition that women's values and experiences have been suppressed within traditional explorations of ethics. Contributors to feminist ethics have proposed alternative models of morality and ethics to correct past biases and create models that are consistent with women's experience. Winnie Tomm (1992) stated that "principles of so-called fairness have entailed discrimination against women and have tyrannized women in the name of justice" (p. 104). This reality is particularly evident when women have sought justice through the legal system after having experienced rape or other forms of violence. Tomm argued that legal procedures and rulings have often been associated with victim blaming and the decrease of women's control over their own lives.

Cultural feminist versions of feminist ethics emphasize the centrality of interdependence over individualism. Relationships, rather than the exercise of individual rights, are the central priority of moral behavior. Two theorists have significantly shaped the focus of this developing field: psychologist Carol Gilligan (1982) and educational philosopher Nel Noddings (1984). Both theorists studied the practical, everyday realities of women, critiqued traditional models that equated morality with individual justice and rights, and stressed the importance of fairness in the application of so-called universal principles of justice (Bartlett, 1992). Carol Gilligan (1982) proposed that many women resolve moral issues through an ethic of care and interdependence:

> The moral imperative that emerges repeatedly in interviews with women is an injunction to care, a responsibility to discern and alleviate the "real and recognizable trouble" of this world. For men the moral imperative appears rather as an injunction to respect the rights of others and thus, to protect from interference the rights to life and self-fulfillment. (p. 19)

Likewise, Nel Noddings (1984) indicated that caring, responsibility, and relationships are cornerstones of an ethic of care. Noddings declared that caring is "feminine in the deep classical sense—rooted in receptivity, relatedness, and responsiveness" (p. 2). Neither Gilligan nor Noddings described ethical decision making as a system of specific principles; instead, they describe it as a process in which human interdependence and responsiveness are crucial to resolving concrete human dilemmas.

Closely related to feminist ethics are influential writings that have focused on women's modes of knowing and experiencing the world. Psychologists Mary Belenky, Blythe Clinchy, Nancy Goldberger, and Jill Tarule (1986) proposed that traditional models of cognitive development are based on a masculine worldview in which knowledge is displayed through argument and debate which sets knowers apart from others. They noted that many women are silenced by this concept of cognitive competence, and proposed that many women prefer a more connected form of knowing which values empathizing rather than critiquing ideas, appreciating diverse perspectives, and learning within a community of thinkers.

In *Maternal Thinking,* Sarah Ruddick (1989) outlined three "demands" of mothers' thinking that contribute positively to women's ethics, activism, and a politics of peace. The activities of mothering include awareness of (1) the need to preserve life, to enhance children's possibility of survival by minimizing their exposure to risks; (2) the complexity of fostering children's intellectual, emotional, and physical growth; and (3) the importance of raising children to behave in socially acceptable ways and in accordance with the values of a reference group. These demands call on women to engage in continuous "disciplined reflection" (p. 24) about their complex roles, and these practices form a foundation for thinking about and creating peace. Ruddick (1989) added both women and men can behave destructively but the central demands of mothering teach women to value activities that enhance the preservation of relationship and life.

Although cultural feminism has represented a powerful force in the consideration of gender and ethics, feminist ethics also encompasses other traditions within feminism. Across various feminist theoretical perspectives, contributors to feminist ethics have exposed the variety of ways in which the study of ethics has been biased and dominated by the moral concerns, issues, and methods that reflected the realities of men's lives (Friedman, 2000). Second, feminists have focused on a diverse range of global and local concerns of women that have often been ignored by ethicists. These issues include discrimination against women, reproductive technology and abortion, violence against women, gendered aspects of family and medical leave, public health care, pornography, comparable worth, AIDS, and immigration policy (DiQuinzio and Young, 1997; Held, 1998). Third, feminist ethicists have challenged traditional dichotomies of reason versus emotion, public versus private domains, abstract versus everyday concerns, and self-sufficiency versus relationality. Whereas traditional approaches to ethics have tended to emphasize the primacy or superiority of the first concept of each of these pairs, feminists have worked toward highlighting the relevance of previously ignored concepts that are more frequently associated with femininity (e.g., cultural feminists) or have proposed ways of integrating these concepts (Held, 1998).

Cultural Feminism and Ecofeminism

In her book entitled *Gyn/Ecology,* Mary Daly (1978) defined ecology as "the complex web of interrelationships between organisms and their environment" (p. 9) and asserted that male efforts emphasizing the separation of the human from her or his environment could not be successful in counteracting the horrors committed against the earth. This concern with the interconnectedness of all things anticipated the emergence of ecofeminism, which has focused on the ways in which the oppression of women has been closely connected to the domination and destruction of the earth through various forms of technology and science. In addition to identifying the negative connection between men and nature, many ecofeminists have paid special attention to the positive connections between nature and women, as is revealed by the following statement: "Nothing links the human animal and nature so profoundly as woman's reproductive system, which enables her to share the experience of bringing forth and nourishing life with the rest of the living world" (Collard, 1989, p. 106). By virtue of their involvement in mothering, caring, and nurturing roles, women may be especially equipped to understand the interconnectedness of people and the natural world.

Three primary principles are central to ecofeminism. First, Western civilization was built in opposition to nature, which interacts with the domination of women. Because of this connection, feminists should be concerned with the struggle of all nature. The fate of human and nonhuman life is inextricably intertwined, and the struggle for social justice for women and other people cannot be achieved apart from care for the earth's resources. Second, all life must be considered part of an interconnected web; hierarchies associated with patriarchy must be rejected. The earth must be seen as having intrinsic value; no one being is more valuable or superior to other beings. Third, a healthy and balanced ecosystem is based on diversity of human and nonhuman experience. The perspectives of non-Western and indigenous peoples who have maintained a close connection with the earth are especially important for showing society how to develop a new relationship to nature (Diamond and Orenstein, 1990; King, 1990; Warren, 2000).

One strand of ecofeminism explored prepatriarchal nature-based feminist spiritualities and promoted the revival of rituals centered on goddess images of deity. Some ecofeminists believe that prior to the emergence of patriarchy and industrialization, the earth was held in reverence, people felt connected to the earth as a living being, and the reproductive and life-giving powers associated with women's bodies were highly valued (Plant, 1989). According to this perspective, returning to these traditions allows people to honor the feminine values of compassion, caring, and nonviolence as part of an earth-based spiritual tradition. In addition, the cycle of life as well as the experiences of birth, growth, decay, death, and regeneration can be celebrated as they coincide with the seasons of the year. Balance among all the different communities that comprise the living body of earth can be established when the rhythms of human, plant, animal, and environmental life are commemorated (Eisler, 1990; Starhawk, 1989).

Ynestra King (1990) noted that much ecofeminist thought is closely related to cultural feminism but suggested that it offers a more complete analysis than most forms of cultural feminism. First, ecofeminism moves beyond cultural feminism's emphasis on personal transformation and provides an important focus for activism. Second, it suggests a new basis for ethics and provides direction for the reconciliation of people and the earth based on hope. Third, ecofeminism acknowledges the interconnectedness of all women, while also recognizing diversity among women. It encourages women of all backgrounds to draw upon the earth-related imagery of their own traditions and to actively contribute to feminist theory.

During the 1990s and the beginning of the twenty-first century, ecofeminist thought has become increasingly connected to varying theoretical perspectives within feminism. Karen Warren (2000) noted that underlying all ecofeminist perspectives is the assumption that the domination of human nature and nonhuman nature is interrelated. However, although some ecofeminists celebrate the connection between traditional feminine qualities and nonhuman nature, others warn that these associations may merely romanticize or reinforce traditional and harmful stereotypes. At present, ecofeminist thought is associated with diverse expressions around the globe in the sciences, arts, literature, philosophy, and grassroots organizing. Ecofeminists focus on a wide range of issues including religion and spirituality, environmental concerns, land management and ethics, social justice, animal welfare issues, and lifestyle choices such as vegetarianism (Warren, 2000).

Cultural Feminism and Feminist Standpoint Epistemologies

Individuals who value cultural feminist thought are also likely to value feminist standpoint epistemologies or approaches to knowledge. Standpoint perspectives are based on the assumption that "men's dominating position in social life results in partial and perverse understandings whereas women's subjugated position provides the possibility of more complete and less perverse understandings" (Harding, 1986, p. 26). According to this view, traditional academic methods are based on an androcentric view of the world that categorizes much of human experience according to a set of polarities: subject-object, mind-body, inner-outer, reason-sense, and public-private domains. These abstract categories are not only inadequate for explaining the experiences of women but have been used by those in power to define women in comparison to and as less complete than men. For example, women have traditionally engaged in work (e.g., housework and mothering) that has not been valued in and of itself; it is valued only because it has freed men to engage in activities valued within the culture. Sandra Harding noted that "women are thus excluded from men's conceptions of culture" and women's experience is "incomprehensible and inexpressible within the distorted abstractions of men's conceptual schemes" (Harding, 1990, p. 95). To correct these biases, those who endorse feminist standpoint epistemologies believe that the role of feminists is to create a "successor science" which can replace the narrow views of traditional analysis with more complete and inclusive analyses. Feminist standpoint theorists argue that "while certain social positions (the oppressor's) produce distorted ideological views of reality, other social positions (the oppressed's) can pierce ideological obfuscations and attain a correct and comprehensive understanding of the world" (Hawkesworth, 1989, p. 536).

Feminist standpoint theories reject dualisms, reductionism, and linear models associated with traditional inquiry and attempt to replace these with more holistic and complex models of experience embedded in women's frames of reference (Hartsock, 1983; Rose, 1983). These approaches question the very methods and nature of intellectual inquiry, such as the assumptions that truth is objective, rational, and ahistorical, and that the inquirer must maintain distance from the subject matter being studied. Standpoint theorists have proposed alternative visions of truth and emphasized the special knowledge and skills that women hold, such as relational thinking and an appreciation for connectedness with others (Harding, 1986; Morawski, 1990). According to this viewpoint, knowledge and truth are also influenced by factors that modify or inform women's special skills and perspectives, such as social identities related to race, class, and other aspects of diversity which shape a person's view of reality and inform knowledge claims. Feminist standpoint inquiry is also grounded in many of the social practices of feminism such as collaboration and consensus as appropriate forms of interaction for devising effective research programs. It seeks to place women at the center of inquiry and erase the boundaries between researchers and the persons studied. As a result, the qualitative, in-depth study of women's lives is viewed as particularly useful for clarifying women's strengths, perspectives, and realities.

The compatibility of cultural feminist perspectives and standpoint epistemologies is self-evident, as noted by the similarity of themes associated with standpoint epistemology and cultural feminism. It is also important to note that standpoint approaches have also been associated with the feminisms of women of color and thus will be revisited in Chapter 5. A discussion of the criticisms of standpoint epistemologies and their differences from feminist empiricism and feminist postmodernism will be addressed in Chapter 7.

Summary of Cultural Feminist Themes

Cultural feminists during the nineteenth and twentieth centuries attempted to achieve broad cultural change by infusing the larger society with "female" values. They have described women's unique cultural and ethical heritage as based on altruistic, cooperative, pacifistic, life-affirming values, and promoted the notion that women have an obligation to better the world through social reform. They believe that through the "feminization" of culture, violence and aggression can be overcome, and the strengths of gentleness, harmony, and peace can be realized (Donovan, 2000). Emotional, nonrational, intuitive, and holistic elements of women's experience have been considered important to the cultural feminist vision. Because holistic experiences are so rarely valued in the larger culture, women must learn to listen to themselves in new ways and affirm their inner strengths. Through identification with other women, new freedoms and visions can be fully developed.

It is sometimes difficult to differentiate clearly between cultural feminism and radical feminism because the boundaries between these two strands within feminism are often blurred. Both radical feminists and cultural feminists have viewed women as holding special ways of understanding and conceiving the world. However, cultural feminists are more likely to identify women as essentially different from men, often embracing the assumption that women are inherently more nurturing, cooperative, and peaceful. In contrast, radical feminists have historically viewed masculinity and femininity as socially constructed characteristics, have provided a more radical critique of traditional concepts of gender, focusing on eliminating a sex-class system, and viewing an ideal world as one in which gender would be irrelevant. Radical feminists call for the eradication of male supremacy in all areas of life and have engaged and fought patriarchy to change the larger society (Echols, 1989). In contrast, cultural feminists are generally viewed as less combative and have sought to instigate social change by creating rich internal, interpersonal, and community lives based on female values.

CULTURAL FEMINIST THEMES
IN FEMINIST THERAPY

Many of the writings of feminist therapists that are most consistent with cultural feminism emphasize women's unique strengths, maternal values, mother-daughter relationships, and the relational capacities of women. This chapter includes a summary of the early contributions of cultural psychoanalytic feminists Karen Horney and Clara Thompson. It then describes feminist theories and therapies that emphasize relational themes, and it concludes with a brief summary of feminist archetypal psychology. Within each section, I identify the strengths and limitations of these applications as well as modifications that increase the multicultural applicability of these models.

Early Cultural Feminist Practitioners:
Karen Horney and Clara Thompson

From the 1920s to the 1940s, Karen Horney and Clara Thompson contributed a series of articles on the psychology of women that anticipated current versions of cultural feminism. Both theorists rejected Freud's biologically deterministic views and emphasized the way in which culture influences women's sense of self. Karen Horney ([1926] 1967) stated,

> Like all sciences and all valuations, the psychology of women has hitherto been considered only from the point of view of men. It is inevitable that the man's position of advantage should cause objective validity to be attributed to his subjective, affective relations to the woman, and . . . the psychology of women hitherto actually represents a deposit of the desires and disappointments of men. (p. 56)

Horney noted that power differences between men and women significantly influence their development and commented: "Historically the relation of the sexes may be crudely described as that of master and slave. . . . In actual fact a girl is exposed from birth onward to the suggestion . . . of her inferiority" (Horney, [1926] 1967, p. 69).

Horney was especially critical of Freud's use of concepts such as penis envy to reinforce the inferior status of women in society. She declared, "In fact, there is scarcely any character trait in woman which is not assumed to have an essential root in penis envy" (1939, p. 104). Within Freud's model, traits attributed to penis envy included women's presumed sense of vanity, physical modesty, limited sense of justice, and jealousy. Horney suggested that Freud's use of penis envy to explain women's feelings of inferiority represented a "simple" (1939, p. 107) solution that ignored complex social factors. Instead, women's envy of men "may be the expression of a wish for all those qualities or privileges which in our culture are regarded as masculine, such as strength, courage, independence, success, sexual freedom, right to choose a partner" (1939, p. 108).

According to Horney, women had unconsciously learned to adapt to men's perceptions and had learned to see themselves "in the way that their men's wishes demanded of them" ([1926] 1967, p. 57). She noted ways in which women were encouraged to engage in a "flight from womanhood" ([1926] 1967, p. 54) because female strengths were assumed to be inferior to men's strengths. Women had been trained to overvalue that which is male and to compete with one another for relationships with powerful men, thus encouraging women to ignore positive skills and qualities within themselves. Socially prescribed roles encourage women to please men through the pursuit of a "cult of beauty and charm" and to depend on men for care, protection, love, and prestige (Horney, [1934] 1967; O'Connell, 1980).

As a part of her efforts to revalue women's experiences, Karen Horney posited the existence of unique female and mothering instincts. She suggested that womb envy in men is as significant a factor in men's lives as penis envy is in women's lives (Horney, [1933] 1967; O'Connell, 1980). In contrast to men's need to prove their masculinity through erections, women do not need to prove themselves in a similar way, a reality that fills men with both admiration and resentment as well as anxiety about their physical inferiority (Horney, [1932] 1967). This position, which suggested women's life-giving biological superiority, represented a departure from her sociological perspective and a reliance on biological determinism reminiscent of Freud's work. This version of women's "special nature" or "differentness" has been criticized by some feminists for "essentializing" women's characteristics, exaggerating differences between women and men, and supporting stereotypes that legitimize differential treatment of men and women (Garrison, 1981).

During the second stage of her career, Karen Horney developed an inclusive theory of development and neurosis and postulated three major modes of dealing with the world: moving toward others, moving against others, and moving away from others (Horney, 1945). Her descriptions of these styles and the family factors that influence their development provided a foundation for recent feminist theories that focus on how early experiences reinforce relationship-oriented identities in women and more separate, disconnected identities in men (e.g., Chodorow, 1978; Gilligan, 1982; Jordan and Surrey, 1986).

Clara Thompson was influenced by the interpersonal school of psychoanalysis, which emphasized the centrality of relationships in development. She did not propose new theories about the causes of women's difficulties but sought to clarify how women had coped with awareness of their cultural inferiority. As with Karen Horney, she rejected the notion that penis envy is biologically based and proposed that it represents "a picturesque way of referring to the type of warfare which so often goes on between men and women" (Thompson, 1971, p. 74). She noted that physiological/sexual differences between men and women are easily distinguishable and thus become the focus of "derogation in any competitive situation in which one group aims to get power over the other" (p. 75). In a patriarchal culture, the penis becomes the symbol of power, and "the restricted opportunities afforded woman, the limitations placed on her development and independence give a real basis for envy of the male quite apart from any neurotic trends" (1971, p. 77). In contrast, Thompson proposed that the breast would become the symbol of power if Euro-American culture were matriarchal. Although male power is associated with aggression, power associated with the breast would stand for "life-giving capacity rather than force and energy" (p. 74).

Clara Thompson (1971) encouraged women to avoid accepting the dominant male model of mental health, which she termed the "masculinity complex" (p. 91), and challenged women to define themselves on the basis of their own strengths. She believed that women would lose connection with their own interests if they tried to mold their lives after men. Both Thompson and Horney anticipated the many contemporary cultural feminists who have encouraged women to develop a psychology based on women's ways of being and knowing.

Contemporary Feminist Critiques of Traditional Personality Theories

Jean Baker Miller (1976) and Carol Gilligan (1977) noted that most personality theories were based on androcentric models of maturity, embedded in empirical research on white, middle-class men, and generalized to the lives of women (e.g., Kohlberg, 1981; Levinson, 1978). They also criticized mainstream theorists for equating separation, autonomy, and individualism with positive mental health. The role of relationships in women's lives was often ignored or portrayed in negative ways. Several examples follow.

Erik Erikson (1968) proposed that for men, identity precedes intimacy; for women, identity and intimacy tasks are fused. He also asserted that the interpersonal nature of female development glosses over the most vital issues of identity, which he described as the selection of an ideology and the choice of an occupation. Contrasting women with men, he concluded that whereas women's activities are oriented toward valuing harmonious activities associated with their "vital inner potential" (p. 275) and the "inner space" (p. 270) of women's reproductive organs, men pursue activities associated with independence, assertiveness, and "outer space" (p. 270). Erikson viewed women's capacity to maintain relationships as positive attributes, but he also saw women's relational skills as impeding clear identity formation characterized by independence and autonomy.

Ruthellen Josselson's (1987, 1996) study of women's identity formation has provided an important corrective to Erikson's restricted view of women's identity formation. Her longitudinal study of thirty women who graduated from college in 1972 found that women's life paths are marked by diversity and ongoing revision, and are not defined by "inner space." She used the terms *connection* and *competence* to depict life priorities, and prefers these words to *love* and *work*, which were originally identified as key life tasks by Freud. She proposed that whereas love and work are more specific, bounded, and perhaps more indicative of male identity formation, connection and competence go beyond these fairly restricted domains. She stated, "Competence includes the sense of having meaningful import in others' lives and connection embraces skill in making deep and abiding ties. Most of the time, these themes are interlaced" (Josselson, 1996,

p. 179). Josselson's work reframed relationship themes in more positive and flexible ways than traditional theories such as Erikson's.

The emphasis of much personality theory on the singular and self-defined self is also present in humanistic psychology. Although Abraham Maslow (1956) depicted the self-actualizing person as capable of more profound interpersonal relationships than others, he also described this individual as a "self-contained" person who is "independent of the good opinion of other people" (Maslow, 1956, p. 176). For Carl Rogers (1956), genuine, congruent, empathic relationships provided the medium for self-affirmation and prizing of the self. According to his model, however, one's mental health is ultimately expressed through an internal locus of evaluation. Individual experience is construed as the highest authority, and evaluation by others is not considered an appropriate guide for behavior.

Another problem is that many mainstream personality theories were based on formative empirical research with homogenous groups of relatively privileged men. As a result, women have often been evaluated according to the level of their pursuit of the dominant goals of privileged men: achievement, individualism, self-determination, mastery, and personal success (Enns, 1991; Gilligan, 1982). Cultural feminist perspectives within psychology have offered important correctives to the deficiencies of previous theories, which are summarized next.

Feminist Relational Theories of Development and Personality

Carol Gilligan: In a Different Voice

Feminist relational theorists have not only criticized androcentric biases but also proposed theories that revalue relational qualities of women which have been previously ignored by psychologists. Perhaps the most influential of these theories has been that of Carol Gilligan, whose groundbreaking study of moral development was among the first efforts to correct the biases of androcentric theory. Her work has been widely recognized across disciplines and has had a significant impact on the development of feminist ethics and cultural feminist theory (see the previous section on feminist ethics). It has also been a catalyst for the development of other relational theories of women's identity.

Gilligan's (1982) findings about women's capacity to maintain significant attachments were integrated within her model of connected moral development, which she proposed as an alternative to Kohlberg's (1981) morality of justice and fairness that was based on the study of the evolution of moral thinking in the lives of boys and men. The primary source for this relational theory of moral development came from Gilligan's abortion decision-making study, which examined the reproductive choices of women from diverse social, ethnic, and marital backgrounds. She proposed that a morality of care develops through three major phases which represent a modification of the stages proposed by Kohlberg's (1981) model, which emphasized abstract principles of justice. At stage one, morality is based on individual survival and self-interest, which is often formed as a response to feelings of powerlessness. At stage two, individuals define morality as responsibility toward others, meeting others' needs, and self-sacrifice. Finally, at stage three, ethical behavior is defined as a morality of nonviolence that allows women to balance self-nurture with care and concern for others. According to Gilligan, Kohlberg's model did not account for the complicated and rich ways in which relationships may influence decisions as one's sense of connectedness becomes increasingly mature. Kohlberg devoted minimal attention to the potential role of relationships for facilitating positive growth throughout the developmental process. Gilligan argued that women's ethical decisions are not only dictated by abstract principles of justice but embedded in a web of relationships which influence a morality of care and nonviolence.

The implications of Gilligan's (1982) work extend beyond the domain of moral development and also hold significance for the ways in which people define themselves. Nona Lyons (1983) noted that relationships play a role in all people's lives but take on different meanings for persons who define themselves in separate and/or connected ways. For persons with a more separate self, reciprocity, rules, and roles take center stage. Issues are negotiated through the application of impartial and objective rules that are embedded in one's obligations to fulfill specific roles. For persons with a more connected self, the strict application of rules is less important than considering issues within context. This orientation involves "seeing others in their own terms, entering into the situations of others in order to know them as the others do, that is, to try to understand how they see their situations" (Lyons, 1983, p. 135). In contrast to the heightened role of reciprocity, rules, and roles, the relational self focuses more extensively on responses to others, care, and interdependence.

Because women spend significant time enhancing their skills in relational realms (e.g., families, friends, and significant others), they may be more likely than men to assume personal blame for relationship failures, thus leaving them more vulnerable to disorders such as depression and low self-esteem (Jack, 1987, 1991). Building on Carol Gilligan's (1982) model of moral development, Dana Jack (1991) suggested that depression is often associated with the middle phase of moral development, which defines the "good woman" as behaving in self-sacrificial ways. Learning to care for oneself as well as for others is often a necessary step toward creating a healthy self. Rather than defining depression negatively, Dana Jack stated that women's depression reveals "the vulnerabilities of a relational sense of self within a culture that dangerously strains a woman's ability to meet basic needs for interpersonal relatedness, while maintaining a positive sense of self" (1987, p. 44).

Although the literature on the "ethics of care" (e.g., Gilligan, 1982; Lyons, 1983) has revalued the relational self, women of color note that they are often marked by "color blindness" (Thompson, 1998). Audrey Thompson (1998) argued that models such as Gilligan's do not pay adequate attention to "the cultural specificity of what counts as caring" (p. 527). These models tend to pattern "caring" after ideal mother-child relationships enacted in white, middle-class environments and chart a development of an ethic of care that is consistent with the stresses and strengths of a private nuclear household. For Black women living in a racist society, caring is often embedded in community and social activist networks and is associated with not only private ethical issues but also "bringing about justice for the next generation" (p. 533). A Black feminist ethic of caring is associated not only with affectionate or sacrificial images of mother love but also with the practical task of earning enough money to ensure the survival of a household. This pragmatic aspect of caring also leads to another act of caring: teaching one's offspring about the racism that may threaten their well-being. Thus, the evolution of the ethic of caring is not limited to movement from selfishness to self-sacrifice to a balance of self and other concerns but encompasses the use of power, competence, and social action on behalf of one's community.

In addition to exploring ethical development among girls and women, Carol Gilligan and colleagues studied the evolution of identity in adolescent girls (Brown and Gilligan, 1992; Gilligan, Lyons, and Hanmer, 1990). Their studies of adolescent girls, who were primarily from white, middle-class backgrounds, concluded that although young girls typically express their ideas and opinions with confidence, they begin to silence themselves during adolescence rather than express open disagreement or conflict. Because of the fear of endangering relationships, they begin to monitor their own responses and often avoid expressing their true feelings. This change in behavior is an outcome of girls' awareness of cultural expectations about what it means to be a "good" woman in the dominant society. However, a qualitative study of adolescent urban girls, who were predominantly of color and from poor and working-class backgrounds, revealed that many of these girls maintained the ability to speak their minds and to express both disagreement and traditional caring in relationships (Way, 1995). Niobe Way (1995) suggested that the ability to speak out may be a result of the unique caring mother-daughter relations which are evident in many families of color. For example, women of color are often encouraged by adult models to be strong and independent. To survive in the world, these young women learn that they must speak out: "Inner-city adolescent girls, especially girls of color, may realize that they will be offered little, if anything, if they do not speak up for what they want" (pp. 124-125). These findings demonstrate the importance of exploring the ethics and development of caring by women of color on their own terms.

Ongoing research on relational models of personality and moral reasoning suggests that the self-structure as well as moral and ethical reasoning of women may not be as different from men's experience as the original model suggested. In general, Gilligan's (1982) model has encouraged therapists to think about women's relationships as a source of empowerment. However, Sara Jaffee and Janet Shibley Hyde's (2000) meta-analysis of 113 studies of moral reasoning found only a small overall tendency for females to favor care reasoning and males to favor justice reasoning. The specific content of dilemmas and the context in which dilemmas occur are likely to influence both men's and women's moral reasoning. For example, one study found that men's and women's responses to both hypothesized and real-life parenting issues were remarkably similar, suggesting that situational demands are likely to influence the moral reasoning of both men and women (Clopton and Sorell, 1993). Jaffee and Hyde (2000) concluded that men and women use a combination of care and justice reasoning, and that "the field should move beyond the debate about gender differences in moral reasoning and focus instead on how individuals integrate justice and care reasoning and under what conditions they determine which is a more adequate basis for moral action" (p. 721).

Women's Ways of Knowing

Mary Belenky and colleagues (Belenky et al., 1986) developed a theory of cognitive development that expanded on models which traced the development of "separate" knowing, which focuses on the development of traditional methods of objective, impersonal evaluation and analysis. They found that rather than relying primarily or exclusively on separate knowing, women often used connected knowing, which is more contextual in orientation and focuses on the importance of understanding another person's view, learning through experience, and connecting ideas and theories to personal events and relationships. Connected learning occurs primarily through participant observation, personal immersion in situations, and understanding various perspectives from another person's point of view. Connected knowers tend to value support and confirmation throughout the educational experience and may feel isolated when they receive feedback only at the conclusion of their work.

The authors of *Women's Ways of Knowing* (Belenky et al., 1986) described a series of developmental phases that women often experience as they approach learning. During the earliest stages of development, women often feel silenced and learn to overvalue the voice of authorities and separate knowing, which they referred to as "received" knowing. As women become aware of the limitations of external knowledge, they emphasize the importance of subjective, personal knowledge and connected knowing. At a final phase of development, women become constructed knowers and integrate separate and connected knowing. Throughout the process of intellectual development, women's relationships remain important.

In a more recent commentary about this model, Nancy Goldberger (1996) noted that authors had focused originally on women as a single category. Further reflection and research revealed that the model needed to be more attentive to the ways in which contexts, culture, class, and history influence the ways in which people know. For example, she noted that silence, which she and her co-authors conceptualized as "not knowing" and as "a way in which women protect themselves and hide from dangerous authority" (p. 343), may hold positive meanings in some cultural contexts. In some cultures, silence holds value and can be seen as a sign of maturity. In some Native American cultures, silence often means that one is not wasting time in foolish talk, or is engaging in respectful and active listening. In more collectivist cultures that emphasize interdependence more than personal autonomy, silence is often the most appropriate response because "who speaks to whom" may be regulated by one's place in various statuses and relational circles. Silence and speech are also modified and influenced by stereotyping, racism, and other oppressions. For example, a Native American woman who chooses silence may be stereotyped as a quiet stoic Indian; if she chooses to talk, however, she may be labeled as a "mouthy militant" (Goldberger, 1996, p. 344). Tactical or strategic silence may also be a useful tool for creative survival in an oppressive environment.

Nancy Goldberger (1996) also noted that within the original model of women's knowing, the phrase *received knowers* is often used to refer to individuals who accept external authority in an unreflective manner. In some cultures, such as many African-American spiritual communities, individuals may choose to listen actively and receive knowledge, which provides an important source of support. Furthermore, God's authority is often seen as collaborative, not merely as "received." God's authority also coexists with a strong sense of self that empowers one to act within one's community (Collins, 2000). In some situations, one's willingness to defer to "authority" is a strategic choice that supports a person's ability to cope with or endure a situation over which she or he may have no influence. This acceptance of authority does not imply resignation but a deliberate choice to save one's words for those occasions when others will listen. To be useful for women other than those who identify themselves as white and middle class, this model has been modified to be more attentive to diversity of cultures, oppressions, and knowing experiences.

Nancy Chodorow's Object Relations Model

Object relations theories emphasize the ways in which one's relationships with early caretakers are internalized and form the basis for a self-concept and relationships with other people. Internalized images of others become the basis for mental representations of oneself and others. These mental representations of others may resemble actual people but may also be based on distorted perspectives that become the foundation for the defensive processes of

1. *splitting,* or separating people into strict good and bad categories;
2. *projection,* which involves attributing denied aspects of the self to others;
3. *projective identification,* or projecting disowned aspects of oneself on other persons who unconsciously absorb these qualities and react in accordance with expectations; and
4. *introjection,* which entails incorporating an aspect of another person or the external world within oneself.

Object relations theories focus on how one's mental images are played out in current issues and relationships (Okun, 1992). Traditional object relations theorists view separation and individuation as the primary outcomes of healthy development. In contrast, feminist object relations theorists have emphasized the centrality of relationships in women's lives, the means by which relational qualities and strengths are developed, and the role of relationships in supporting women's well-being.

Nancy Chodorow's (1978) influential theory proposed that in capitalist industrialized family societies in which mothers play primary parenting roles, boys are encouraged to disconnect themselves from a primary identification with their mothers, but girls are encouraged to maintain more connected, fluid relationships. Boys, who recognize themselves as biologically different from their mothers, learn to view themselves as different from their mothers and begin to define themselves as separate from their mothers. Girls, who see the similarities between themselves and their mothers, learn to define themselves in more relational ways. Many cultural feminists use Chodorow's analysis to describe why men often define themselves in more separate terms and women in more relational terms. In her recent work, Chodorow (1999) has sought to more fully integrate culture and personal meanings associated with gender.

The strength of Chodorow's work is that she discussed the importance of viewing mothering in social context (Segura and Pierce, 1993). However, she devoted limited attention to how parenting might be modified by class, race, and ethnicity. One of the principles originally proposed by Chodorow (1978) was that the sexual division of labor, especially as it relates to mothering, is reinforced by a split between private and public work realms in capitalistic society. Women are responsible primarily for relational work in the private domain of family while men are responsible for work that establishes them as autonomous beings in the public domain.

Nancy Chodorow's original model was predicated on the assumption that women's mothering occurs primarily within the nuclear family, that there is a strict division of labor between adult men and women, and that girls' relational selves are based on their perceived similarities to their mothers. However, for people of color, race and ethnicity may be more powerful or salient sources of perceived similarity or difference than gender. Thus, a mother who is a woman of color may feel a strong sense of sameness to both her male and female children based on their shared ethnic and racial background. Rather than proposing that gender identity is either relational or separate, it may be more productive to speak of multiple selves which are enacted in different social contexts. Elizabeth Spelman (1988) noted,

> Because mothering may be informed by a woman's knowledge of more than one form of dominance, the development of gender occurs in a context in which one learns to be a very particular girl or boy, and not just simply a girl or boy. (p. 97)

The dangers of proposing universal mothering roles or activities are illustrated by an example of how mothering varies by culture. The notion of motherhood as woman's highest calling is embedded within white Eurocentric culture. Black Afrocentric views are more flexible. Patricia Hill Collins (1991) identified several aspects of Eurocentric thought that are problematic for understanding mothering within an African-American context: (1) mothering occurs in the context of a private, nuclear household; (2) strict gender-role segregation separates male and female spheres of influence; and (3) to be a "good" mother, one must stay at home and make motherhood a full-time occupation. Within many Black communities, however, the boundaries that differentiate biological mothers from other women who provide care and nurture of children are less rigid and more fluid than in many white communities. As noted earlier in this chapter, mothering is not only associated with the private realm of the home but involves the integration of economic and caregiving roles. Providing economically for children is seen as a significant part of mothering. Because mothering is associated not only with the nuclear family but also with service to other children, Black women often develop a sense of social activism based on their sense of accountability to the larger community of children (Collins, 1991; Trotman, 2000). These realities suggest that Chodorow's analysis of mothering is based primarily on white, middle-class realities and is inadequate for understanding the variations of family and individual identities.

Denise Segura and Jennifer Pierce (1993) noted that the structure of Chicana/-o families also shapes personality. A prominent feature of Chicana/-o families is *campadrazgo,* which refers to relationships with godparents that serve to enlarge the family and create connections between families. Extended household and networks that cross generations are often central to the family and identity development. Attachments with multiple mother figures, such as godmothers and grandmothers, shape the nature of gender-related behaviors. Consistent with Chodorow's theory, Chicanas often develop strong relational selves. However, the relational self is influenced not only by an exclusive mother-child relationship but also by multiple mothering individuals, and collective cultural values that call for children to "think and act communally—for the good of the family and the community" (Segura and Pierce, 1993, p. 81). Thus, the meaning of the relational self may be somewhat different for Chicanas than for most white women.

Luise Eichenbaum and Susie Orbach's Object Relations Theory

Similar to Nancy Chodorow's theory, Luise Eichenbaum and Susie Orbach's (1983) model of women's development provided an important foundation for feminist object relations and psychodynamic approaches. Eichenbaum and Orbach described how women's difficulties are related to the unconscious internalization of patriarchal norms and cultural requirements. One powerful mandate requires women to defer to others and articulate their needs only in relationships. Because they are not the main characters in their own lives, women learn to feel "unworthy, undeserving, and unentitled" (p. 7). A second requirement is that women should shape their lives in relationships to others, which results in the loss of self, feelings of neediness, and insufficiency.

According to Luise Eichenbaum and Susie Orbach, cultural mandates are transmitted primarily through the mother-daughter relationship. The mother unconsciously projects on her daughter the same negative culturally prescribed feelings that she has about herself, including the repressed aspects of the mother's needy self which she has learned to deny and dislike in order to survive. Because the mother experiences conflict and ambivalence about her role, she unconsciously creates frustration and gratification patterns that lead the daughter to feel insecure and rejected. The daughter learns to identify with her mother's caretaking role, gives up her expectations of being cared for by others, and instead develops emotional antennae that are highly sensitive to the needs of others. As the daughter absorbs information from her mother, she learns to respond to other people's needs as a way of dealing with her own unmet needs. The daughter represses the "little girl" inside, develops false ways of relating to others and the world, and develops difficulty in forming personal boundaries and articulating her own needs. The woman denies she is needy because she believes that her psychological needs will never be met, but she also searches in vain for a nurturing relationship which will result in personal fulfillment.

Through a positive psychotherapy relationship, the woman learns to acknowledge her own neediness and unmet dependency needs, works through these issues, and eventually integrates needs for closeness and autonomy. Eichenbaum and Orbach (1983) concluded that "feminist therapy is about learning to love the little girl inside that patriarchy has taught us to fear and despise; it is about allowing her to grow up and become part of an autonomous woman" (p. 107). This new woman successfully integrates self-care with other care.

The work of Luise Eichenbaum and Susie Orbach emphasizes how women's problems may be embedded in well-intentioned but harmful mother-daughter relationships. They view feminist therapy as the context in which early painful lessons can be replaced. Many of the same strengths and limitations of the relationship models that were discussed in previous sections are relevant to their model of development.

Relational/Cultural Theory and Therapy

Contributors to the relational cultural model use Jean Baker Miller's (1976) often-quoted work, *Toward a New Psychology of Women,* as a foundation for their thinking. Miller was one of the first contemporary feminist psychologists to describe the importance of women's capacities for empathy, nurturance, and affiliation, and to note how these qualities are distorted and denigrated in a culture dominated by men. She also articulated how women's anger and aggression are suppressed in male-dominated societies and are expressed in many of the psychological problems women experience. As a result, clinical work should center on revaluing women's core relational selves as well as identifying ways of expressing anger and assertion in self-affirming ways.

In contrast to Eichenbaum and Orbach's (1983) emphasis on the ways in which mother-daughter relationships transmit negative patriarchal values and limit girls' abilities to develop an integrated sense of self, the self-in-relation model (now referred to as the relational/cultural model), emphasizes the positive impact of the mother-daughter dyad on women's relational self. The mother-daughter relationship contributes to a more "encompassing" or complete self that can be contrasted with "the more boundaried, or limited, self that is encouraged in boys from a very young age" (Miller, 1991, p. 15). Rather than viewing the successful outcome of identity development as separation and individuation apart from others, this model identifies "relationship-differentiation" (Surrey, 1991, p. 38), "mutual inter-subjectivity" (Jordan, 1991, p. 82), or "agency within community" (Miller, 1991, p. 16) as central to women's identity development. It takes issue with such terms as *merger, symbiosis,* or *fusion* that are used in traditional object relations theories to describe early infant-mother relationships, and suggests that mother-child relationships are more complicated, complete, and rich than traditional object relations models imply (Miller, 1991).

The relational/cultural model underscores four positive motivational and structural aspects of the mother-daughter relationship that mold the self, including

1. an early emotional attentiveness between mother and daughter,
2. the experience of mutual empathy and affective joining between mothers and daughters,
3. the expectation that relationships are a major source of personal growth, and
4. mutual empowerment, which involves seeing relationships as an important context in which to experience further growth and maturation (Jordan and Surrey, 1986; Kaplan and Surrey, 1984).

Women's positive connections to others validate their capacities as relational beings; provide the necessary foundation for personal beliefs about autonomy, competence, and self-esteem; and are central to helping women experience continuing growth and well-being. Problems in women's development do not occur because women experience a failure to separate from others but because they have difficulties asserting a distinct self-concept which is both differentiated from that of others and also connected to others (Kaplan, 1986).

During recent years, the authors have renamed what was originally known as the self-in-relation models as relational/cultural therapy. The shift in wording is related to several factors, especially the increasing emphasis of the theory's authors on relational themes in psychotherapy and the recognition that cultural and sociopolitical forces influence perceptions of the "self" (Jordan, 2000, 2001; Jordan and Hartling, 2002). The phrase *self in relation* may be seen as overemphasizing "an individualist, separate-self perspective" (Jordan and Hartling, 2002, p. 55). For example, women from collectivist cultures may not see the "self" as a separate entity, but as rooted in interdependence with others (Louie, 2000; Kashima et al., 1995).

According to a relational-cultural perspective, connection is essential to growth, and disconnection is the major cause of suffering (Jordan, 2000; Jordan and Hartling, 2002; Miller and Stiver, 1997). Connections lead to growth through mutual empathy, which is defined as a relationship in which all parties participate as fully as possible in dialogue that leads to mutual empowerment. Mutual empowerment consists of at least five major features:

1. *Zest,* or a type of vitality and energy that come from positive interactions
2. *Action,* which is informed in a more complete way because of the interplay between individuals
3. *knowledge,* or the more complete picture individuals have of themselves through interpersonal communication
4. *a sense of worth* which comes from feeling worthwhile in an authentic relationship
5. *the desire* to form more empowering connections

These features of empowerment are markers of power-with rather than power-over or power-against, which mark many disempowering experiences in daily life (Miller and Stiver, 1997).

Disconnection, or isolation and the absence of connection, is hypothesized as the major cause of psychological distress. Disconnection does not necessarily involve the dissolution of a relationship. It represents the ordinary as well as ongoing and traumatic conflicts that result in separation and disempowerment, which may lead to decreased energy, paralysis, low self-esteem, and the avoidance of relationships (Jenkins, 2000). The main function of relational/cultural therapy is to help individuals move from disconnection to connection through a mutually empathic therapeutic relationship. Judith Jordan (2000, 2001) proposed that mutual empathy implies much more than traditional therapeutic definitions of empathy as a facilitative or supportive feature of therapy. She defined mutual empathy as the knowledge that "both people are affected by the other and that this knowledge is valuable to both people" (2000, p. 1008). She added, "The patient must be able to see, know, and feel (empathize with) the therapist being impacted, touched, and moved by him or her" (Jordan, 2000, pp. 1008-1009). Jordan also noted that relational/cultural therapy "is not so much about technique but about attitude, values, and point of view" (2000, p. 1014). Although this attitude is refreshing, Ellyn Kaschak (1998) also noted that the lack of clear definition of many concepts (e.g., growth, connection, disconnection) may decrease the usefulness of these concepts.

Concepts such as transference, countertransference, and resistance are reframed in relational/cultural therapy (Miller and Stiver, 1997). Relational/cultural therapy replaces Freud's notion that objectivity and neutrality are necessary for transference relationship with the belief that an empowering and empathic relationship provides more "fertile ground" (p. 139) for transference which helps clients modify old images of relationships that constrict their lives. In its most positive manifestation, countertransference can represent a therapist's genuine and empathic response to a client's pain, and can deepen the possibility for connection. Finally, resistance is reconceptualized as a fear of connection rather than deliberate efforts on the part of the client to avoid movement toward health. These redefinitions provide a foundation for therapeutic attitudes that can enhance the psychotherapy relationship.

Speaking of its limitations, Kaschak (1998) proposed that although recent writings on relational/cultural theory have identified the importance of considering the larger social context and its impact on relationships, these writings also tend to use the word *woman* without noting the other social identities that influence the experience of being a woman. Although this model was based initially on the experiential base of white, middle-class women, efforts to extend this model to more diverse groups of women are increasing. Several authors have noted that the concept of connection as a basis for empowerment is useful for diverse groups of women (e.g., Jenkins, 2000; Turner, 1997). However, developing connection may be more challenging because of the powerful disconnection women of color may face as they deal with racism as well as sexism. For many women of color, connection cannot be sought from all people, because survival and protection are sustained by maintaining distance and disconnection from groups and experiences that inflict pain. Yvonne Jenkins (2000) indicated that although growth may be complicated by the need to first destroy and challenge stereotyped cultural myths and images of African-American women (e.g., mammy, matriarch, and welfare mother), abundant examples of empowering relational images in the African-American women's community can be used to support mutual empathic growth among women of color. Therapists who make efforts to facilitate mutual empathic growth must recognize the complex realities of women from diverse backgrounds. In noting the relevance of relational/cultural theory to the lives of African-American women, Yvonne Jenkins (2000) quoted the following African proverb: "I am because we are, and since we are, therefore I am" (p. 78). With sensitivity to culture and daily challenges of women of color, the relational-cultural themes of this model can be integrated with African-American values that emphasize interdependence, collective goals, and a unifying spiritual orientation.

Limitations and Critiques of Feminist Relational Models

Although the authors of relational theories provide important advances over traditional psychological theory, some feminists believe that these theories may contribute to artificial dichotomies between the identities of men and women, overemphasizing the role of mothering and ignoring the role of fathering in providing nurture and growth-enhancing support (e.g., Lerner, 1988; Mednick, 1989; Okun, 1992). Generalizations such as "women's basic orientation is toward caretaking" (Jordan and Surrey, 1986, p. 100), and "women define their identity through relationships of intimacy and care" (Gilligan, 1982, p. 164) may encourage individuals to think of autonomy and relatedness as caricatures of maleness and femaleness (Lerner, 1988). Although the revaluing of relatedness is central to creating inclusive models of personhood, the tendency to define women as having affiliative capacities and men as having instrumental capacities may deflect attention from the ways in which the capacities to be independent and nurturing are available to all individuals as well as the ways in which personality qualities are socially constructed (Hare-Mustin and Marecek, 1986). The more theories emphasize the importance of women's nurturing and caring capabilities, the less likely men will identify and act on their own skills in this area, further reinforcing gender inequities.

Gaining skills of autonomy or relatedness is largely an outgrowth of one's location in the social structure (Hare-Mustin and Marecek, 1986). Women's economic dependence and their responsibility for child care continue to rule out independence for some women, and pressures to be a "good provider" and to attain individual accomplishments rule out affiliative roles for many men. Furthermore, the relationship strengths ascribed to women have historically been associated with subordinate groups (Kerber, 1986; Lerner, 1988). If articulations of the relational capacities of women are not adequately connected to an analysis of the impact of power, domination, and subordination on behavior, old stereotypes that attribute gender differences to inherent qualities rather than social categories and cultural influences may persist.

As noted within specific sections of this chapter, important critiques of the relationship models have come from feminists of color who note that the authors of these models have often paid inadequate attention to race, class, and situational factors which interact with gender. Oliva Espín (1990) noted that women's "universal" characteristics of connectedness, empathy, nurturance, and affiliation may merely reflect white, middle-class women's methods for dealing with their own oppression. Although applications of relational models for women of color are emerging (e.g., Jenkins, 2000; Turner, 1997), additional discussion of how the relationship models can be relevant to women who are dealing with the multiple consciousness required by multiple social identities (e.g., race, ethnicity, nationality, class, sexual orientation) is important.

Within most individualistic cultures, the relational self is generally defined as an orientation that exists within the individual and becomes a vehicle for self-expression. The person who defines herself or himself in relational terms values a sense of emotional connectedness to others. In cultures based on more collectivist values, the notion of a distinct personal self-concept may not be as relevant. The self may not exist apart from the social systems in which the person participates; it is flexible and defined differently in specific social situations that call for specific role-related responses. This self is influenced by relationships but does not operate in the same manner as a relationship-oriented person within most dominant Western cultures. Within collectivist cultures, the relational self is not merely a vehicle for self-expression but is based in a sense of interdependence, unity, and harmony with others as well as with the physical world (Bradshaw, 1990; Comas-Díaz, 1994; Kashima et al., 1995; Louie, 2000; Markus and Kitayama, 1991). Since the early 1990s, the relational/ultural model (Jordan and Hartling, 2002) took its new name (originally the self-in-relation model) to acknowledge the reality that the self, including the relational self, varies across cultures. Similar modifications within other relational theories will increase their applicability to and compatibility with more collectivist, group-oriented cultures.

To date, the relational models have focused primarily on the implications of mutual empowerment for individual growth. Authors have not generated recommendations about how the relational models and connections among women might inform social change. The feminisms of women of color may be useful in expanding these models into the domain of social change. For example, Black feminism identifies relationships among women, mothering, and othermothering as important foundations for social action. One's commitments as a person in relation extend beyond concerns for the empowerment of one's immediate family or circle of relationships. Growth in relationships can also become important catalysts for fighting injustice and supporting the growth of an entire community (Collins, 2000).

Jungian Archetypal and Goddess Psychology

Feminist archetypal psychology is also embedded in cultural feminist ideals about the unique qualities of women. Because it emphasizes women's relational qualities in a less central way than other approaches discussed in this chapter, I briefly summarize salient themes of archetypal psychology in this separate section. Jungian archetypal psychology has been adopted as a theoretical orientation by some feminist therapists who believe that contemporary women have been pressured to "do it all," and have found their deep feminine values to be questioned and devalued (Nelson, 1991). These feminist counselors and psychotherapists have embraced archetypal psychology because it defines receptivity and feminine instincts as valuable assets for making meaning of one's life (Rowland, 2002; Wehr, 1987; Young-Eisendrath, 1984). Archetypes can serve as role models that help women identify the goddesses within themselves and expand their emotional and behavioral repertoires (Bolen, 1984; Gomberg, 2001).

Jung's belief that an unconscious man exists within the woman (animus) and that an unconscious woman exists within the man (anima) implies that masculinity and femininity can be united in a balanced relationship. Although Jung's notion that mentally healthy persons have a well-developed anima or animus seems consistent with feminist goals, Jung associated masculinity with rational thought and viewed it as superior to femininity. He attributed a "magic authority" (Jung, [1954] 1959, p. 82) to the "feminine." In contrast to a man's "decisiveness and singlemindedness," however, Jung associated femininity with characteristics such as "indefiniteness," "passivity," and "feelings of inferiority which make her continually play the injured innocent" (Jung, [1954] 1959, p. 90). Some feminist counselors and psychotherapists believe that although some of Jung's notions about masculinity and femininity were misguided (Romaniello, 1992; Rowland, 2002), many of his concepts can be integrated with feminist principles. Consistent with feminist ideals, Jung emphasized that symptoms represent a healthy struggle toward wholeness and an effort of the psyche to regain balance. He viewed individuals as essentially self-regulating and believed that persons move toward maturity through a natural and continuous exchange between the conscious and unconscious. Jung also de-emphasized the authority of the analyst and accentuated the centrality of the client's experience, self-understanding, and insights (Lauter and Rupprecht, 1985). Each of these values is consistent with feminist psychotherapy principles.

One of the major challenges for feminist Jungian therapists is to generate woman-centered archetypes that provide concrete and empowering visions of women's social economic, political, and personal behavior. Many of the archetypes, myths, and symbols used by Jungian therapists are based on patriarchal myths that undervalue women's experience and reinforce traditional visions of masculinity and femininity. The typical motif in fairy tales depicts the man as engaging in a heroic task, rescuing a woman, and sweeping her into an idyllic existence. Thus, some feminists have sought to identify pre-patriarchal archetypes and goddess images to avoid contaminating images associated with more recent, patriarchal mythologies. According to Riane Eisler (1988), early matriarchal societies were based on egalitarian, nonviolent, earth-centered values that included reverence for the Great Mother and other goddess figures. Humans lived in harmony with one another during these eras, and women exercised greater social power than they did during patriarchal societies that have been associated with widespread "spiritual bankruptcy" (Woolger and Woolger, 1989, p. 17). In general, liberating archetypes consistent with feminist values can be found in diverse sources such as women's poetry, writing, painting, needlework, dreams, and quilts.

Although associated with patriarchal society, some Jungian feminists have used Greek mythology to identify empowering goddess archetypes (e.g., Hera, Athena). Although the goddesses of Greek mythology typically experienced lower status than male gods, they also demonstrated greater power and diversity of behavior than women have historically exercised in Western culture. They also used creative means for counteracting the negative aspects of male gods' power (Bolen, 1984; Woolger and Woolger, 1989). Thus, knowledge of the psychic life of Greek goddesses can help women understand themselves and their relationships, as well as what motivates, frustrates, and satisfies them. The different styles and personalities of goddesses can also help women appreciate diversity among women and their various means of achieving fulfillment (Bolen, 1984; Gomberg, 2001).

The task of feminist archetypal therapy is to revalue women's strengths of all kinds and to "disentangle feminine archetypes from the masculine warp of culture" (Lauter and Rupprecht, 1985, p. 19). To accomplish this task, women learn how confining images have been internalized by men and women and how these images have become misconstrued as objective, universal facts. By exploring these issues, women gain awareness of the specific behavior patterns that women have used for many generations to cope with their lower status (Wehr, 1987). Through this form of "unconsciousness raising" (Pratt, 1985), women gain insight about how their past behavior patterns have allowed them to cope with their lower status, which then releases them from self-blame for acting on cultural imperatives. Women also gain insights that allow them to transcend narrow roles, explore new emotional and behavioral alternatives, and implement plans for achieving equality (Gomberg, 2001).

Feminist therapists whose work is inspired by Jungian perspectives have redefined many of Jung's concepts in ways that are consistent with feminist perspectives. However, the Jungian definition of archetypes as universal can encourage individuals to view masculinity and femininity as qualities that are fixed and lodged within the individual psyche. In addition, the person who believes that the internal anima and animus provide information about the full range of masculine and feminine experience may ignore the significance of external circumstances, such as socialization, sexism, and violence, and assume that women's difficulties are caused by internal deficiencies or women's inability to balance feminine instincts and the masculine animus (Pratt, 1985; Romaniello, 1992). Some of the feminist revisions of Jungian archetypal psychology have consistently emphasized the importance of seeing all archetypes as socially constructed and caution against essentializing masculinity and femininity (e.g., Lauter and Rupprecht, 1985). Nevertheless, the revisions of archetypal psychology that are often referred to as goddess psychology frequently emphasize the special and unique qualities or "instincts" (Estes, 1992) that are presumed to be a part of women's essence (Enns, 1994; Romaniello, 1992).

As noted in this chapter, efforts to revalue traditional strengths of women can be used inappropriately to create new stereotypes of "woman's nature" (Mednick, 1989). Nancy Goldenberg (1976) cautioned that any fixed or highly defined archetypes or goddesses may limit the behavioral alternatives of women by establishing new boundaries on women's experience which can be as constricting as traditional female archetypes. Women can continue to internalize oppression by attributing relational, nurturing skills to innate qualities rather than viewing them as survival mechanisms that help women find meaning in a world in which they hold lower social status (Wehr, 1987). Approaches that focus exclusively on helping women look inward to recover buried images of strength may result in women's lowered expectations for external and social change and an overemphasis on changing the self (Enns, 1994; Romaniello, 1992; Walters, 1993).

A final limitation of archetypal/goddess psychology is that women from multicultural backgrounds may feel invalidated, excluded, or marginalized by a psychology that is based solely on Greek mythology and the history of white women (Enns, 1994; Lorde, 1983). Reiko True (1990) noted that it is difficult for minority women to identify with "blond, blue-eyed goddesses" (p. 483) and thus women should be encouraged to draw on their own rich heritages of mythologies which include powerful female images. Culturally meaningful images can be used as role models to help women contend with the oppressive aspects of sexism in their cultures as well as the racism of dominant white culture (e.g., Allen, 1989; Kingston, 1976; Larrington, 1992; Lorde, 1983). Many women of color look to spirituality that is embedded in their own traditions as a form of renewal; culture-specific archetypes can be used to enhance the power and relevance of this spirituality (Comas-Díaz, 1991).

CONCLUDING COMMENTS

Cultural feminism was first inspired by feminists who envisioned a transformation of culture in accordance with a uniquely matriarchal vision. Cultural feminists defined women's experiences as distinctly different from men's experiences and sought to revere and valorize traditional feminine strengths. Contemporary cultural feminists have less frequently assumed that women's strengths are innate than early cultural feminists, and they are less likely to emphasize a utopian, romantic vision of the world than were their predecessors. However, they continue to focus efforts of revaluing "female" strengths and a unique moral and ethical vision of women (Donovan, 2000). These themes, then, are reflected in cultural feminist adaptations of feminist therapy.

Cultural feminist views were especially influential during the 1980s and early 1990s. At a subjective level, a cultural feminist perspective offers a "ring of truth" for many women. The cultural feminist vision provides validation and comfort by conveying to women that they are not flawed and that they do not need to give up the relational skills with which they may feel most comfortable. This is perhaps the greatest strength of cultural feminism as it is applied to feminist therapy.

The most frequent criticism of cultural feminism is that it is "essentialist" (Bohan, 1993). Although authors of relational models of personality and psychotherapy do not propose that women are inherently different than men, the models often imply that gender is "resident within the individual" (Bohan, 1993, p. 6). Relational skills are qualities of individuals or "fundamental attributes that are conceived as internal, persistent, and generally separate from the on-going experience of interaction with the daily sociopolitical contexts of one's life" (p. 7). In contrast, social constructionist views conceptualize gender as occurring within interactions; gender is a verb rather than a set of personal qualities. If relationship qualities are seen as personal qualities rather than as outcomes of social arrangements, one's views of gender become less flexible, the diversity of women is less frequently considered as important, and women may be less likely to explore options outside of relational domains. Social change becomes a less salient mandate; the inner self becomes a more important focus of attention than the social structures that shape the relational self (Bohan, 1993).

A future challenge is the integration of relational models with social constructionistic perspectives. According to a constructivist framework, identity is shaped by social context which is influenced by relationships, power, and privilege (Marecek, 2002; Suyemoto, 2002). At the relational level, relational traits can be conceptualized as components of a connected or a relationship self-schema, or a set of beliefs about the self that influence self-perceptions, perceptions of others, basic cognitive processes, and one's activities in the world (Bem, 1993; Markus and Oyserman, 1989). In addition, many factors, including socialization, cultural factors, patriarchy, power structures, and experiences of privilege and oppression, contribute to the development of a connected or separate self-schema. By viewing the relational and separate selves as types of socially constructed self-schemas embedded in a larger social context, one can describe the relational and separate selves in rich terms and also maintain awareness that each type of self is constructed and shaped by myriad factors. Such integration can help feminist therapists view the relationship models of personality, ethics, moral development, and psychotherapy as descriptive and flexible models rather than as prescriptive models.

Chapter 5

Women-of-Color Feminisms and Feminist Therapy

Some of the most important changes since the mid-1980s emerged from critiques of feminisms associated with the "new" feminist movement. Women of color have been influential in voicing these critiques and creating more inclusive feminisms. The perspectives of women of color are important for clarifying the complexities and intersections of women's social identities that are influenced by gender, race, ethnicity, sexual orientation, age, nationality, and class. Women of color have been attentive to these interdependent aspects of identity and have made rich contributions to feminist theory and psychotherapy.

As a white, middle-class woman, I am aware that my efforts to be inclusive may be limited by my own experiences and perceptions. As a result, I rely whenever possible on discussions of feminist therapy that are written by feminist therapists of color and for women of color. The first section of this chapter reviews racism and ethnocentrism of early and second-wave feminisms, and is followed by a brief overview of three strands of feminisms created by women of color: Black feminisms, Chicana feminisms, and Asian-American feminisms. Each of these feminisms is marked by a rich set of ideas and traditions, as evidenced by a variety of anthologies that have sought to collect essential historical writings relevant to Black women (e.g., Guy-Sheftall, 1995), Chicanas (García, 1997; Trujillo, 1998) and Asian-American women (Asian Women United of California, 1989, 1997; Chin, 2000; Lim, Tsutakawa, and Donnelly, 1989). In addition, women-of-color feminisms have been characterized by coalition building among and between specific groups. Several anthologies summarize the outcome of these collaborative efforts (e.g., Moraga and Anzaldúa, 1983; Anzaldúa, 1990; Anzaldúa and Keating,

2002). Following a discussion of women-of-color feminisms, this chapter discusses implications for feminist psychotherapy.

Throughout this chapter and the rest of this book, I have chosen to capitalize references to specific identities and feminisms of women of color, such as Black feminism and Asian-American feminism. In contrast, the labels *white* and *women of color* are not capitalized because they refer in general to the wide range of women who are associated with majority culture and dominant traditions in North American (white women) and the diverse group of women who identify themselves as nonwhite (women of color).

WOMEN OF COLOR AND FEMINISM

To use the following items as a form of self-assessment, respond to each statement with a "yes" or "no."

_____ 1. Traditional feminisms have often promoted simplistic views of feminism that overemphasize the importance of gender while ignoring significant social identity variables such as race, ethnicity, class, and sexual orientation.

_____ 2. White feminists have often reinforced inequality among women by defining issues according to the views of middle-class white women and assuming that, with only minor adjustments, these perspectives can be applied to the lives of women of color.

_____ 3. For a theory of feminism to be complete, it must be pluralistic and recognize the complex and interlocking social identities of women. These include but are not limited to race, gender, sexual orientation, age, ethnicity, culture, religion, and nationality.

_____ 4. The lives of diverse groups of women must be understood from their own standpoints; women of color must be involved in theory development at all levels.

_____ 5. As individuals with "outsider" status, women of color often have greater awareness of the complex manifestations of oppression than do most middle-class white women.

Agreement with these statements suggests that your views are consistent with the major concerns and contributions of many feminists of color. Although women-of-color feminisms are represented by diversity of thought and perspective, the following themes and trends have been especially salient:

1. The creation of feminisms that are informed by the struggles against discrimination and racism experienced by many women of color
2. A critique of the narrowness of many feminisms proposed by white feminisms
3. An emphasis on the intersections of race, class, gender, language, immigration, and other aspects of social identity
4. The creation of inclusive women-of-color feminisms (e.g., that address the specific needs of women of color who are lesbian or from different social classes)
5. The development of epistemologies or standpoints unique to the experiences of specific groups of women of color

A Legacy of Racism Within Feminism

Early feminist efforts by white women in America were associated with the rise of the industrial era, the loss of middle-class women's central economic roles within the home, and increased leisure time for middle-class women. With increased time and leisure, white women invested time in social reform, and through their involvement in antislavery efforts many early feminists became acquainted with the nature of oppression and the ways in which it resembled their own experiences. During these early years, feminist activists such as Angelina and Sarah Grimké believed that women would not achieve freedom apart from Black people and worked toward achieving a "common dream of liberation" (Davis, 1981, p. 45).

When placed against these hopeful beginnings, the racism and ethnocentrism of nineteenth-century feminism is particularly disappointing. The ethnocentrism of American feminism was revealed as early as the 1848 Seneca Falls Convention, when delegates articulated the frustrations of middle-class women and ignored both the condition of Black women in slavery and the oppression of white working-class women who were contending with long hours and inhumane working conditions. Sojourner Truth played a significant role in exposing the classism and racism present within feminism during these early years, and along with many other Black women, invested energy in feminist and antislavery efforts on behalf of both men and women (hooks, 1981). However, these efforts did not eradicate white supremacist ideas within the feminist movement.

With the outbreak of the Civil War in the United States, many women's rights leaders directed their energies in support of the Union cause, and the Women's National Loyal League, which called for the "civil and political rights of all citizens of African descent and all women" (Gurko, 1976, p. 211). Angelina Grimké was especially vocal about the importance of connecting the struggle for women's equality with Black liberation. She stated, "I want to be identified with the Negro. Until he gets his rights, we shall never have ours" (Lerner, 1971, p. 354). During postwar years, however, it became apparent that legislators in Washington were not inclined to grant suffrage to both Black men and women. Notable feminists backed away from their earlier commitments and revealed their unwillingness to promote Black liberation if white women would not also gain immediate benefits. They argued that it was more important for white women than Black men to earn the vote. Elizabeth Cady Stanton ([1865] 1881) stated,

> The representative women of the nation have done their uttermost for the last thirty years to secure freedom for the negro; and as long as he was lowest in the scale of being, we were willing to press his claims; but now, as the celestial gate to civil rights is slowly moving on its hinges, it becomes a serious question whether we had better stand aside and see "Sambo" walk into the kingdom first. (pp. 94-95)

Despite this rhetoric, the Fourteenth and Fifteenth Amendments, which entitled all male citizens to the ballot and prohibited disfranchisement on the grounds of race, color, or other forms of servitude, were passed without the inclusion of women's rights (Davis, 1981). As the struggle for women's rights continued at the turn of the century, suffrage organizations adopted white supremacist and racist arguments that were fueled by the eugenics movement. Women's suffrage was viewed by white organizations as central to purifying and redeeming "the Race." Many white suffragists supported racial segregation, harbored racist stereotypes of Black women as morally impure, and rejected efforts of Black women activists to build bridges and foster cooperation (hooks, 1981). Despite their efforts to create a multiracial movement, women of color "were betrayed, spurned and rejected by the leaders of the lily-white suffrage movement" (Davis, 1981, p. 148).

Despite racism and exclusionary efforts, Black women remained actively involved in the fight for women's rights. For example, Mary Church Terrell, Josephine St. Pierre Ruffin, Fannie Barrier Williams, Anna Julia Cooper, Ida B. Wells, and Frances Ellen Watkins Harper worked tirelessly for women's suffrage and defined and addressed issues on Black women's terms. They organized to counter stereotypes of Black women and to focus on many immediate issues such as poverty, care of the elderly, prostitution, and suffrage. Josephine St. Pierre Ruffin stated, "Our woman's movement is a woman's movement that is led and directed by women for the good of women and men, for the benefit of all humanity, which is more than any one branch or section of it" (1895, cited in hooks, 1981, p. 164).

The passage of the Nineteenth Amendment in 1920, which granted women the vote, resulted in little or no change for Black women. In the South, election managers and the Ku Klux Klan worked actively to prevent Black people from voting. Segregation and oppression deepened as white supremacy denied Black people full citizenship. Many Black activist women became disillusioned with the promise of women's rights per se and shifted their attention to other important issues such as campaigns to eradicate lynching (hooks, 1981).

Racism and Ethnocentrism Within the "New" Feminist Movement

Given the racism associated with feminism throughout its early history, it is not surprising that women of color were skeptical when white women activists during the 1970s repeated a claim that had been made over a century before: that the oppression of women resembled the oppression of minority groups in America (hooks, 1981). According to bell hooks, this comparison represented a form of racism based in narcissism and egocentrism. Toni Morrison (1971, quoted in Giddings, 1984) charged that white women's description of "woman as nigger" was "an effort to become Black without the responsibilities of being Black" (p. 308). Linda LaRue (1970) added that although white women experience suppression, "Blacks are oppressed . . . and there is a difference" (p. 61). The assumption that white women and Black women experience a similar oppression did not acknowledge the basic reality that the social experiences and status of white women and women of color have been vastly different. Attention is also deflected from the ways in which women of color are simultaneously exposed to other oppressions, such as racism, classism, and sexism.

In addition to resenting comparisons to women of color, Paula Giddings (1984) expressed frustration and anger that the predominantly white women's movement would "reap the benefits that the Black movement had sown" (p. 308). White women would use the human rights climate of the civil rights movement to gain prominence and power which they would then reserve for themselves, thus preserving the "historical servant-served relationships where white women have used power to dominate, exploit, and oppress" (hooks, 1989, p. 179). Linda La Rue (1970) stated, "One can argue that Women's liberation has not only attached itself to the Black movement but has done so with only marginal concern for Black women and Black liberation" (p. 60).

The writings of the "new" feminist movement were not overtly racist but often ignored the presence of women of color by implying that "the word woman is synonymous with white woman" (hooks, 1981, p. 138). For example, Betty Friedan's ([1963] 1983) analysis of "the problem with no name" was based on the realities of white, middle-class housewives who had become dissatisfied with their stereotyped roles and lack of opportunities for self-fulfillment and achievement. Friedan's assessment ignored the realities of those women who had always worked outside of their homes, struggled to survive economically, and did not have the luxury to claim "the problem with no name." Beginning with slavery and persisting today, compulsory labor has permeated all aspects of many Black women's identities (Davis, 1981). As noted by bell hooks (1984), oppression involves an absence of choices. The ability to choose whether one will or will not work is a form of liberation that many women have never experienced (hooks, 1984; Húrtado, 1989, 1996; Spelman, 1988). Aída Húrtado (1996) also noted that although class issues are also experienced by white women, women of color are more likely to be sole providers for their families, to live in poverty, and to experience low levels of compensation for their work; they "bear more economic burdens than any other group in this country" (p. 5), and this reality influences their experiences of oppression. Gerda Lerner (1979) stated,

> White society has long decreed that while "woman's place is in the home," Black woman's place is in the white woman's kitchen. No wonder that many Black women define their own "liberation" as being free to take care of their own homes and their own children, supported by a man with a job. (p. 82)

The prominent slogan of the feminist movement, "the personal is political," encouraged all women to define their own realities. However, the perspectives of women of color were often ignored, and "the personal is political" became "the politics of imposing and privileging a few women's personal lives over all women's lives by assuming that these few could be prototypical" (King, 1988, p. 58). When individuals invoke the phrase "the personal is political," they tend to presume that all women experience a clear distinction between private and public worlds (Húrtado, 1989, 1996). However, although private and public realms have often been sharply divided for white, middle-class women, the economic realities of many women of color have not allowed this division to exist. Because external forces and the government have altered the private lives of many people of color and poor people, they often have had difficulty creating a private life on their own terms. Aída Húrtado indicated that for people of color, it would be more accurate to state that the "public is *personally* political" (1989, p. 849). The concerns of women of color and white women are likely to differ because of this reality.

White women have been particularly concerned about issues that appear in the private arena but are also relevant for the public domain, such as unequal division of labor in the household, identity issues, equality in personal interactions with men, and the tenacity of socialized gender differences. In contrast, many women of color have directed their activism toward public issues such as desegregation, affirmative action, inadequate housing, poverty, welfare, and prison reform, issues that point out how public policy has limited personal choice. These issues are related to basic survival needs, while middle-class white women have often focused on personal fulfillment (King, 1988).

Early feminist analyses of violence against women were also characterized by a narrow focus. Angela Davis (1981) and bell hooks (1981) stated that feminists have devoted inadequate attention to the ways in which the rape of Black women during slavery and later generations influenced contemporary attitudes about violence against Black women. Although Susan Brownmiller (1975) noted the negative impact of institutionalized rape in women's lives during slavery, she failed to acknowledge that "it led to a devaluation of black womanhood that permeated the psyches of all Americans and shaped the social status of all black women once slavery ended" (hooks, 1981, p. 52). A primary image that remains today is that of the Black woman as "fallen" woman, whore, or slut (West, 2000). Continued exploitation of Black women has undermined the morale of those who must still contend with an image that is imposed on them and limits their capacity to develop positive self-concepts. Furthermore, contemporary feminism has attended primarily to violence in interpersonal relationships. Discussions of cycles of violence elaborate the stages of escalation and contrition that occur between two people (e.g., Walker, 1979). A more comprehensive analysis of violence considers the systemic cycle of violence as it begins at work and other social institutions, where it is also influenced by racism and classism (Davis, 1981; hooks, 1981).

The reproductive rights campaigns that emerged in the 1970s tended to frame women's rights to control their own bodies in white women's terms, and early analyses conveyed a lack of understanding of the legacy of sterilization abuses, the eugenics movement of the early twentieth century, and the role of abortion during slavery. Angela Davis (1981) noted that abortion during slavery did not result in increased freedom but represented "acts of desperation" (p. 205) that were intended to avoid bringing children into the world who would know only forced labor and slavery. During the eugenics movement at the turn of the century, birth control advocates argued for compulsory birth control and the sterilization of lower classes. Recommendations that the birth rates of minority and lower-class groups should be restricted were motivated by efforts of white Americans to maintain superiority of numbers and power. When understood in terms of these realities, the notion of "abortion rights" does not bring up images of freedom but may elicit images of genocide or remind women of color of the demand to limit family size to avoid greater oppression or poverty. Programs associated with limiting family size are often imposed by outside groups looking in on the communities of color and thus represent another form of external pressure rather than liberation.

When white feminists focused energy on reproductive rights, they tended to view voluntary motherhood as an important way to ensure that women could pursue their career and self-development dreams. However, these dreams may not seem relevant to working-class women and women of color who are struggling to survive and who may feel compelled to resort to abortion in order to increase the likelihood of basic survival. If white feminists had worked with women of color from the outset and had arrived at mutually useful definitions of issues, a more comprehensive program of social activism could have been devised (Davis, 1981).

Author bell hooks (1984) also faulted white feminists for providing an overly narrow analysis of the family. Early radical feminists recommended that the family in its current forms should be eradicated without considering the differential impact of this statement on various groups of women. Middle-class women often have the financial resources that allow them to reject traditional family life without giving up options for receiving care and nurture. Furthermore, although white, middle-class feminists often experienced the family as the primary source of oppression, the family provided many women of color with a haven from external oppression. Although sexism exists within families of color, many women of color experience greater self-worth and dignity within their families than in the outside world, where they must face multiple oppressions. The family provides a context in which men and women of color share a common past, culture, religion, and tradition, and gain mutual support for dealing with racism and classism (hooks, 1984; Húrtado, 1989).

Finally, white women have tended to identify men as enemies rather than as potential allies, thus fueling antagonism between white women and women of color and limiting the attractiveness of their analysis to diverse groups of women. The legacy of many women of color includes shared resistance with men against racism and/or slavery. Angela Davis (1981) noted that all members of slave families were oppressed and all members worked as economic providers. As a result, male supremacy was not as evident in many Black families as it was in middle-class America. Although sexism is also a factor in the lives of women of color, they are also aware of the hardships that men of color face and feel compassion for them. Radical feminist separatist views are especially likely to alienate women of color. According to this view, patriarchal values are so strong and overpowering that it is impossible to successfully resist male supremacy while maintaining personal connections with men. The mandate for separatism does not acknowledge the shared oppression of men and women of color but instead suggests that Black women should form an alliance with white women. However, white women are the very persons who have been instruments of oppression in the lives of many women of color.

Many women of color worked simultaneously for the rights of their racial/ethnic group as well as women's rights and understood the need for a connection between civil rights and feminism. Paula Giddings (1984) stated, "In times of racial militancy, Black women threw their considerable energies into that struggle—even at the expense of their feminist yearnings" (p. 7). In less militant times, Black women also demanded rights in their relationships with Black men. These demands were not "seen in the context of race *versus* sex, but as one where their rights had to be secured in order to assure Black progress" (Giddings, 1984, p. 7). These dynamics have also characterized the experiences of many Chicana and Asian-American feminists.

Ethnocentrism in Feminist Theory

The previous section identified ways in which the political activities of mainstream feminism excluded women of color; this section identifies how academic theory has also excluded the perspectives of women of color. Radical feminists of the 1970s proposed that gender oppression is the fundamental form of oppression (e.g., Firestone, 1970; Millett, 1970), thus implying that the most important form of oppression is discrimination on the basis of sex. If sexism is seen as more "fundamental" than other "isms," privileged women can ignore the roles they may play in perpetuating racism. Conceptualizing sexism in this way can also lead to "white solipsism," which entails the tendency "to think, imagine, and speak as if whiteness described the world" (Rich, 1979, p. 299). If gender oppression is viewed as essential for understanding all other oppressions, women of color may feel forced to identify primarily as women and to ignore their race and minority status as a source of pride.

For many women of color, racism is a far more visible, virulent, and everyday experience than sexism. In noting the different experiences of white women and women of color, Aída Húrtado (1989, 1996) stated that whereas women of color were the objects of rejection, white women were the objects of seduction. White women are "seduced into joining the oppressor under the pretense of sharing power" (Lorde, 1984, pp. 118-119). Speaking more specifically about this dynamic, Húrtado (1996) stated,

> Women of Color are not needed by white men to reproduce biologically pure offspring and therefore have been subordinated through rejection, whereas white women have been seduced into compliance because they are needed to reproduce biologically the next generation for the power structure. (p. vii)

The possibility of sharing power or privilege was never an option for women of colonized peoples and slaves. Evelyn Higgenbotham (1992) concluded that the gender identity of women of color and white women is constructed in radically different contexts. Because of the salience of race in American culture's constructions of class, gender, and sexuality, race is inextricably linked to one's sense of self as a woman.

Some of the early statements that recognized the unique concerns of women of color spoke of the double and triple jeopardy experienced by women of color (e.g., Beale, 1970). The notion of double and triple jeopardy implied that various discriminations can be interpreted "as equivalent to the mathematical equation, racism plus sexism plus classism equals triple jeopardy" (King, 1988, p. 47). If this were the case, each type of oppression would have an independent and direct impact on one's status, and the contributions of each would be readily apparent. However, by attempting to separate sexism from other forms of oppression, our understanding of the interlocking, interactive aspects of various oppressions is limited (hooks, 1984; Spelman, 1988). When racism and sexism are seen as additive, the most likely conclusion is that all women are victimized by sexism and some women are also oppressed by racism. This thinking fails to acknowledge the differing contexts in which white women and women of color experience gender oppression. It also implies that a woman's ethnic or racial identity can be subtracted from her larger identity, when in fact these aspects of experience may be inseparable; bell hooks (1984) concluded: "Suggesting a hierarchy of oppression exists, with sexism in first place, evokes a sense of competing concerns that is unnecessary" (p. 35). A major contribution of women-of-color feminists is an understanding of the complex interactions of social identities that contribute to one's sense of self.

BLACK FEMINISMS

Although many Black feminists experienced exclusion by white feminists, it is important to note that many Black women did not reject feminism but created organizations that directly reflected their concerns as Black women of color. These organizations operated parallel to many predominantly white feminist organizations and became a rich source for activism and theory building (Guy-Sheftall, 1995; Springer, 2001). Although some Black women chose the term *feminist* to reflect their commitments, other Black women and women of color have preferred to use the term *womanist* rather than *feminist* to highlight the uniqueness of their commitment to women of color as well as to demonstrate their rejection of approaches that propose gender-based dichotomies or a "false homogenizing" (Higgenbotham, 1992, p. 273). Alice Walker (1983) defined *womanist* as "a black feminist or feminist of color" (p. xi). *Womanist* also refers to women who love other women, appreciate women's culture, women's strength, and women's emotional flexibility. A womanist is committed to the "survival and wholeness of entire people, male *and* female." Finally, a "womanist is to feminist as purple is to lavender" (Walker, 1983, p. xii). These definitions underscore the strength, resiliency, and capacity of women of color.

One of the earliest and most widely read statements of radical Black feminism was written by members of the Combahee River Collective (1982). The collective was formed in 1973 in response to the racism and elitism that limited the involvement of Black women in feminism. The collective's manifesto noted that the pervasive nature of racism had not allowed many Black women to examine the ways in which sexual oppression is a "constant factor in our day-to-day existence" (Combahee River Collective, 1982, p. 14). Members committed themselves to address sexism, racism, heterosexism, and economic oppression within capitalism. They noted that contemporary Black feminism is built on a legacy of Black women's resistance, sacrifice, and activism directed by generations of both prominent and unheralded Black women. Furthermore, Black women have never passively succumbed to oppression but have demonstrated "an adversary stance to white male communities in both dramatic and subtle ways" (p. 14). They articulated

1. the interconnections between race, class, and sex oppression;
2. solidarity with progressive Black men and a rejection of separatism;
3. a commitment to eradicating capitalist structures by raising consciousness about "the real class situation of persons who are not merely raceless, sexless workers, but for whom racial and sexual oppression are significant determinants in their working economic lives" (p. 17); and
4. the importance of expanding the definition of "the personal is political" to include issues of race and class.

The Combahee River Collective identified several key issues as the focus of their activism:

1. Commitment to issues for which race, sex, and class oppression operate simultaneously
2. Identification of racism within white feminism
3. A commitment to collective discussion and continual examination of their personal politics (The Combahee River Collective, 1982)

During the 1980s and 1990s, feminist theory by and about women of color became increasingly more visible, especially the writings of Black feminists (e.g., Collins, 1986, 2000; hooks, 1981, 1984). Barbara Smith (1985) underlined the relevance of feminism for Black women by exposing five myths: the notions that

1. Black women are already liberated due to their need to take on a wide range of roles in an effort to cope with oppression,
2. racism is the only or primary oppression experienced by Black women,

3. feminism is about hating men and detracts from Black women's coalition building with men,
4. women's issues are apolitical and narrow whereas Black people must face a larger challenge, and
5. all outspoken feminists of color are lesbians.

She also highlighted strengths of Black feminism, including

1. a commitment to a multi-issues approach to liberation,
2. an emphasis on being Black *and* female,
3. leadership in day-to-day activism and grassroots organizing,
4. contributions to important issues such as reproductive rights and violence against women,
5. the development of solidarity with women around the globe, and
6. the creation of Black feminist literary, musical, and cultural contributions.

Patricia Hill Collins (1986) noted that African-American women play a particularly important role in the development of feminist theory because they have been exposed to "insider" information and the "intimate secrets of white society" (p. S14) while also maintaining an outsider (and often marginalized) status that allows them to develop a unique standpoint and insight about behaviors that remain invisible to dominant members of society. Black feminists use their relationship to dominant society to develop a standpoint "of and for Black women" (p. S16). This standpoint assumes that Black women share some common perceptions and experiences as a group and thus can articulate a unique perspective about Black women. However, their different experiences due to age, region, sexual orientation, and class mean that these commonalities will be expressed in different ways (Collins, 2000).

Many features and themes are especially central to Black feminist thought, including the importance of self-definition and self-valuation by and for African-American women, as well as the honoring of Black women's legacy of struggle and the reclamation of their intellectual and artistic heritage and culture (Collins, 2000). Self-definition is particularly important in light of historical distortions and stereotypes of African-American women. Black feminists seek to identify the power dynamics that have led to these distortions and redefine and "value those aspects of Afro-American womanhood that are stereotyped, ridiculed, and maligned in academic scholarship and the popular media" (Collins, 1986, p. S17). Black feminists explain and redefine the significance of Black women's culture, as well as revealing previously unexplored aspects of African-American women's experience. This scholarship often reveals ways in which women have expressed themselves in concrete ways through the church, family, and political and economic activity. It also includes previously unexplored aspects of Black women's interpersonal relationships as expressed through sisterhood and mothering, as well as the role of creative expression and creative arts in "shaping and sustaining Black women's self-definitions and self-valuations" (p. S23). The exploration of Black women's culture reveals the unique and complex ways in which Black women have resisted oppression over time, points to limitations in traditional notions of activism, and redefines women's everyday activities as forms of activism (Collins, 1986).

A second important feature of Black feminism is an analysis of the interlocking factors and "simultaneity of oppression" (Smith, 1983, p. xxxii) (e.g., due to race, class, gender, sexual orientation) as well as the recognition that despite common challenges and standpoints as a collective group, "there is no essential or archetypal Black woman whose experiences stand as normal, normative, and thereby authentic" (Collins, 2000, p. 28). Collins elaborated further, noting that "an essentialist understanding of a Black women's standpoint suppresses differences among Black women in search of an elusive group unity. . . . Black *women's* standpoint eschews essentialism in favor of democracy" (2000, p. 28). A third feature is represented by a dialogical relationship between action and thought such that "a self-defined Black feminism occurs through an ongoing dialogue whereby action and thought inform one another" (p. 30). This tradition of activism is complex, wide-ranging, and often occurs within antiracist social justice projects. Gaining knowledge for the sake of understanding Black women's oppression is not enough; a commitment to resisting oppression and bettering the lives of oppressed persons is essential.

Flowing from this dialogic relationship is the activity of Black feminist scholars, who integrate everyday actions with their theoretical and conceptual work. Collins (2000) argued that "the commonplace, taken-for-granted knowledge shared by African-American women growing from our everyday thoughts and actions constitutes a first and most fundamental level of knowledge" (p. 34). Concrete experience is melded with Black theoretical scholarship, which is produced by Black intellectuals with diverse class, educational, and generational experiences, and who complete their work within the academy as well as within a wide range of coalitions and communities of activism. Related to this flexibility and inclusiveness with regard to the formation of knowledge is the recognition that Black feminism must respond to the changing social conditions and issues that African-American women face in their roles and work. The topic areas that have received the most extensive attention in Black feminist thought are work, family, sexual politics, and political activism. Final features of Black feminism are its emphasis on human solidarity, its valuing of a wide range of social justice projects, and its interest in eradicating all forms of discrimination (Collins, 2000).

Patricia Hill Collins (2000) summarized the four elements of a Black feminist epistemology, noting that it places emphasis on the concrete, everyday experiences of Black women and values the testing of all ideas in everyday life as "a criterion of meaning" (p. 257). Second, it is based in the belief that knowledge claims must be embedded within dialogue, and that empowerment occurs in the context of community. Third, it is supported by an ethic of care that is characterized by the valuing of individual uniqueness and personal expressiveness, an appreciation for emotion as a sign that "a speaker believes in the validity of an argument" (p. 263), and a capacity for empathy. Fourth, the person who proposes knowledge claims must endorse an ethic of accountability that includes an evaluation of the character, values, and ethics of the person proposing knowledge. The person's verbal commitments need to match her or his actions.

CHICANA FEMINISMS

Chicana feminisms hold much in common with Black feminisms, and the concerns of Black women and Chicanas overlap. However, in order to develop feminisms that are relevant to specific groups of women, the diverse historical, cultural, and everyday experiences of Black women and Chicanas need to be uncovered, honored, and integrated within theory and practice. While Black feminists contended with a history and legacy of slavery, Chicana feminists experienced colonization, the consequences of land theft, and racial discrimination associated with immigration. Although the family was important to both Black and Chicana feminists, many family dynamics associated with religious belief (e.g., Catholicism versus the Black church) and cultural beliefs (e.g., machismo) represent unique challenges for these groups of women (Rosen, 2000).

During the civil rights years of the 1960s and 1970s, the Chicano movement *(el movimiento)* became the voice of Mexican-American activists who challenged racism as well as social and economic inequality. The term *Chicanismo* emphasized nationalistic cultural pride and encouraged solidarity among divergent voices and groups that resisted the internal colonialism, domination, and exploitation experienced by Mexican Americans within the United States. Building on a tradition of Mexican women's resistance and outcry against poverty, political oppression, economic displacement during the Mexican Revolution and throughout the twentieth century (Mirandé and Enríquez, 1979), Chicanas became major participants in all aspects of *el movimiento*'s social protests and activism related to welfare rights, farm workers' rights, health and immigration issues, legal issues, antiwar concerns and campus activism, and community organization (Moya, 2001; Rosen, 2000; Ruiz, 1998). Their experiences as women also motivated them to point out sexism, male domination, and contradictions within the larger society, within the Chicano movement, and within the foundational concept of *Chicanismo* (García, 1997). They opposed the narrowly defined image of the Chicana as someone who struggled with social injustice by being strong and long-suffering, providing for her family in the safe haven of the home, and, in so doing, ensuring cultural survival. They also resisted traditional representations of Chicana womanhood such as the Virgen de Guadalupe, who represented sexual denial and submission, and La Malinche, who was sold into slavery, became the mistress of Spanish conquistador Cortés, and later "sold out" to foreign domination. When Chicana feminists expressed explicit feminist convictions, called for platforms that emphasized egalitarian relationships and access to birth control and child care, or resisted their relegation to gender specific tasks within *el movimiento* (e.g., cooking, cleaning) they were often criticized for focusing on issues that were secondary to racial or class oppression. They were sometimes referred to by men in the Chicano movement as *malinchistas* or *vendidas* (sellouts), accused of being bought out by white feminists (Women Libbers or *agringadas*), or labeled as lesbians (García, 1997; Moya, 2001; Ruiz, 1998; Segura, 2001).

Although Chicana feminists began to work with white feminist organizations during the late 1970s, they found that many white feminists had "blank spots" regarding their own race and privilege, and showed limited willingness to uncover race and class biases that were present within many white feminist organizations. During the 1980s and early 1990s, Chicana feminists sometimes identified themselves as "third world" feminists and made connections with women from other racial minority groups who had encountered similar issues and dynamics as they contended with complex intersections of racism, classism, sexism, and homophobia within ethnic nationalist movements and within predominantly white feminist organizations (see Anzaldúa, 1990; García, 1997; Mirandé and Enríquez, 1979; Moraga and Anzaldúa, 1983).

Chicana writers and activists have placed significant emphasis on raising consciousness about the following issues that restrict their lives and self-concepts:

1. Religious mythologies that reinforce patriarchy and constrain women from enjoying their sexuality
2. Familism and the pressures placed on marriageable women (often by other women) to practice submission to men and to be silent in men's presence
3. The tracking of women into paid labor that represents a continuation of the work they do at home
4. Violence against women (Kafka, 2000)

In response to these issues, Chicana feminists are rewriting traditional myths and folklore in order to disassemble patriarchal values and provide new models of strengths by

1. documenting and preserving Chicana history,
2. speaking out about violence and encouraging women to rebel against sexism and oppression,
3. encouraging women to own their sexual freedom and challenge power relations in the home and work, and
4. facilitating opportunities for women to reach out to other women for support (Anzaldúa, 1987; Kafka, 2000; Mirandé and Enríquez, 1979; Trujillo, 1998).

Like Black feminists, Chicana feminists have also proposed approaches that generate and legitimize knowledge about Chicanas that is "probably not visible from a traditional patriarchal position or a liberal feminist standpoint" (Bernal, 1998, p. 560). A Chicana feminist epistemology honors the diversity of Chicanas while also emphasizing the similarities of Chicana experiences, which are rooted in an indigenous mestiza-based cultural group. Some of the unique issues and experiences that are central to Chicana experience include language, such as bilingualism and/or limited English proficiency; immigration and migration experiences; generational status and generation of residence in the United States; and religion, including both the positive features and contradictions associated with Catholicism. As noted by Dolores Delgado Bernal (1998), embedding one's perspective within Chicana experience "means that we deconstruct the historical devaluation of Spanish, the contradictions of Catholicism, the patriarchal ideology that devalues women, and the scapegoating of immigrants" (p. 562).

Also unique to Chicana feminism are concepts such as borderlands, *Xicanisma,* and mestiza status, or being a woman of mixed ancestry who "straddles cultures, races, languages, nations, sexualities, and spiritualities" (Bernal, 1998, p. 561). The term *borderlands* refers to emotional, psychological, and geographical spaces on the borders between cultures, and the sixth sense that is required to juggle cultures and contradictions associated with these spaces (Anzaldúa, 1987). *Xicanisma* refers to feminisms that are relevant to and developed within "our work place, social gatherings, kitchens, bedrooms, and society in general" (Castillo, 1995, p. 11) and that represent "an uncompromising commitment to social justice rooted in a woman-centered indigenous past" (Ruiz, 1998, p. 125). Anzaldúa (1987) encouraged women to "live *sin fronteras* [without borders]/be a crossroads" (p. 195) between three cultures of relevance to Chicanas: the Indian, white, and Mexican cultures.

Chicana feminists have also described personal skills and standpoints that are central to Chicana epistemology. Chéla Sandoval (1991) proposed the construct of differential consciousness, which is defined as a personal subjectivity or set of survival skills of persons facing multiple oppressions (e.g., U.S. third world feminists). Differential consciousness allows one to emphasize specific aspects of personal identity to achieve important goals. For example, the third world feminist working within a race-based group learns to strategically privilege race-related issues but also has the capacity to highlight gendered aspects of identity when working with mainstream feminist organizations. Third world feminists develop flexibility and strength, and often become adept at "shifting their ideologies and identities in response to different configurations of power" (Moya, 2001, p. 461). They become skilled at moving between groups with different ideologies and political strategies. Gloria Anzaldúa (1987) proposed that women of color develop *la facultad,* a survival tactic which is based on knowledge of one's own painful experiences of marginalization and discrimination. *La facultad* is defined as an intuitive perceptiveness of power dynamics in everyday experiences and allows one to "adjust quickly and gracefully to changing (and often threatening) circumstances" (Moya, 2001, p. 469). The concepts of differential consciousness and *la facultad* emphasize the unique consciousness that women of color bring to feminist and multicultural issues and the in-depth perspective they can offer for developing a more comprehensive understanding of women's lives.

Chicana feminism is characterized by diversity. Beatriz Pesquera and Denise Segura (1993) identified three major positions:

1. Chicana liberal feminism, which emphasizes improving the status of women by focusing on access to employment, education, health care services, and political opportunities for women
2. Chicana insurgent feminism, which focuses on the intersections of race, class, gender, and sexual orientation and calls for the revolutionary change of social institutions and international solidarity with other people who are oppressed
3. Chicana cultural nationalist feminism, which focuses on gaining gender equality while also preserving *la familia,* and maintaining allegiance to Chicano culture and cultural nationalism

To this list, Chéla Sandoval (1998) added two other feminisms:

4. Chicana separatism, an alternative chosen by some Chicana lesbian feminists
5. *Chicana Mestizaje* approach, which calls on Chicanas to live at the "borders" and to "function as a working chiasmus (a mobile crossing) between races, genders, sexes, cultures, languages, and nations" (p. 352)

Sandoval proposes that this final "syncretic form of consciousness" (p. 352) has been most widely recognized and adopted by Chicana feminists.

The work of Chicana lesbian feminists represents another important contribution to feminist activism and theory. Carla Trujillo (1991) argued that Chicana lesbians are perceived as posing a threat to the Chicano community "because their existence disrupts the established order of male dominance, and raises the consciousness of many Chicana women regarding their own independence and control" (p. 186). Lesbians contradict the message given to Chicanas by the Church and culture to "suppress our sexual desires and needs by conceding all pleasure to the male" (p. 186). Carla Trujillo also noted that Chicana identity has often been tied to women's connection to a man (as daddy's girl, wife, mother, or girlfriend) and that overcoming the pressures to conform to this "parasitic identification" (p. 187) is not easy. Overcoming internalized self-hatred and developing self-love and love for other women pose significant tasks to Chicana lesbians, who have experienced resistance from the larger Chicano movement and have been described even more frequently than heterosexual Chicana feminists as *vendidas* or "sellouts." In general, Chicana lesbians have provided insight about the specificity of oppression experienced by women with diverse life experiences and sexual orientations, and have called for an inclusive homeland "where Chicanos and Chicanas of all colors, classes, and sexualities work together in the service of decolonization" (Moya, 2001, p. 459).

This brief overview has been limited to one of many Latina or Hispanic feminisms: Chicana feminism. My goal has been to provide an example of one of many rich Latina feminisms, and to provide a sample of issues that are significant for feminists whose cultures have intersected with Spanish language and culture. Many other distinctive and culture-specific contributions have been offered by women of color with roots in Latin America, Puerto Rico, and South America, and the reader is encouraged to explore this rich heritage of voices.

ASIAN-AMERICAN FEMINISMS

The Asian-American Movement (or the Movement) emerged in the late 1960s in the wake of Vietnam War protests. The 1960s became the first decade in which the numbers of college-age Asian Americans reached a critical mass; as a result, the concerns of these students began to coalesce (Chow, 1996; Wei, 1993). The Movement focused on challenging stereotypes of Asian Americans; overcoming a legacy of legalized racism and discrimination marked by exclusion, economic exploitation, restrictive immigration policies, and prohibitions that barred persons of Asian origin from participation in many sociopolitical activities (e.g., prohibitions against land ownership and marriage with non-Asian persons, as well as exclusion from many professions); and establishing a positive Asian-American identity. Women were actively involved in this movement but were often ignored or expected to play support roles (Chow, 1996; Wei, 1993).

Asian-American women met in "rap groups" or study groups in which they discussed experiences of sexism within their communities and the fact that they were often relegated to secondary positions in the Movement. Some of these groups explored radical Marxist readings and applied these analyses to the class challenges and exploitation experienced within their ethnic communities. As the twenty-first century begins, some Asian-American women continue to use socialist and revolutionary perspectives to inform their feminism (Yamasaki, 2000). More formal groups of Asian-American women were founded during the 1970s and helped sustain activism that focused on the intersections of race, gender, and class (Wei, 1993). The writings of most European-American feminists were of limited interest or appeared irrelevant to many Asian-American women. For example, Betty Friedan ([1963] 1983) recommended employment as a solution to middle-class women's frustrations with their home-based roles. In contrast, many Asian-American women had experienced a legacy of economic exploitation, were often working in low-wage roles to ensure the economic survival of their families, and gained a sense of self-image and self-esteem from cultures that valued the family and extended family in defining the self. Asian-American women also found that predominantly white feminist organizations contributed to a polarization of the sexes, emphasized individualistic causes, showed limited appreciation for obligations to others and connectedness to a culture, and showed limited receptivity to Asian-American women's concerns and presence (Chow, 1996; Wei, 1993).

Asian-American women were active in establishing educational programs, engaging in community activism and antipoverty programs, challenging stereotypes of Asian women, establishing women's centers and health services for women, and producing a variety of literary and autobiographical writings about their experiences (Asian Women United of California, 1989). Asian-American women faced significant challenges, such as

1. the ethnic diversity among Asian groups and difficulty achieving solidarity;
2. Asian-American women's invisibility within the larger culture;
3. stereotypes of Asian women as prostitutes, picture brides, or compliant romantic partners;
4. Asian-American women's limited time for activism because of their essential commitments to economic survival;
5. Asian-American women's segregation from each and the larger society in colonies such as Chinatown and Little Saigon; and
6. lack of funding for activist causes.

Asian-American women also experienced criticism from men in the Movement for diluting resources, weakening an Asian male identity, threatening Asian solidarity, contributing to a loss of identity within the Asian community, destroying working relationships between women and men, and selling out to the larger society (Chow, 1996).

Despite many challenges, Asian-American feminists have developed coalitions with other Asian-American women's groups (e.g., Asian Women United and the Organization of Pan Asian American Women) and have relied heavily on the use of literature, poetry, artistic expression, and public performances to express their identities and political visions as well as raise consciousness about the concerns and experiences of Asian-American women. Organizations such as Unbound Feet provided support for writers who both wrote and performed works with the goals of expressing their art and voices as social activists, thus challenging traditional roles and relationships, dismantling the invisibility of Asian-American women, making Asian-American women's art and culture more accessible, and linking women's experiences around the world (Wong, 2000). The products of Asian-American women's collaborations include a variety of influential anthologies of Asian-American women's writing (e.g., Asian Women United of California, 1989, 1997; Lim, Tsutakawa, and Donnelly, 1989; Lim-Hing, 1994). Helena Grice (2000) described these anthologies and other Asian-American women's writings as textual swords or as a "countercultural medium in which to express their own versions of identity and experience in opposition to dominant versions and paradigms" (p. 183). Asian women writers have provided unique insights about Asian-American women's history, immigration, and challenges of survival; and the wrongs of racism, sexism, and colonialism. They have also conveyed a sense of Asian-American women's community by integrating many genres, voices, and cultural traditions within their work, as well as incorporating literary and oral traditions associated with their cultures of origin within creative works. Asian-American women's writings have also contributed to the revision of Western feminist theories (e.g., of mother-daughter relationships) (Grice, 2000).

THE FUTURE: NEW IMAGES OF SISTERHOOD

The previous sections have summarized ethnocentric aspects of traditional feminisms and articulated important features of several women-of-color feminisms. Author bell hooks noted that some of the ethnocentrism of contemporary feminism emerged out of the failure of white women activists to address the conflicts between women of color and white women and the racism of early feminism. White feminists have often failed to understand how their privileged standpoints sometimes perpetuated the very abuses that they attempted to eradicate. They often ignored differences among women, leading bell hooks to assert that white feminists' emphasis on the common oppression of all women provided white women with a "vehicle to enhance their own individual, opportunistic ends" (1981, p. 150) and to reinforce patronizing attitudes toward women of color. When women of color were invited to cooperate with white women, they were often invited to do so within the parameters established by white women, thus limiting opportunities for productive and mutual exchange (Húrtado, 1989). When women of color have declined to participate in narrowly defined causes, their choices have been misread as lack of interest in women's liberation rather than lack of interest in a movement that is defined by and for white women.

The skepticism that women of color hold toward white women persists. Evelyn Higgenbotham (1992) suggested that although white feminists have largely rejected the notion of a homogenous woman, they "pay hardly more than lip service to race as they continue to analyze their own experience in ever more sophisticated ways" (pp. 251-252). The task of building bridges between white women and women of color is complicated. It was suggested by bell hooks (1984) that we must continue to forge definitions of feminism that focus less on equality of the sexes and more on the diversity of women's experiences. Feminism is not only about gaining equality with men, nor should it "privilege women over men" (hooks, 1984, p. 26). Feminism needs to challenge the philosophical structures that support white supremacist institutions. In addition, feminism needs to transcend the boundaries of academic life and be integrated with a mass-based movement whose goals are not only communicated through writing but also through word of mouth and action (hooks et al., 1993). If women from diverse backgrounds are to feel a sense of solidarity, feminism will need to be based on shared resources and strengths, as well as the willingness to tolerate discussion, confrontation, and criticism. White women need to be willing to confront racism directly and move beyond feelings of guilt to commitment to action. Conversely, it is important for women of color to confront the ways in which they have absorbed beliefs based in white supremacy (or internalized racism) in order to free themselves from racist stereotypes and contribute fully to feminist theory and social action.

Critical Race Feminisms: Toward Coalition Building

Some of the promising integrative developments within feminism are referred to as *critical race feminisms* (Wing, 2000, 2003). Influenced by a variety of strands of thought, such as legal theory, postmodern thought, and postcolonial theory, this orientation to feminism emphasizes multiple consciousness and multiplicative identity. A key feature of this approach is the assumption that liberal Eurocentric thought is not neutral, rational, objective, or universal. Instead, all knowledge is influenced by power and value systems, and even "neutral" approaches contribute to inequality. Furthermore, oppressions are seen as embedded in the basic structures of society (e.g., legal systems, school systems) and must become a focus of social change. Global critical race feminisms also use the experiential knowledge of women of color throughout the world to help explain the complex ways in which various forms of oppression and privilege influence women's lives. Finally, a commitment to coalition building and social action across groups is essential for challenging powerful structures of society that reinforce the status quo.

Women from all regions of the world experience multiple forms and levels of discrimination and privilege that are influenced by a wide range of social identities such as nationality, ethnicity, color, class, sexual orientation, age, religion, education, occupation, minority status, and language (Wing, 2000, 2003; Worell and Remer, 2003). It is the interaction of relevant social identities that shapes a person's unique and complex identity. The person's identity is indivisible; each aspect of identity (e.g., ethnicity or nationality) influences the experience of another aspect of identity (e.g., gender). Second, some aspects of one's identity may contribute to discrimination and oppression and other aspects to privilege. For example, a woman of color may experience discrimination because she is nonwhite, but she may experience privilege because she is a member of the middle class or is highly educated. Third, the specific context also influences the degree to which a specific aspect of identity is relevant, a source of privilege, or associated with disadvantage. Fourth, for some individuals, gender may only rarely become the most significant marker of identity but may be filtered through or modified by other social identities such as race, ethnicity, or class. Finally, each person may be both the target of discrimination as well as a perpetrator of oppression. For example, a white, middle-class woman may experience sexual harassment that is perpetrated by a male co-worker in the workplace, but she may in turn show subtle forms of racism in her interactions with a woman of color who works as her secretary.

Because of limited space, this chapter's review of women-of-color feminisms has been limited to brief summaries of Black, Chicana, and Asian feminisms. These frameworks are useful for explaining experiences that are shared by a significant group of women and for understanding many of the intersecting dynamics of race, gender, and other aspects of social identity. Each standpoint, while valuable, holds limited or partial explanatory power. Global critical race feminisms provide insights about how we can recognize the diversity of women across all racial and ethnic groups. This recognition of diversity and complexity will facilitate coalition building among and between women.

WOMEN OF COLOR AND FEMINIST THERAPY

Early Critiques of Feminist Therapy

Laura Brown (1994) opened her chapter on diversity in feminist therapy by stating, "Feminist therapy cannot arise from a theory that would require someone to choose which aspect of her identity is the one to be liberated while others lie silenced, unattended to, or rendered marginal" (p. 69). A multicultural analysis of behavior and an integrated analysis of oppression are especially important for establishing a framework or model of viewing diversity as a central and defining characteristic of feminist therapy. Using this framework, gender must be understood within an integrated analysis of oppression (Kanuha, 1990).

In large part, feminist therapy was developed originally "by and with White women" (Brown, 1990a, p. 3), and early statements on feminist therapy made only brief references to issues influenced by poverty, homophobia, racism, or classism. Landmark descriptions of feminist therapy (e.g., Greenspan, 1993; Rawlings and Carter, 1977; Sturdivant, 1980) were based primarily on the realities of middle-class white women, and only occasional references were made to the types of oppression and life experiences that poor women and women of color encounter (Brown, 1990a). Even during the mid-1980s, the *Handbook of Feminist Therapy* (Rosewater and Walker, 1985), which heralded the "coming of age" of feminist therapy, included no discussion of the perspectives of women of color.

As feminist therapy matured, feminist therapists expressed concern about the inattention of feminist therapy and theory to the issues of women of color (e.g., Brown, 1990a; Comas-Díaz, 1991; Espín, 1990, 1994, 1995). However, efforts to be more inclusive often fell short of including the perspectives of women of color in a fully integrated and central manner (Espín, 1995). Beverly Greene (1995) commented, "White feminists as a group have continued the American traditions of their foremothers in presenting a slowly changing but still frequently arrogant and unexamined white, middle-class perspective on what issues are important to all women" (p. 306). These critiques have contributed to increased understanding that attending appropriately to diversity is essential to the relevance, vitality, and growth of feminist therapy.

The following discussion of women of color and feminist therapy begins with the limitations of feminist research and feminist personality theories that have emerged since the mid-1970s, as well as commentary about some necessary correctives. It is followed by a discussion of the value of antiracism or antidomination training for white feminist therapists. The final section of the chapter describes the work of several feminist therapists of color who have contributed substantially to theory and practice in feminist therapy. This chapter focuses primarily on general principles for working with women of color. For in-depth discussion of specific populations, I recommend Lillian Comas-Díaz and Beverly Greene's (1994) edited book, *Women of Color*, and Leslie Jackson and Beverly Greene's edited book, *Psychotherapy with African American Women* (2000). For in-depth discussion of guidelines for antiracist practice in feminist psychology, I recommend Jeanne Adleman and Gloria Enguídanos' (1995) edited book, *Racism in the Lives of Women: Testimony, Theory, and Guides to Antiracist Practice.*

Developing an Inclusive Psychology of Women: The Research Foundation

When the subject of psychology of women was born in the early 1970s, psychologists successfully challenged a wide range of theories and research practices that held up the lives of privileged white men as normative and evaluated all other groups in comparison to this group. During the 1970s and 1980s, a substantial amount of research was conducted on the lives of women; it focused on topics such as work, achievement, intimate relationships, violence against women, attitudes toward women, and gender socialization during childhood and adolescence. However, most of this research was conducted by white feminist researchers, and most research participants were traditional undergraduate students from primarily white, middle-class backgrounds. The initial body of knowledge that emerged was a psychology of women based largely on the lives of white women (Vaz, 1992; Yoder and Kahn, 1993).

Janice Yoder and Arnold Kahn (1993) noted that feminist psychology's reliance on traditional empirical methods and traditional comparison groups has sometimes contributed to ethnocentrism. For example, if the researcher is studying women's attitudes toward some issue, the researcher is most likely to compare a group such as African-American women with white women. Such comparative research is very useful when it "debunks misconceptions and undermines harmful stereotypes about group differences" (Yoder and Kahn, 1993, p. 848). However, this form of research becomes harmful when white women are seen as "women in general" (p. 848), the normative group, or the baseline from which other groups deviate. This type of bias can be described as "the tendency to make one's own community the center of the universe and the conceptual frame that constrains all thought" (Gordon, Miller, and Rollock, 1990, p. 15). Too frequently the attitudes and behaviors of women of color have been measured or assessed according to their similarity and divergence from white women's values and attitudes. Such attitudes can lead to dichotomous comparisons between women of color and white women, which may reinforce stereotypes and erase or obscure information about differences within specific groups of women. In other words, feminist psychologists have inadvertently practiced forms of ethnocentrism that parallel the biases of the traditional male psychologists whom they have criticized.

As an illustration of this point, Karen Wyche's (1993) review revealed that much of the applied research on African-American women consisted primarily of comparative studies and studies of poor single mothers. This narrow focus ignored the diversity of African-American women and sometimes resulted in inappropriate generalizations from one subgroup of women to African-American women in general. In addition, white researchers have often assumed that the life experiences of women of color have the same meaning as they do for white women, which further contributes to biased understanding and knowledge. Finally, past research has tended to focus on the negative or dysfunctional behaviors of women of color rather than their positive coping mechanisms.

Efforts to create an inclusive research foundation have increased in recent years, but they are sometimes inadequate. For example, when researchers use an "additive" framework, the perspectives of women of color are merely added to existing frameworks and research questions. The assumptions underlying research are not challenged, and white, middle-class norms remain central. In a second model, the relationships between class, gender, race, and culture are studied as parts of a complex equation. Although offering an improvement over an additive model, groups such as middle-class, Black, heterosexual women are still likely to be seen as a "homogeny of heterogeneous types" (Morawski and Bayer, 1995, p. 118). Jill Morawski and Betty Bayer (1995) contended that neither an additive nor an interactive approach sufficiently challenges the centrality of a white, middle-class perspective. White, middle-class individuals remain the norm; other groups are treated as "special cases" or as "fixed social categories" (p. 121), and the status quo is maintained. It is important for feminist researchers to consistently consider how the experiences of individuals are socially constructed, how they shift and change over time, and how they are shaped by history and social relationships. For each woman, the various social locations (e.g., gender, race, ethnicity, class, religion) that influence identity and life experience intersect in complex, unique, and multiplicative ways, and often contribute to a multidimensional identity. Furthermore, within the same person, some aspects of social identity may be associated with oppression and other aspects with privilege (Wing, 2000). The use of nontraditional research methods may be necessary for exploring many of these multiplicative and shifting identities.

It is also crucial for feminist psychologists and researchers to expand the range of topics they explore. Pamela Trotman Reid and Elizabeth Kelly (1994) noted that white women are generally viewed as having no race. Researchers should examine the impact of ethnicity on all women (see also Frankenberg, 1993). Second, women of color need to be studied as "enactors, not victims" (Reid and Kelly, 1994, p. 483; Wyche, 1993). An examination of the survival strategies and strengths of women of color is necessary for viewing groups of diverse women as complete individuals. Third, research on women of color needs to focus on the issues, definitions, and perspectives that women of color identify as relevant to their lives. The contributions of women of color must be considered as central to defining feminist theory, therapy, and research (Espín, 1995).

Antiracism/Antidomination Training for White Feminist Therapists

To implement inclusive methods, feminist therapists need to be aware of their own values. White feminist therapists are not likely to be aware of their subtle ethnocentric or racist beliefs unless they examine their own experiences of white privilege and become educated about the lives and histories of diverse women (Brown, 1991a, 1993, 1995; McIntosh, 1989; Frankenberg, 1993). bell hooks (1984) argued that the basis for solidarity among white women has been shared victimhood. Ironically, white women are the very women who experience higher levels of power and privilege than most other women in society. In contrast, "women who are exploited and oppressed daily cannot afford to relinquish the belief that they exercise some control, however relative, over their lives" (hooks, 1984, p. 45). When white women view themselves primarily as victims, they are conveniently absolved of responsibility for confronting the ways in which they may help maintain and perpetuate racism, classism, and sexism.

Feminists of color have noted that white feminists who are unaware of the context of the lives of diverse groups of women are often guilty of condescension. For example, Gloria Anzaldúa (1983) compared some of the activities of white feminists to "the monkey in the Sufi story, who upon seeing a fish in the water rushes to rescue it from drowning by carrying it up into the branches of a tree" (p. 206). Merle Woo (1983) added, "I have seen how white women condescend to Third World women because they reason that because of our oppression, which they know nothing about, we are behind them and their 'progressive ideas' in the struggle" (p. 143). Both statements reveal the importance of listening to women of color on their own terms and respecting their leadership and insight about the issues relevant to them.

Patricia Collins (1991) indicated that women of color have typically developed intimate knowledge of the dominant culture in order to survive in it, while members of white society often remain oblivious to issues of diversity. Judit Moschkovich (1983) added, "As a bilingual/ bicultural women, I live in an American system, abide by American rules of conduct, speak English when around English speakers, only to be confronted with utter ignorance or concocted myths and stereotypes about my own culture" (p. 80). It is necessary for feminist therapists to acquire knowledge of the cultures of their clients in order to deal effectively with those individuals whose cultures are different from their own. This practice is especially crucial for white therapists because, unlike most women of color, they have not needed to become educated about other cultures in order to cope with the social roles they enact. By becoming aware of the cultures of women of color, white feminists are also more prepared to explore their unexamined perceptions about the presumed universality of some life experiences.

One of white women's most common sources of information about diversity comes from their knowledge of exceptional women of color. This information is often gained through media reports, academic experiences, or biographies/autobiographies. The lives of exceptional women of color provide rich information about how individual women have overcome sexism, violence, and racism. However, accounts about exceptional women can sometimes be used to support white supremacist notions that although racism exists, it is not a particularly significant factor if women are determined to achieve and willing to "pull themselves up by their bootstraps" (Crawford and Marecek, 1989). Thus, it is important for white feminist therapists to become aware of the everyday struggles of women of color.

Another potential problem that merits attention is the danger of inadvertently romanticizing the lives of women of color. As white feminists become aware of the rich traditions of women of color (rich spiritual traditions, healing rituals) they may desire to incorporate some of these experiences within their own experience. However, if these practices are borrowed merely as forms of convenience that are not matched with knowledge and appreciation of the full significance of these traditions, white feminists may engage in a form of colonization or objectification of people of color. One form of romanticizing women of color may occur when white feminists emphasize the strength of women of color without acknowledging the very real struggles they encounter. An overemphasis on strength does not allow for images of women of color as human or as persons who experience ordinary stresses and strains of living. For example, Carolyn West (1995) indicated that the mammy stereotype reinforces the image of the notion that Black women are able to "selflessly meet the needs of others" (p. 461). The stereotype does not give Black women permission to experience genuine vulnerability and fear when it is appropriate. bell hooks (1981) elaborated on this issue:

> When feminists acknowledge in one breath that black women are victimized and in the same breath emphasize their strength, they imply that though black women are oppressed they manage to circumvent the damaging impact of oppression by being strong—and that is simply not the case. . . . They ignore the re-

ality that to be strong in the face of oppression is not the same as overcoming oppression, that endurance is not to be confused with transformation. (p. 6)

Laura Brown (1991a) observed that when white people grow up in the dominant white culture, they are likely to be either covertly or overtly racist to some degree. To eradicate nonconscious racism, which is often marked by the tendency to define normalcy in terms of one's own experience, feminist therapists can benefit by antiracism training designed to increase awareness of how white privilege often perpetuates power differentials (Adleman and Enguídanos, 1995; Boyd, 1990; Brown, 1990a, 1991a, 1993, 1995; Cross et al., 1982). Peggy McIntosh (1989) suggested that just as men have difficulty recognizing male privilege and power, white feminists have difficulty recognizing white privilege or the "invisible package of unearned assets which I can count on cashing in each day, but about which I was 'meant' to remain oblivious" (p. 10). These unearned privileges resemble a "weightless knapsack" of special tools and blank checks that are accorded to people who have greater social and economic power. In order to raise consciousness, Peggy McIntosh illustrated privileges that white people can expect to receive, such as

- being able to count on skin color adding to rather than detracting from perceptions of personal reliability,
- being able to accept a job with an affirmative action employee without individuals being suspicious that the job was awarded on the basis of race versus competence, and
- being assured that educational materials will give ample attention to the existence of one's race.

In addition to examining privilege, it is important for feminist therapists to be aware of modern racism and its manifestations. Racism is apparent in activities such as

1. dysfunctional rescuing, or assisting women of color based on the belief that they do not have the background or knowledge to help themselves;
2. blaming the victim, or ignoring the impact of systemic racism on people's lives, and blaming women of color for not acting on their own behalf;

3. avoiding contact with women of color for various reasons, including fear or unwillingness to learn about the experiences of women of color; and
4. denying that racial, social, political, and economic differences between people have political significance (Essed, 1991; McIntosh, 1989).

Philomena Essed (1991) elaborated on three behaviors that support everyday racism: marginalization, containment, and problematization. Through marginalization, the "other" status of people of color is perpetuated by denying women access to power, considering the perspectives of people of color to be irrelevant, ignoring problems of racism, or ignoring the contributions of people of color. Through containment, the efforts of people of diversity to achieve equality, justice, and power are suppressed through denial of racism or verbal aggression. Through problematization, people of color are viewed as deficient and responsible for the very problems they experience. For example, a woman of color who expresses anger may be labeled as too emotional, and the problem of oppression may be denied and defined as an individual problem.

Despite the long-standing distrust between women of color and white women, bell hooks (1989) suggested that opportunities do exist for rapprochement and cooperation. If the goal of feminism is merely to gain the type of power that white men hold, relationships between white women and women of color are likely to remain divisive because this form of power is based on gaining power at the expense of others. White feminist therapists will need to counter white privilege and supremacy, refuse to accept myths and stereotypes about women of color that separate women, listen to women of color on their own terms, engage in honest discussion about similarities and differences, and engage in truly collaborative problem solving and activism.

Knowledge of Social Identity and Racial Identity Development Models

Both the feminist therapist's and client's levels of identity development regarding their experiences of oppression and privilege are likely to influence the therapy experience. Since the late 1970s, multiple "minority" identity development approaches have been proposed, including models of feminist identity development (Downing and Roush, 1985; Moradi, Subich, and Phillips, 2002), womanist identity development (Helms, 1990; Ossana, Helms, and Leonard, 1992), gay and lesbian identity development (Cass, 1979; McCarn and Fassinger, 1996), African-American identity development (Cross, 1991; Cross and Vandiver, 2001), ethnic minority identity development (Sue and Sue, 1999), multiracial identity development (Wijeyesinghe, 2001), and white identity development (Hardiman, 2001; Helms, 1995).

With the exception of white identity development, each of these models explores the evolution of a healthy identity among those who experience one or more nondominant statuses (e.g., as a lesbian, feminist, or member of a racial or ethnic minority group). Prior to entering phases of active exploration, individuals typically accept and internalize the stereotypes about their group that are held by the dominant culture. As they encounter injustice, however, they experience a form of "revelation," begin to question societal assumptions, and often feel anger and other negative emotions toward people and institutions who promote stereotypes, racism, and other "isms." They often immerse themselves in their minority cultures and learn to appreciate experiences and traditions that have been devalued by society. Following a period of awareness building and reflection, they develop a positive and holistic sense of themselves. Core processes associated with ethnic, feminist, or lesbian identity include the positive definition of one's minority identity and the integration of this transformed identity with the entire constellation of developmental and life experiences that are important to personality (Adams, 2001).

In contrast to identity models that focus on nondominant statuses, white identity development models (e.g., Hardiman, 2001; Helms, 1995; Tatum, 2002) focus on how white persons become aware of the ways in which they have adopted the stereotypes and prejudices of the culture about nondominant groups, learn to transcend their negative learning, and develop a healthy nonracist white identity. At early phases, white persons tend to experience naive forms of color blindness and do not think of themselves as having a cultural heritage or a color. As they become aware of the reality and implications of racism, they may feel overwhelmed by the enormity of racism, feel the need to reduce dissonance associated with this new awareness, and have difficulty acknowledging that their whiteness is associated with privilege. To absolve themselves of guilt or reduce internal conflict, they may become concerned about the "plight" of minorities and adopt a rescuing mode, distort reality and deny racism, or avoid contact with persons who hold racial minority status (Tatum, 2002).

If and when individuals move beyond denial or a "guilty white liberal perspective," they begin to explore racism and other "isms" as systems of advantage, and accept responsibility for the roles they have played in perpetuating racism and other oppression. They also consider ways of becoming allies with rather than rescuers of persons with nondominant statuses. They develop a positive nonracist identity, integrate their whiteness with other aspects of identity, and commit themselves to activism directed toward empowering others and challenging the racism of other white people.

A therapist's knowledge of her or his own racial identity development is important for ensuring that the counselor does not unconsciously bring biases and stereotypes into the feminist therapy relationship. In addition, the feminist therapist's knowledge of a client's social identity development is crucial for understanding the way in which the client interprets oppression that she or he encounters or observes. For example, during early phases marked by limited awareness of oppression, clients may not respond to direct critiques of various "isms." In such situations, feminist therapists may focus on raising awareness by gently asking questions designed to help clients discover the impact of sexism, racism, and homophobia on their development. During phases when the client is actively gaining awareness of injustice in her or his own life, feminist therapists may need to provide additional support and encouragement as clients gradually move from seeing themselves as victims of discrimination to active coping ages. Finally, feminist techniques such as power analysis, self-disclosure, and group work may be especially useful when individuals are both aware of the discrimination around them and are solidifying a nonracist, nonsexist, nonhomophobic identity.

Feminist Therapy with Women of Color

Despite some of the ethnocentrism present in the first forms of feminist therapy and the difficulties creating truly inclusive forms of theory and practice, feminist therapy is well suited to the needs of women of color. Feminist therapy is especially useful for helping women of color

1. acknowledge the harmful and interactive effects of racism, sexism, and classism;
2. explore feelings of anger and self-degradation related to racism and ethnic minority status;
3. recognize themselves as competent, powerful individuals with the capacity to enact solutions to problems;
4. clarify the interaction between the sociocultural environment and their internal experiences; and
5. identify and implement opportunities to change social and institutional responses (Comas-Díaz, 1988, 1991; Raja, 1998).

The following two sections describe important features of feminist therapy for women of color as defined primarily by Lillian Comas-Díaz (1991, 1994, 2000); Oliva Espín (1994), and Beverly Greene (1986, 1990, 1992, 1994; Jackson and Greene, 2000).

Feminist Therapy As Decolonization

People of color often have a personal and cultural history that has been influenced by colonization. People of color have been obligated to accommodate themselves to the norms of a dominant, colonizing culture that has demanded the sacrifice and eradication of their cultures of origin. Lillian Comas-Díaz (1994, 2000) indicated that *colonization* is a more useful term than *oppression* to conceptualize the unique experiences of people of color because the term implies that people of color have been required to accept the norms of the dominant culture in order to survive. Although groups such as the elderly, the disabled, white women, and gay people have experienced oppression and discrimination, only people of color have experienced the suppression of their own cultures through colonization due to race and culture. Some of the personal consequences of colonization include victimization, alienation, self-denial, identity conflicts, assimilation within the dominant culture, and/or ambivalence about oneself and the dominant culture. Comas-Díaz (2000) used the phrase "post-colonization stress disorder" to name the consequences of contending with a legacy of cultural imperialism and racism. She contends that this terminology does not pathologize individuals but depicts the repetitive trauma experienced by many people of color and signifies "adaptive reactions in contending with profound social pathology" (p. 1321).

Colonized peoples often become convenient scapegoats for social problems and the recipients of narrow stereotypes. Women of color are especially vulnerable to being blamed for family problems and stresses that are the product of institutional racism (Greene, 1990). Women of color have also been perceived as the colonizer's bounty and individuals who can be enslaved or sexually abused (Comas-Díaz, 1994). They experience sexual objectification, are viewed as oversexual or asexual beings, or are confined to polarized or narrow images. For example, the concept of *marianismo,* based on the image of the Virgin Mary, confines many Hispanic women to images of women as virgin and Madonna who are spiritually superior to men and capable to surviving all suffering at the hands of men (Comas-Díaz, 1988). Similarly, Black women are often seen through the lenses of three stereotyped images: "as angry, volatile, castrating bitches, as nurturing, pious, caring mammy figures, or as morally loose and sexually promiscuous 'whores'" (Greene, 1992, p. 20). The psychological wounds of forced assimilation and imposed stereotypes can be extensive. As a result, feminist therapy for women of color may be best understood as a process of decolonization, which involves the restoration of personal dignity and the transformation of oneself and the world. Through decolonization, women experience the recovery of themselves, develop an autonomous self-identity, and engage in action that results in change of themselves and/or the conditions they experience as colonized individuals (Comas-Díaz, 1994, 2000).

Conscientizacao, or the development of a critical consciousness (Freire, 1970), is a central component of feminist therapy for women of color. Through consciousness raising, the woman becomes aware of the nature of colonization and the internalized racist beliefs associated with it, the impact of these beliefs on the self, and methods for countering these beliefs. In the case of Black women, for example, the dominant culture's standards of beauty that idealize Caucasian features and devalue African features are especially harmful (Greene, 1992). Black women are rewarded for attempting to replicate Caucasian standards, and the internalization of these standards is reflected in many Black women's concerns about body type, facial characteristics, hair texture, and skin color. The narrow range of cultural images of Black women (as mammy, sexually loose, or angry woman) may also be internalized and severely restrict women's self-perceptions, contribute to high levels of stress, and limit women's capacity to enact authentic roles (West, 1995). Although Black women are criticized for fitting stereotypes associated with these images, they are also often criticized by the wider society for undermining Black men when they choose to adopt more diverse roles. This type of double bind is especially painful. Awareness of these types of issues and their consequences is important as a precursor to challenging these images and developing a healthy self-concept (Greene, 1992; West, 1995).

Lillian Comas-Díaz (1994) indicated that helping clients develop an understanding of the personal consequences of colonization is important for transcending it. That which is associated with the dominant culture is often seen as good, even by colonized peoples, and that which is associated with the minority or colonized culture is seen in negative terms. Deconstructing polarized images and finding ways to understand oneself and the world in more meaningful ways is challenging. As a part of self-recovery, clients need opportunities to express anger about confining images and correct cognitive distortions that are a consequence of the narrow images promoted by society. The expression of anger is complicated by the fact that the expression of strong feeling outside of psychotherapy may result in becoming the target of institutional racism. The legitimate expression of anger may be labeled as the misplaced expressions of an "angry minority" (Comas-Díaz and Greene, 1994b). Thus, working through anger within the therapy relationship and finding productive methods for anger expression in daily life are especially important activities.

As women of color become aware of the impact of the interactive impact of racism, gender, and/or classism on their lives, they are likely to become aware of how self-hatred and/or ambivalence toward themselves and their cultures of origin are reactions to or methods of coping with colonization. This awareness forms the foundation for more flexible and positive thinking about themselves. Lillian Comas-Díaz (1994) also indicated that it is helpful for clients to differentiate between the ways in which they experience discrimination from external sources and how their internalized negative images influence behavior. This process helps women make informed decisions about what they can change as individuals and what desired outcomes will require social change and organized action.

Following this awareness stage and recovery of the self, decolonization therapy focuses on the creation of an autonomous, integrated, and healthy identity that is "independent of the colonizer's idealized White female standard" (Comas-Díaz, 1994, p. 291). An exploration of the positive aspects of womanhood associated with one's personal culture may be especially useful. For example, although the concept of *marianismo,* which is embedded in the Catholic and colonial tradition, may be confining and limiting, the concept of *hembrismo* may provide a rewarding and freeing alternative (Comas-Díaz, 1987, 1988). *Hembrismo* "connotes strength, perseverance, flexibility, and an ability for survival" (Comas-Díaz, 1988, p. 45). This image, based in indigenous Puerto Rican matriarchal culture, conveys an image of women who are powerful but not oppressive and whose influences are reinforced through spiritual leadership.

Yvette Flores-Ortiz (1995) noted that Chicanas often feel pressured to simultaneously fulfill multiple roles such as mother, sister, spouse, and comrade *(companera)* in the political struggle. While attempting to fulfill these multiple roles, Chicanas may struggle with the demands of being "La Superchicana" and/or may feel alienated from both the mother culture and the dominant white society. Sorting out these conflicts, finding ways to balance roles, and choosing what roles to emphasize are important to the formation of an autonomous, integrated identity.

Comas-Díaz (1994, 2000) also suggested that asking clients to tell their personal and cultural stories, including information about their ethnocultural group's origins, migration, and identity, may be especially helpful in developing and reinforcing healthy personal identities. Storytelling about mothers or other significant persons, which involves providing recollections of significant others, how they dealt with racism and sexism, and/or how they negotiated life tasks, can form the foundation for further clarification of personal hopes and dreams. Drawing on culturally relevant myths, legends, and spiritual traditions may also represent a rich source of positive images for women of color (Comas-Díaz, 1991; LaFromboise, Heyle, and Ozer, 1990; True, 1990).

The development of an integrated identity includes building skills to deal with discrimination and channeling anger into social action. A final aspect of decolonization involves planning healthy action on behalf of oneself and others, including challenging the social structure in which one lives. In other words, advocacy, political action, and other methods of improving the conditions and opportunities of people of color are crucial features of a fully integrated approach to feminist therapy with women of color. Comas-Díaz (2000) summarized her approach in the following way:

> Therapeutic decolonization entails raising consciousness of the colonized mentality, correcting cognitive distortions, recognizing the contexts of colonization (including post-colonization stress disorder), affirming reformulated individual and collective identities, increasing dignity and self- and social mastery, and working for personal and collective transformation. (p. 1322)

Ethnospecific Feminist Therapy

Many feminist therapists believe that a female-female therapeutic dyad is important for effective feminist therapy. Oliva Espín (1994) took this concept one step farther and articulated the advantages of a feminist ethnospecific approach, which is defined as therapy in which the therapist and client are from the same ethnic or racial background. The positive aspects of an ethnospecific approach are multiple. First, the therapist is aware of the client's language and culture through firsthand experience. Espín cautioned that when the therapist is white and the client is a woman or man of color, the client is often expected to inform the therapist about her or his racial or cultural traditions, which detracts from the focus of therapy. Second, a therapist from the same racial background as the client serves as a more powerful role model than a white feminist therapist. Through her presence with the client, the woman of color feminist therapist raises the client's consciousness about the possibilities available to her. Third, there is greater likelihood that power will be equalized. Because of racial and cultural similarity, it is less likely that a relationship of dominance and submission will be re-created. When the therapist is white, her or his greater power than the client is magnified: she or he holds greater power due to expertise as well because of dominant status in society at large. The therapeutic relationship can resemble the colonizer-colonized relationship in which the less powerful position of the woman of color is reinforced (Comas-Díaz, 1994). Fourth, "the therapist is more likely to be invested in the client's success in therapy and life" (Espín, 1994, p. 276). Although there is some danger that the therapist may overidentify with the client, it is more likely that similarity will be an advantage.

As individuals who have experienced multiple forms of oppression (e.g., both racism and sexism), feminist therapists of color often develop a heightened sense of awareness of their clients' needs, which Virginia Hammond (1987) referred to as "conscious subjectivity." Conscious subjectivity operates in several ways. First, through mutual identification points the feminist therapist is able to note common or shared experiences with the client, which allows the therapist to both validate the client's perceptions that racism exists and model the reality that it is possible to survive and transcend oppression. Second, the therapist helps the client understand that many internalized racist or sexist beliefs evolved as tools for coping with a racist society. This discussion further validates the client and her inherent strengths. Timely therapist self-disclosure facilitates both of these activities. Third, because of their own experiences with racism and sexism, feminist therapists of color may be especially aware of how to act as an advocate or power agent on behalf of the client as she or he negotiates institutions or systems that have often limited her or his options. Fourth, by teaching specific skills, the therapist helps the client develop mastery and competence. The feminist therapist's actual encounter with multiple forms of oppression helps her or him engage in effective teaching (Trotman, 2000). Frances Trotman (2000) also noted, however, that a woman-of-color therapist working with a client of color may become overidentified with the client as a victim of racism and may "aid her in denial of the responsibility for her own life" (p. 259). Alternatively, the therapist of color can become dissociated from her or his own culture and convey forms of internalized racism that may be harmful to the client. Thus, self-awareness is crucial to all therapists.

Skin color is a highly visible difference between individuals and may evoke transference and countertransference issues in more pronounced ways than other differences (Greene, 1986; Shorter-Gooden and Jackson, 2000). Racial-ethnic similarity between therapist and client decreases the number of differences that the therapist and client need to transcend and may help the counselor and client establish an initial relationship of trust. However, even when the therapist and client share a common racial heritage and/or commonalities that may be defined by language, religion, and/or culture, many differences between women exist. Hispanic women, for example, identify themselves in many ways: as Cuban, Spanish, Hispanic, Puerto Rican, Chicano, Mexican, Mexican-American, or Latina. To deal effectively with differences among and between groups of women, it is important for feminist therapists to be knowledgeable about historical influences such as colonization and unique cultural values, the client's level of acculturation and/or experience with immigration, and the client's relationship with language, such as Spanish. In addition, variables such as class, professional status, and sexual orientation are also crucial aspects of a client's identity (Comas-Díaz, 1988; Espín, 1986, 1987; Trotman, 2000). Thus, even ethnospecific approaches must be informed by knowledge of diversity within racial and ethnic groups.

Despite the many advantages of an ethnospecific approach, many women of color who seek out a feminist therapist will eventually work with a white feminist therapist or a feminist therapist whose social identity is substantially different from her own. At its best, therapy between a white therapist and a woman-of-color client can provide a useful context for learning to deal effectively with similarities and differences (Espín, 1994; Trotman, 2000). When the therapist is white and the client is from an ethnic minority group, it is possible that the fear, anger, and tension present in the wider society will influence the relationship in some way. The effective white feminist therapist strives to be cognizant of any legacy of distrust that may exist between her or his racial group and the client's ethnic or racial group, and works toward interacting as genuinely as possible with the client. It is also important for the therapist to recognize that the client may bring a healthy "cultural paranoia" to psychotherapy. On occasions when the client tests a therapist's trustworthiness, it is useful to frame the client's behaviors as representing healthy and productive survival skills that may reflect methods the client has used to protect herself or himself from additional discrimination within the social world.

When the social identities (e.g., race, ethnicity) of a client and therapist are different, the process of forming a therapeutic alliance is often more complex than when both persons share many identities or experiences (Shorter-Gooden and Jackson, 2000). At times, white therapists' desires to appear "color-blind" or their anxieties about acknowledging difference may contribute to ineffective interventions. Although color blindness is dangerous because it may lead to the avoidance of critical issues, it is equally dangerous for therapists to uncritically comply with a client's belief that "one's discriminated status justifies a failure to take into account the feelings or needs of others" (Greene, 1986, p. 54). Because of anxiety, guilt feelings about racism, or fears that their own racism may influence the psychotherapy experience, white feminist therapists may fear confronting the client about the clients' behaviors that may have been hurtful to others. Frances Trotman (2000) also indicated that a European-American therapist with limited self-awareness may act out roles that range from being a "self-appointed advocate" to a "self-effacing sympathizer" (p. 259). The self-appointed advocate acts in paternalistic ways and shows a lack of respect for the client. In contrast, the self-effacing therapist becomes trapped by feelings of guilt and the symbolism of her or his white skin and thus cannot be genuine or fully available to the client. The self-aware therapist is able to facilitate a nondefensive exploration of issues related to difference, which provides a productive foundation for empowering work with clients (Greene, 1986).

Consistent self-monitoring on the part of therapists is important for guarding against minimizing the impact of race or ignoring factors other than race and ethnicity that the client and therapist need to confront. It is also important for white feminist therapists to recognize occasions when they are not able to adequately empathize with clients of color. Lillian Comas-Díaz (1994) suggested that although therapists in cross-cultural dyads may understand the client's experience from a cognitive perspective, they may have difficulty empathizing at an affective level. She suggested that the collaborative efforts between a white therapist and person of color can be enhanced through "empathic witnessing" in which "the therapist recognizes his or her ethnocultural ignorance of the client's reality and reaffirms, through empathic witnessing, the client's experience and reality" (pp. 294-295).

To summarize, the therapist's self-explorations and understanding of the following dimensions are critical to effective work with women of color:

- The therapist's feelings and knowledge of her own interlocking social identities (e.g., race, class, ethnicity, language, religion, privileges) and her willingness to use this self-awareness to learn about the multiplicative identities of her clients
- Her comfort level with the language, traditions, values, and behavioral styles of women of color
- Her ability to be both vulnerable and powerful in her interactions with women of color
- Her ability to hear and affirm the anger and pain of women of color without becoming defensive, paralyzed, or ridden with guilt (Adams, 2000)

Ethnospecific Therapy and Indigenous Therapies

An ethnospecific approach to feminist therapy can sometimes be enhanced by integrating indigenous therapies with feminist therapy. For example, Lily McNair (1992) and Matthew Taylor (1999) recommended using a synthesis of Afrocentric and feminist therapy. Although many feminist models do not adequately attend to cultural issues and Afrocentric models may not attend to issues related to gender, the combination of these approaches may be especially suited to the needs and values of many African-American women. The following summary will briefly describe the central features of one form of Afrocentric psychotherapy that can be used to enhance feminist therapy. Afrocentric values and therapy are based on the core principles of

1. harmony, the spiritual belief that unity of mind, body, and spirit allows individuals to align themselves effectively with the basic forces of life;
2. balance, the process by which seemingly competitive aspects of experience are combined in a holistic manner;
3. interconnectedness, the notion that all experience is linked and creates a bridge between internal and external experiences;
4. authenticity, or the valuing of spontaneous, genuine, and intention relationships within a community; and
5. cultural awareness, or the importance of discovering one's identity as it is influenced by Afrocentric values.

Underlying these principles is an affective epistemology that places significant value on emotional self-knowledge and well-being. Whereas a Eurocentric worldview tends to emphasize individualism, control over nature, and material versus spiritual values, an Afrocentric approach places priority on collective responsibility and cooperation, harmony and unity with nature, and the equal valuing of spiritual and material aspects of living (Jackson and Sears, 1992; Phillips, 1990; Taylor, 1999; Thomas, 2001).

Anita Jackson and Susan Sears (1992) suggested that the application of an Afrocentric worldview to women's concerns is especially positive for several reasons. First, an Afrocentric approach provides clients with knowledge about their history, gives relevance to Black women's heritage, and fosters self-worth and a positive identity. Second, Afrocentric values provide a framework from which to counteract negative images of Black women in the dominant culture. Third, the holistic and multidimensional approach associated with Afrocentric psychology forms a foundation for stress management and problem solving, and helps women cope with and transcend difficult circumstances. Finally, this approach fosters a communal orientation and the development of positive support networks. These principles are highly consistent with feminist therapy's emphasis on empowerment, women's strengths, and the enhancement of women's functioning rather than a focus on deficits and pathology.

Although the integration of indigenous therapies with feminist principles is often valuable, some cultural/indigenous therapies are embedded in social values that maintain a patriarchal social structure. The feminist therapist must be careful not to romanticize culturally defined therapies that reinforce male domination and minimize the realities of women's oppression (Bradshaw, 1990; True, 1990).

Ethnospecific Therapy and Support Systems

Many women of color come from cultures that value collectivism, community, and interdependence (Louie, 2000). For example, the Japanese value of *amae* emphasizes the centrality of reciprocity, belongingness, and indebtedness between individuals. *Amae* refers to the "indivisibility of subject from object, self from other" (Bradshaw, 1990, p. 73). Relationships within the inner circle of family and relatives are characterized by oneness between persons, unconditional love, affirmation, and indulgence. In many Hispanic cultures, the values of *respeto*, or respect, *familiarismo*, or familism, emphasize the manner in which family members share responsibility for the health and well-being of the extended family (Comas-Díaz and Duncan, 1985). Many Black women value an Afrocentric worldview, which underscores the importance of collective responsibility, extended kinship systems, and harmony between humanity and nature (Greene, 1992, 1994; Jackson and Sears, 1992). Native American women often experience their identity as an extension of the extended family, the tribe, and a spiritual perspective that stresses the interconnectedness of people and their environments (LaFromboise, Berman, and Sohi, 1994).

Given the importance of interdependence to many women of color, culturally relevant consciousness-raising groups, support networks, and self-help networks that build on these values may be especially productive forms of feminist therapy. Such experiences are likely to strengthen women's historical, ethnic, and cultural identities; emphasize issues that are primary concerns of their specific ethnic group; provide concrete assistance and emotional support to each other; and empower women to make changes in their lives and in the larger community (Fulani, 1988; True, 1990; Vasquez, 1994). For example, Teresa LaFromboise, Joan Saks Berman, and Balvindar Sohi (1994) recommended several types of groups for American Indian women. Culturally sensitive time-limited workshops of skills groups can be used to focus on specific issues such as sexual abuse, self-esteem, or alcoholism. Groups may also be built on traditional healing practices. The "talking circle" incorporates aspects of ritual, prayer, role-playing, and modeling, but does not require direct interaction between members. The "four circles" option involves discussion of issues associated with four levels of interaction which include (1) the Creator at the center; (2) one's spouse or partner; (3) the immediate family; and (4) the extended family, community, and tribe. Finally, family network therapy allows for the re-creation of a clan network for the purpose of mobilizing social support system for an individual or family.

Spirituality and religious experience represent additional support systems for women of color. Toinette Eugene (1995) and Jacqueline Mattis (2002) indicate that spirituality and the Black church provide important therapeutic benefits as well as an impetus for social activism in the lives of Black and African-American women. For example, the singing of spirituals and gospel songs is a way of articulating suffering and also becomes a way of protesting and confronting evil. Prayer, singing, and other expressions of spirituality allow individuals to name the oppression that faces them. This expression of suffering can facilitate a powerful emotional release, healing, and the ability to transcend difficulties. In general, spirituality and religion often validate Black women's experiences, facilitate insight and personal growth, support the exploration of existential questions of meaning, contribute to increased self-esteem, decrease isolation and self-blame, and provide a sense of purpose and destiny. These activities are consistent with Alice Walker's (1983) definition of a womanist identity, which emphasizes the importance of Black women's commitment to the wholeness and survival of other women and an entire people. In summary, feminist therapists should value women's diverse expressions of themselves in communal environments as central components of healing.

CONCLUDING COMMENTS

Although it is easy to give lip service to the importance of a multicultural perspective in feminist therapy, the implementation of inclusive, antiracist practice is difficult. Oliva Espín (1995) noted the following reality:

> When statements are made about the "need to include" women of color in theories or organizations, in the very statement of the need for their inclusion the assumption is being made that some other group (meaning, of course, *white* women) "owns" and defines the movement in which the women of color are to be included. (p. 128)

For feminist psychotherapy to transcend this historical problem, antiracist multicultural practice will need to become a cornerstone of all feminist psychotherapy practice. Attention to diversity should be central to all theory building and practice. Feminist psychologists Beverly Greene and Janis Sanchez-Hucles (1997) defined diversity as "(a) openness to differences among/between people; (b) the cultivation, appreciation and nurturance of different perspectives; (c) a receptiveness to and respect for others; (d) valuing difference; and (e) a noun and a verb in which we are all subject and object" (p. 185).

The following goals are central to forming inclusive and diverse approaches to feminist therapy. First, feminist therapists work toward explicitly identifying their unconscious assumptions that have supported ethnocentrism. Feminist therapists also work toward destroying the myth of the "universal woman" and stereotypes about women of color by examining the complexity and diversity of women's lives. Feminist therapists engage in ongoing efforts to increase their understanding of the multiple experiences, multiple realities, multiple truths, and multiple oppressions that individuals experience. Feminist therapists seek to listen to and understand women of color on their own terms, and to see the experiences of women of color as lived and embodied rather than as statistics and generalizations about women.

An inclusive feminist therapy is based on comprehensive knowledge about how the inner and outer lives of women are intertwined, how women's lives are socially constructed, and how political forces influence the inner experiences of the self. A feminist therapy that respects diversity is also based on an understanding of the myriad coping skills and strengths of women of color. This knowledge includes awareness of how women resist the limitations placed on their lives by race, gender, and class, and how women reinvent their lives in response to the challenges they face.

Women of color have helped to demonstrate that although "all women are women, there is no being who is only a woman" (Spelman, 1988, p. 102). Furthermore, "There is no *woman's* voice, no *woman's* story, but rather a multitude of voices that sometimes speak together but often must speak separately" (Baber and Allen, 1992, p. 19). It is not possible to isolate gender from other complex aspects of experience; gender can only be effectively understood in its multiple manifestations and as it is modified by individual difference, cultural/ethnic values, class, race, and sexual orientation.

Chapter 6

Global/Transnational Feminisms and Their Implications for Feminist Therapy

Some of the most exciting recent developments in feminist theory and practice have their origins in a wide range of countries around the world. In general, feminisms with an international focus include those which emphasize transnational communication and cooperation among feminists from many nations, and local or indigenous feminisms which focus on the unique needs of women in a specific country (Basu, 1995, 2000). The breadth of these theories and movements is vast, and this summary is cursory at best. This chapter begins with a general definition and discussion of global, transnational, and local indigenous efforts. It is followed by an overview of feminist activism, theory, and therapy in the country of Japan. Rather than providing vast generalizations about a variety of indigenous feminisms, I hope to provide readers with enough information about one country's feminisms and feminist practices to convey the reality that many other countries have spawned myriad approaches that rival the complexity of thought and activism present in North America. I have chosen Japan as an example for several reasons. Like the United States and Canada, Japan is a highly industrialized country; however, unlike its North American counterparts, it is a more collectivist or group-centered society. The similarities and differences between Japan and North America make it an interesting example of feminist theory and activism. In addition, feminist therapy has become increasingly important in Japan and provides a useful example of the international practice of feminist therapy.

GLOBAL AND TRANSNATIONAL FEMINISMS

To use the following items as a form of self-assessment, please respond to each statement with a "yes" or "no."

_____ 1. Transnational and global feminisms, which examine the impact of women's choices on other women around the globe, are important for increasing sensitivity to interconnections and differences among women.

_____ 2. "Gender" oppression is often a less salient concern of women around the world than are other human rights, economic, and political issues. "Women's concerns" need to be identified by and for women of a given country and/or region.

_____ 3. Becoming informed about and challenging government and transnational corporation practices that influence the economies and political systems of other countries represents important components of education and activism for ensuring a sustainable future of all global citizens.

_____ 4. The lives of women around the world are often romanticized or exoticized, and a key aspect of global feminism involves exposing and deconstructing these stereotypes.

_____ 5. Western feminists can learn much from global and transnational feminists about how indigenous and grassroots practices can be integrated with feminist therapy in culturally sensitive and empowering ways.

_____ 6. A major challenge facing feminist and human rights activists around the world is how to challenge culturally relativistic viewpoints that condone violence against women and other human rights violations in the name of "cultural difference" without engaging in invasive activity that implies the superiority of Western models, priorities, and agendas.

Global Feminisms: General Themes

Global feminisms with a transnational focus have emerged out of efforts to examine women's experiences within and across national boundaries, analyze their interdependencies, and build linkages and coalitions among feminists around the world. To understand interconnections among women, it is important to explore the interplay between classism, racism, sexism, economics, religion, colonialism, nationalism, multinational systems, and gender (Saulnier, 1996; Tong, 1998). Transnational feminists have generally placed less emphasis on developing unifying theory and more emphasis on creating global perspectives that recognize the diversity of women's experience.

Many transnational feminists operate from the assumption that the circumstances, choices, and experiences of women in one part of the world have an impact on women in other regions. For example, Western women's efforts to ban harmful birth control methods may be successful in removing them as alternatives in the West, but an unanticipated consequence may be the imposition of these devices on women in other, less wealthy parts of the world. It is important for local feminist efforts, such as those that are centered in the United States, to take into account the global implications of feminist activities (Burn, 2000; Saulnier, 1996; Tong, 1998).

Global feminisms also challenge Western feminists to recognize that each woman lives under a unique system of oppression and to acknowledge that Western feminisms have often promoted the intrusive, patronizing, or disrespectful treatment of women around the world (Burn, 2000; Lips, 2003; Ward, 1998). One ethnocentric practice of Western women has been the tendency to view women in other parts of the world as passive victims who need Western women's expertise and insight to overcome oppression. In reality, many successful and culturally sensitive grassroots feminist efforts are being enacted around the world, and Western feminists can learn much by observing these activist efforts, gaining information about the powerful impact of feminist efforts around the world, and forming coalitions and alliances with these women's groups (Anderson, 1999; Basu, 1995, 2000; Burn, 2000; Lips, 2003; Peterson and Runyan, 1999; Tong, 1998).

An example of Western women's limited perspective is their tendency to view a religion such as Islam as a monolithic entity that is highly oppressive to women. Such a conceptualization distorts the views of Islam and hides or erases the complexity and diversity of Islamic women's lives. In the minds of many Western feminists, the veil is often associated with Islamic traditions that signify the seclusion, segregation, and subordination of women. However, Islamic women hold a wide range of views about the importance or the veil or the role of the veil. Although some Islamic women see the veil as oppressive, others see the veil as promoting self-responsibility and modesty, as protecting one from the stares of men, or as providing practical protection from environmental elements. Some women also argue that the separation signified by the veil also unifies women and promotes intimacy among women. At times, feminists around the world also express frustration with Western feminists who state their outrage about practices such as female circumcision or genital mutilation but resist seeing the role that multinational corporations, which have roots in their own Western countries, play in the exploitation and oppression of women (Ward, 1998).

Economic issues and the impact of multinational systems on women are especially important to many global feminists with both transnational and local interests. Multinational business practices and international monetary policies have a significant impact on the social structure of many so-called third world countries. For example, multinational companies have often chosen developing countries as locations for major factories because they are able to pay workers low wages. Health, safety, and pollution standards are often minimal, and sexual harassment issues often accompany these problems. Women are often disproportionately affected by multinational business practices because they make up a large proportion of the factory workforce. Another major economic issue is related to the monetary lending and repayment policies of powerful institutions such as the World Bank and the International Monetary Fund. Debt repayment policies are often associated with required structural changes that may trigger wage reductions and cutbacks in public services. These issues have very significant consequences for many women, who are typically responsible for practical matters related to family survival. Although interventions that influence macroeconomic levels are essential for combating these issues, many nongovernmental organizations (NGOs) have also focused on methods of increasing women's access to economic resources through diverse mechanisms such as land ownership and inheritance rights, as well as access to natural resources and credit institutions. These economic issues are of particular importance to women, who make up 70 percent of the people around the world who live at the absolute poverty level, and also represent two-thirds of the world's illiterate (Basu, 2000). In summary, women around the world often see general economic and political issues as more critical to their oppression than issues that are traditionally defined by Westerners as gender issues (Burn, 2000; Peterson and Runyan, 1999; Saulnier, 1996).

Amrita Basu (1995) introduced her volume on global feminisms with the statement that "few social movements have flourished in as many parts of the world as *women's movements* have" (p. 1). She added, however, that although these movements share some broad commonalities, they also "differ radically" (p. 1) on some dimensions. The first Western feminist efforts to build global feminist thought (e.g., Morgan, 1984) tended to critique "patriarchal mentality" across cultures as well as to assume a common worldview and common condition shared by women. However, they tended to ignore the degree to which women's movements are locally situated. Although many global feminist efforts do focus on transnational concerns, "women's identities within and across nations are shaped by a complex amalgam of national, racial, religious, ethnic, class, and sexual identities" (Basu, 1995, p. 4). These identities shape the scope and focus of women's movements within specific countries. Basu called on contemporary feminists to be less preoccupied by relationships between first and third world women; to pay attention to both women's suffering *and* strengths within postcolonial local feminist movements; and to recognize what indigenous movements have achieved and failed to achieve, and the challenges they face.

Unique local and national concerns often shape the face of feminism in a given country (Basu, 1995). In many countries, particularly those with a colonial history, the concerns of women have often been linked to democratization, human/civil rights, and working-class issues; in other countries (including those with or without a colonial past), feminists and women's movements have emphasized issues that are more likely to influence the private world of women. For example, feminists in India have placed significant emphasis on women's issues such as rape, dowry death, and amniocentesis related to sex selection. One of the issues that feminists from many countries address, albeit in different ways, is violence against women.

Global, transnational efforts against gendered violence have been supported by the 1993 United Nations Declaration of the Elimination of Violence Against Women. The exploitation of women through sex trafficking, prostitution, and sexual violence has been an important emphasis of global feminism in recent years. Sex tourism is a major economic enterprise and often intersects with modernization, capitalism, and colonialism in supporting the oppression of women. Developing countries often benefit financially from sex tourism and trafficking, and thus the governments of these countries often overlook or sanction these forms of oppression against women. Global feminists seek to provide refuge to women and to challenge governments to create policies that can protect women from these abuses. A related issue is the use of rape as a weapon of war to destabilize a country, reinforce the domination of one group over another, or accomplish ethnic cleansing (Anderson, 1999; Saulnier, 1996; Walker, 1999). Basu (2000) concluded that global campaigns have been relatively effective in challenging physical and sexual violence. In contrast, efforts challenging structural violence against women, especially as they relate to economic rights, have been less effective.

Similar to some women-of-color feminists, many women from non-Western countries prefer labels such as "womanist" or "female-ism" (Basu, 1995) over the label "feminist"; such labels imply a broad commitment to rebuilding society rather than a narrow definition of women's issues (Saulnier, 1996; Tong, 1998; Ward, 1998). The term *feminism* has a negative connotation in some countries that have experienced histories of colonization by the West (e.g., African countries) or long-standing conflict with the West (e.g., many Muslim countries). In other countries (e.g., some Latin American countries), feminism is often associated with middle-class, elitist, imperialistic, or antimale values and thus has had limited appeal for women who content with racism, economic exploitation, or governmental repression (Basu, 1995; Burn, 2000). To define feminism on their own terms, women from many countries have identified symbols of women's power that have origins in precolonial periods. Thus, women are able to divest themselves from images of femininity associated with colonizers and create images of autonomy and strength embedded in their indigenous cultural traditions (Basu, 1995; Burn, 2000).

A major unresolved issue is the degree to which global feminists should adopt the values of cultural relativism. To what degree does one culture or group of women hold the right to judge the acceptability of another culture's standards? A major challenge facing feminists is to find some balance that allows for the transcendence of ethnocentrism but the rejection of the form of relativism that seems to condone virtually any behavior as long as it is acceptable within a specific culture. These behaviors include acts such as female circumcision, domestic violence, sexual violence, bride burning, or honor killings of women who have been "dishonored" by rape. Global feminists focus on the importance of respecting difference but are still struggling to deal effectively with cultural differences that contribute substantially to the oppression of women (Burn, 2000; Tong, 1998; Ward, 1998).

The global feminisms reveal that liberatory theory and activism need to become multinational, focusing not only on the needs and issues of ethnic minority groups within the United States but also on the concerns of women and men around the world. Feminist theory and activism should be based on knowledge of the interdependency of members of the global village, the manner in which the individual decisions of persons in the industrialized West may affect persons in less privileged countries, and how some Western practices may oppress persons around the world. Many international feminisms challenge the ethnocentrism of "advanced" societies and encourage Western feminists to listen and learn from women and men around the world. By becoming informed about feminisms and social activism around the world, Western feminists are likely to gain further insight about the limitations of Western psychologies and feminisms as well as information about successful international strategies that can be adapted and applied to challenges faced in the West. As telecommunications, transportation, international events, and economics continue to change, people's lives around the world will be inevitably more connected, and building coalitions across cultures will become increasingly important.

THE EXAMPLE OF JAPAN

Feminism and Feminist Theory in Japan

To provide an example of how culture may influence feminist theory and practice, as well as to communicate what North Americans can learn from feminists around the world, I provide a brief overview of important themes and issues within Japanese feminism. Like many of the feminisms described in this book, Japanese feminism is marked by a diversity of perspectives, goals, and theoretical perspectives that are centered in Asian and Japanese experience.

A major theme within the relatively individualistic feminisms of North American feminists is an emphasis on self-fulfillment, self-esteem, and personal achievement. Within more collectivist cultures such as Japan, group identity, fulfilling social roles effectively, and working to build a positive future for the collective group of women often takes priority over individual self-definition (Markus and Kitayama, 1991). Speaking about Japanese culture, Merry White proposed, "Fulfillment is never regarded as the individual's alone, but is enjoyed by the family or group. Personal gain does not enter into the Japanese model of satisfaction and benefit to the individual" (1987, p. 161). Although there is wide variation in the degree to which Asian and Asian American individuals are influenced by the value of interdependence, Cathie Louie (2000) concluded that interrelatedness remains an important cultural value for Asian and Asian-American individuals. Compared to the profiles of white women, Asian-American women defined themselves in more interdependent ways.

A number of features of recent Japanese culture and history have influenced feminist theory and activism. One is twentieth-century capitalist corporate culture, which contributed to Japan's economic miracle while also severely constricting the lives of many persons, especially Japanese men, who participated in it. A second feature is the presence of highly differentiated gender roles, which are related to Japan's adoption of Confucian values during Japan's modernization process (Iwao, 1993; Kumagai, 1995; Miyaji and Lock, 1994). Another important feature of Japanese feminism has been its efforts to address a history of nationalism and imperialism, which led to the oppression of other Asian women by members of the Japanese military (Aoki, 1997). Japanese feminists have also created alliances with women from other Asian countries to share resources and challenge such practices as sex trafficking.

Japanese feminists note that the subordination of Japanese women is a relatively recent phenomenon. During premodern eras, women enjoyed positions of relative equality with men. Matrilineal descent and matriarchal authority were practiced, husbands and wives disposed of property independently, women were actively involved in commerce and production, and family relationships were "remarkably flexible" (Miyaji and Lock, 1994, p. 99). The erosion of women's rights in Japan was associated with the emergence of Confucian philosophy and the "three obediences," which dictated women's obedience to one's father as a child, to one's husband when married, and to one's male children in old age. Male authority and power was further reinforced by the modernization period (1868-1912) when new laws dictated a more male-dominated, vertically structured society and placed greater power in the hands of adult males (Iwao, 1993; Kumagai, 1996). Following World War II, women earned the right to vote. However, Japan's strategy for capitalistic success in the post–world war era was predicated on the availability of men to work long hours and women's availability at home to support and educate the next generation of leaders and citizens (Dickensheets, 1996). Thus, highly differentiated gender roles were reinforced.

The following sections identify some of the unique features of Japanese feminism as related to three key issues: (1) work, (2) reproduction, and (3) violence against women. Knowledge of the specific ways in which these issues are experienced in Japan and other countries can help challenge ethnocentrism as well as increase appreciation for the perseverance and strategies used by women around the world.

Women, Work, Family, and Definitions of Equality in Japan

Although Western feminists, especially liberal feminists, have seen gender-role differences as a deterrent to gender equality, many Japanese feminists have worked toward preserving and honoring difference. To Westerners, the role differences between men and women appear to signify Japanese women's lack of power. In reality, this role separation does not necessarily result in women's greater dependency and subordination, but sometimes promotes women's greater independence from men, especially in the domain of personal relations. Women are less likely to assume that men will meet their emotional needs and are more likely to maintain close, nurturing relationships with other women (White, 1992).

The role of mother and housewife is an important role in Japan, and it is a source of pleasure as well as a source of stress. Japanese women are less likely than their American counterparts to see themselves as "just housewives," "in service to" or dependent on men than

American women. Rather, they are household executives who manage all financial matters, act as their children's educators, and serve as political activists who work toward increasing the quality of life of their families and communities (Dickensheets, 1996; Iwao, 1993; LeBlanc, 1999; Noguchi, 1992; Sato, 1995; White, 1992). Thus, the housewife role, which often signifies limited opportunity and a restricted life to North American feminists, may actually be the source of "self-enhancing productivity" (White, 1987, p. 159) for many Japanese women. It is possible that Japanese women's high status in the home, even though it is traditional, may confer greater equality to women than that experienced by women in the United States, who experience inequality both in the home and in the workplace (Dunn and Cowan, 1993).

The valuing of gender difference in Japan is related, at least in part, to the reality that the alternative, constricting, and inflexible roles of men in corporate culture are seen as offering few rewards. Feminist theorist Chizuko Ueno (1997) noted, "Our primary goal is not be like men but to value what it means to be a woman" (p. 280). Shimomura (1998) elaborated on Ueno's perspective, stating that "the average Japanese woman doesn't want to be like a Japanese man. Women have no interest whatsoever in getting caught in that crazy trap of working all the time for the corporation. . . . It's a lifelong trap" (p. 62). As implied by these statements, Japanese feminists have often viewed the economic miracle that characterized Japan during the last half of the twentieth century as being built on an oppressive male work structure and have not viewed the integration of women into men's spheres as a panacea. Instead, they have often provided a cultural critique of striving for economic success at all costs and have often supported the dismantling of male-constructed standards and supported equality with protection (Khor, 1999).

Several historic issues within Japanese feminism exemplify questions of equality and difference. Debates about "motherhood protection" explored the degree to which it is possible for women to achieve economic independence and equality in a system in which women's mothering and nurturing roles are protected and valued. Shimomura (1998) stated,

> Women are the only gender capable of reproduction—which is a social, not just a personal act. If our momentous contribution to society is to create the next generation, the society must pay

the costs of that contribution: child-rearing leave, flexible work schedules and child-care facilities. (p. 65)

Closely related to these issues, the "housewife debate" and "work versus living" debates have focused on whether women should seek independence through the workforce or through other essential human activities that support values such as social welfare and a healthy physical and interpersonal environment. Some feminists have argued that formal, paid employment limits a woman's ability to make a real difference in community and peace movements. These debates juxtapose the traditional oppressive workforce culture with more holistic values of living that entail creating new types of organizations and ventures which value women and their strengths (Fujieda and Fujimura-Fanselow, 1995). The centrality of these and related issues have led some to characterize Japanese feminism as "woman-centered" and as similar to some forms of Western cultural feminism. In her efforts to inform Western feminists of the value of Japanese feminists' positions, Diane Khor (1999) stated,

> Denying the distinctiveness of women's experiences in the context of a gender-segregated society where everything—from the food one eats, the language one speaks, the hobbies one has, and the life course one can anticipate—is gender-coded is a refusal to grapple with everyday politics. (p. 652)

Other factors that have influenced women's attitudes toward work have been a variety of legislative and legal efforts during the 1980s and 1990s. The 1986 Equal Employment Opportunity Law called for the equal treatment of men and women in work settings, methods for resolving grievances, and maternity and child care leave. Although it called on companies to "endeavor" to treat women equally with regard to hiring and promotion, it did not establish sanctions or penalties, and most forms of gender discrimination continued (Molony, 1995; Suzuki, 1996). Even before its passage, many feminists opposed aspects of the law, in part because of the absence of penalties but also because of its inattention to the conditions of work that women would be accepting: the same sixteen-hour workday assumed by many men. As one woman noted, "Japanese companies were able to prosper thanks to the selfless devotion of men who had wives at home full time. Do they now expect women to become male clones?" (Suzuki, 1996, p. 57). Fukuzawa (1995) added, "Opting for the management track means copying men as literal corporate warriors, with no time to spend outside work, and giving up almost all hope of starting a family" (p. 160). Without serious rethinking of the employment system and a readjustment of women's heavy responsibilities at home, many feminists viewed this legislation as giving only "lip service" to equality. Although the bill made some provisions related to family leave, it did not attend to the long-term realities for many women of maintaining a career while raising children and fulfilling Japanese social expectations associated with mothering (Shimomura, 1998).

Despite criticisms of the equal opportunity law, young women who were college graduates and willing to accept the conditions of the corporate world experienced increased access to "elite" work roles. However, some argue that the situation for women actually worsened because many companies circumvented new laws by implementing a "two-track" system for women: a career track and a noncareer track. The career track was made available to select women who were willing to enter the corporate world as it existed, and the noncareer track was made available to all other women who were not willing to accept the confining conditions of corporate Japanese culture. The conditions of equal pay and opportunity applied only to those on the career track. One of the consequences was that the wage gap between elite and nonelite women widened: privileged women gained some ground, but other women received no benefits. Furthermore, even career women experienced limited rewards because equal pay applied only to one's point of entry into the corporation. Men were much more likely to be promoted, leaving women behind. Unfortunately, the gains of "elite" women were also short-lived due to Japan's major recession during the 1990s (Ehara, 2000). Women were the first to be fired, and equality within work settings became even more elusive.

Important revisions to the equal employment opportunity law were implemented in 1999. The changes included

- the removal of protective provisions that prohibited women from nighttime and overtime work;
- a greater commitment to nondiscrimination, accomplished largely through removal of the word *endeavor* from clauses about equal hiring and promotion; and
- a stronger commitment to ending gender discrimination and sexual harassment (Liu and Boyle, 2001).

These changes appear to be contributing to a more positive work climate for women in Japan.

For Japanese women, family and career balance issues remain complex. The high status, respect, and social value associated with women's domestic roles have historically been centered primarily on women's mothering roles, and women who do not fulfill social expectations and become mothers may experience negative social reactions or may be seen as incomplete persons. Motherhood, while conferring status and an independent domain of operation as a household executive, also entails a loss of independence in other domains and a significant narrowing of personal options.

Although younger Japanese generations hold generally positive views about women's employment, a comparative study of seven industrialized countries found that the gender gap in workplace authority is most significant in Japan (Wright, Baxter, and Birkelund, 1995). When working women have children, traditional expectations still tend to dictate that mothers with small children should not be employed or should be employed only part-time, and should devote all of their energies to their children. If women continue their paid work during the early years of the children's lives, they usually retain primary, and often exclusive, responsibility for children and housework (Iwao, 1993; Miyaji and Lock, 1994). Many men are both psychologically absent and physically distant from the family, often working extensive overtime hours. Their emotional distance and disconnection from the family often exacerbate the pressures that women experience and limit their opportunity for social and sexual intimacy with a spouse (Iwao, 1993; Kumagai, 1996; White, 1992).

The Politics of Reproductive Control

Throughout the 1990s, the United States media characterized the lack of availability of the birth control pill for women as a sign of Japanese women's subordinate status. In contrast to the typical priorities of Western feminists, Japanese feminists did not place significant pressure on governmental agencies to approve the birth control pill, and the approval of the low-dosage pill did not occur until 1999 (Kihara et al., 2001). Although the unique cultural events and experiences related to the history and nature of birth control go beyond the scope of this short summary, it is important to be aware of the relevance of these factors to the efforts of Japanese feminists (see Norgren, 2001). The following section discusses alternative feminist views of contraception that are embedded in a more collectivist culture, and points to the importance of seeing women's issues from the "inside out."

Ecological feminists in Japan have argued that the birth control pill is "not a guarantee of liberation" but may represent "an extension of the existing mechanisms of control inherent in so much other scientific and technological progress" (Aoki, 1997, p. 16). The birth control pill may represent one more effort to make women's bodies the object of control, which can be contrasted to the Japanese ideal of "bodily autonomy free from artificial intervention" (Jitsukawa, 1997, p. 179). This ecological feminist perspective must be understood in light of Japanese cultural and religious values, which have contributed to the view that the smooth flow of blood during menstruation is a sign of health which contributes to one's harmony with the natural rhythm of life and nature (Jitsukawa, 1997). Natural menstruation allows women to monitor their own health; altering this flow for contraceptive purposes removes women from their bodily experiences and interrupts the balance of the body interacting with the universe. When taking the birth control pill, one is not experiencing true menstruation but "hormone withdrawal bleeding" (p. 193). One way of viewing the use of the pill is that the woman is giving up control rather than gaining control, because agency is assigned to the pill rather than the person. In light of this perspective, which is held by a significant proportion of Japanese women, it is not surprising that fighting for the approval of the birth control pill was not a preoccupation of many Japanese feminists.

Another reason some feminists were less than concerned about the availability of the birth control pill was the belief of many Japanese women that birth control should occur in the context of a relationship in which responsibility is shared (Kihara et al., 2001). Historically, the most common form of birth control in Japan has been the condom, and use of this method places responsibility on men to be active participants in birth control. Some Japanese women argue that relying on the pill implies that men cannot control their desires and hence requires women to assume complete responsibility for reproductive control. In the case of condom failure, abortion is available, as it has has been more or less on demand since the end of World War II

(Norgren, 2001). Furthermore, condoms provide some measure of protection against sexually transmitted diseases (Kihara et al., 2001).

Although the birth control pill is now available to women in Japan, it has not had a dramatic influence on birth control practices. Viewing issues such as reproductive control from a more complete, culturally informed position is essential. One might argue that the cultural acceptance of abortion on demand has allowed Japanese feminists to be less concerned about alternative forms of birth control. They have been able to conserve and channel many of their energies into other critical issues, such as peace and ecological activism. One might also argue that if Western culture were as "advanced" as Japan with regard to views of abortion and reproductive control, the energy required on the part of North American women to fight for and maintain the basic right to reproductive control could have been invested in many other productive social change activities.

Violence Against Women

As noted in the section on global feminisms, violence against women is a universal concern, but the dynamics of violence are influenced by each culture's priorities and "blank spots." Filial violence, primarily the battering of mothers by their sons, was one of the first forms of domestic violence to be acknowledged in Japan (Kozu, 1999). This form of violence appears to be related, at least in part, to the intense mother-son relationship fostered by Japanese culture and the "totalizing" mothering and nurturing role that women play in their relationships with children, especially with sons (Long, 1996). Mother-child relationships are considered the fundamental social relationship, generally taking on greater significance than husband-wife relationships. Japanese women are expected to place the needs of family members before themselves, and to treat children as *jibun no ichibu,* or as extensions of themselves. The child's difficulties may become the mother's difficulties, and Japanese mothers may feel even greater pressure to assume responsibility or blame for their children's problems than mothers in the United States. The intense mother-child connection can also contribute to women's overinvolvement with their children, especially if spouses are uninvolved in the household (Iwao, 1993; Kumagai, 1995; Shimomura, 1998). The psychological exhaustion and loss of self that women may experience as a consequence of serving others may increase their vulnerability to physical battering.

As is the case in many countries, a great deal of secrecy has surrounded the reality of intimate violence. Similar to many other cultures, the Japanese language does not include words that adequately conceptualize violence against women. For example, rape has often been referred to in the media by euphemisms such as a "violent act," and molestation has been referred to as a "mischievous act" (Kozu, 1999). Since the mid-1980s, Japanese feminists have invested significant efforts in naming violence as well as conceptualizing and raising consciousness about rape, public groping of women, sexual harassment, and domestic violence. Sexual harassment was named as a form of violence in 1989 *(sekuhara),* and since the 1999 revision of the Equal Employment Opportunity Act, work-related sexual harassment has received additional attention. The results of a 2000 survey revealed that 70 percent of female government employees identified as having experienced sexual harassment in the office (Associated Press, 2000a). Offenses included a range of activities such as being subjected to sexual jokes, comments, and nude posters; being forced to entertain men or serve tea; and being pressured to have sex. Several high-profile sexual harassment cases have resulted in prison terms for perpetrators, and these legal actions have increased women's willingness to report sexual harassment and pursue legal methods of resolution. Educational and legal campaigns to combat groping in crowded subways and trains have also contributed to increased recognition of women's human rights (Associated Press, 2000b).

Until the early 1990s, male violence toward women in close relationships was considered primarily a private matter and was infrequently recognized as a form of violence (Fulcher, 2002; Kozu, 1999; Weingourt et al., 2001; Yoshihama and Sorenson, 1994). The 1993 United Nations Conference on Human Rights named domestic violence as a human rights violation, and the UN has had a significant impact on Japan's willingness to name this form of violence and initiate efforts to eradicate it. A 2001 law mandated the provision of services for victims of domestic violence as well as for restraining orders, fines, and prison terms for perpetrators of domestic violence. Although Japan is behind North America with regard to its timetable for combating domestic violence, its recent efforts have been very influential (Fulcher, 2002). More specifically, Japan has conceptualized intimate violence under the United Nations human rights framework, established a cabinet-level office on gender equality, and identified domestic violence as a violation of constitutional rights (Fulcher, 2002). This broad framework may be more effective in structuring a comprehensive approach to challenging domestic violence than the criminal justice and "family values" approach that has been used within the United States.

Consistent with their international worldview, Japanese feminists have also focused on the rights of immigrant women and international sex workers in Japan and have worked toward gaining restitution for the "comfort women" of World War II. An example of Japanese feminists' international perspective can be seen in Yayori Matsui's (1996) statement on domestic violence, which drew connections between the experiences of women throughout Asia, including Malaysia, Korea, Nepal, and China. Japan has been the most common destination for other Asian women who have been sold into sexual slavery, and Japanese women have been active in raising awareness about this issue and placing pressure on governments to make more active efforts to stop violence against women. Japanese feminists have also joined with other Asian feminists to protest sex tours for Japanese men. For example, they have staged demonstrations at various airports at cities throughout Asia that have hosted sex tours for Japanese men (Matsui, 1995, 1996).

Issues arising from the treatment of comfort women, the women from various Asian countries who were forced into sexual slavery by the Japanese military during World War II, remain central to the consciousness of Japanese feminists. Despite the activism of many feminists and the testimony of many comfort women, the Japanese government has remained unwilling to make apologies and restitution to victims. Despite these frustrations, the voices of comfort women are being heard, and Japanese feminists have used their testimony to raise consciousness about the expansion of sex trafficking in the present. Kazuko Watanabe (1999) argued that common to the sex trafficking of both World War II and the sex trafficking of the present is the fact that women have been entrapped, imprisoned, raped, and forced to work as prostitutes. She stated,

> Japanese men's sex tours to other Asian countries is a contemporary version of the Imperial Japanese Army's sexual exploitation of Asian women as comfort women. The only difference is

the way the men dress: instead of military uniforms, they now wear business suits. (Watanabe, 1999, p. 23)

Whereas the World War II motive for sex trafficking was to strengthen soldiers' "fighting spirit" for battle, current motives involve ensuring men's fighting spirit and commitment to the company. As noted by Kazuko Watanabe, "Both the soldiers who were forced to die for the emperor on the battle field and businessmen who frequently die today from overwork *(Karoshi)* were—and are—often rewarded with prostitutes" (1999, p. 23).

Definitions of Feminism and Strategies for Social Change in Japan

Individual rights, freedoms, and gaining access to the same economic opportunities as men have been at the core of much feminist activism in the United States. In contrast, Japanese feminists often voice the belief that achieving the same rights as men will not result in personal freedom but will create different and equally confining constrictions (Iwao, 1993). Rather than asking for equality with men, Japanese feminists have often challenged the very priorities of Japanese society, calling for a more fulfilling and human life characterized by greater sharing of life tasks for both men and women. They have noted that men, whose lives are characterized by long work hours and estrangement from family members, are, in the words of psychologist Sumiko Iwao, "the ones to be pitied" (p. 7). Japanese feminists have invested substantial energy in developing a woman-centered perspective. According to Diana Khor (1999), they have often been more successful than Western feminists in working for the good of women in general.

In general, Japanese feminists' strategies have not been marked by overt expressions of anger but rather by pragmatism, nonconfrontation, and a long-term perspective (Iwao, 1993; Shimomura, 1998; White, 1992). In contrast to Western individualists, Japanese feminists have also been less concerned about lack of fairness among individuals at a given point in time and more concerned about achieving equality and balance over time and across a variety of circumstances. These activities are consistent with the priorities of the interdependent self, which is more common in collectivist cultures, rather than the independent self, which is more typical in Western cultures

(Markus and Kitayama, 1991). The Western emphasis on freedom and personal choice is baffling to some people in Japan, who view Westerners as "exercising freedom but having trouble making commitments to our choices" (White, 1987, p. 160).

Much of the achievement and social change activity of many Japanese women can be seen as role-directed rather than goal-directed (Iwao, 1993). A major focus of the interdependent self, which is more typical in Asian countries, is the fulfillment of role-appropriate behavior; a major focus of the independent self, found more typically in Western countries, is the promotion of specific, personal goals. Consistent with their goal-directed behavior, American women activists tend to work toward specific, short-term outcomes. Although goal-directed activity is essential for achieving social change, a singular focus on specific goals may foster dissatisfaction; one is constantly reminded of the gap between the desired outcome and the reality of the present. In contrast, fulfilling feminist roles to the best of one's ability and looking back occasionally at the progress one has made usually reveals at least some positive movement, which may help sustain commitment to a long-term change (Dunn and Cowan, 1993; Iwao, 1993).

Japanese feminisms and political change strategies are marked by a commitment to equality that also acknowledges differences between men and women, and a willingness to work within culturally prescribed roles to achieve social change. Diana Khor (1999) reminded her readers that working within culturally prescribed roles does not mean that women are trapped by these roles; they are choosing to work within existing systems. Rather than focusing on equality with men, Japanese feminists have tended to identify the limitations of economic independence and seek to structure a more holist vision of independence for women. Khor argued that working within women's spheres allows women to "grapple with differences among women within the country and connect with women beyond the country's border" (p. 653). The efforts of Japanese women activists focus on a wide range of women's and quality-of-life issues, such as care of the elderly, the creation of special care environments for troubled adolescents and handicapped individuals, access to homes for battered women, and such consumer issues as product safety and pollution (Khor, 1999).

Feminist Therapy in Japan

The previous sections have revealed some of the strengths, successes, and distinctive features of Japanese feminists. Likewise, feminist approaches to mental health have been distinctive. The first feminist counseling center in Japan was established in 1980 by Kiyomi Kawano. It was called *Nakama,* which means companion, and this word is used to identify feminist counseling centers on all four main islands of Japan. The word *nakama* also reflects the fact that Japanese feminist counselors do not promote themselves as experts on their clients' problems but as companions who accompany their clients on a journey, act as reflective listeners, and help women resolve the issues they bring to counseling. *Nakama* highlights the egalitarian quality of Japanese feminist counseling and its commitment to sisterhood. In general, Japanese feminist counselors with professional training and those trained as paraprofessionals work together cooperatively and effectively. In 1993, the Japanese Association of Feminist Counselor Practices and Studies was founded (Matsuyuki, 1998). Consistent with its commitment to egalitarianism, this organization is designed to meet the needs of both feminist counselors and former clients of feminist counseling. This diverse group of women meet together at an annual conference gathering (K. Kawano, personal communication, 1999; Matsuyuki, 1998).

Diana Khor (1999) noted that the beginnings of some feminist therapy groups coincided with the emergence of many other women's networking groups during the 1980s. She stated, "Feminist therapy groups provide counseling while operating as consciousness-raising groups, validating women's experiences and perspectives. These groups conduct therapy sessions emphasizing women's independence, decision-making for themselves, and/or counseling from women's perspectives" (p. 637). Feminist counseling in Japan incorporates many of the qualities of counseling that Ellyn Kaschak (1981) referred to as radical grassroots feminist therapy. These characteristics include a strong commitment to "the personal is political," group consciousness raising and egalitarianism, and the training of feminist counselors in alternative, nonacademic settings.

The heading of a brochure of the Feminist Counseling Center in Kyoto displays the phrase "the personal is political." Consistent with this logo, consciousness raising and group work are especially important in Japanese feminist counseling. One of the major texts available for purchase at the Kyoto Counseling Center is a translation of the NOW principles for conducting consciousness-raising groups, which was originally published in the United States during the early 1970s. The prominent office display of this source points to the importance Japanese feminist counselors place on making linkages between the personal and political aspects of women's lives. In addition to their commitment to social change, feminist counseling centers offer self-esteem groups, assertiveness training groups, support groups, academically oriented courses on the psychology of women, and groups on mother-daughter relationships. Individual counseling is another important service provided by feminist counseling centers, and the problems that clients regularly bring to counseling include eating disorders, addiction, sexuality issues, and problems associated with interpersonal trauma and sexual violence.

Perhaps the strong and sustained commitment of Japanese feminist counselors to both personal and political change is due, in part, to the fact that psychotherapy as a profession is not as well established in Japan as it is in North America. Feminist counselors are not required to conform to standards imposed by an outside regulatory body, and Japanese feminist counselors have not felt as compelled as their North American counterparts to seek legitimation by traditional institutional structures and professions. Compared to feminist practitioners in North America, Japanese feminists appear to be less likely to use traditional diagnostic labels and are less likely to feel compelled to use psychological theories and practices that tend to decontextualize problems and define problems in intrapsychic terms. It is important to note, however, that the absence of external regulation also has costs; Japanese feminist counselors are not eligible to receive reimbursement for services from the national health care system, limiting both client access to service and counselor access to support and funding. Feminist counselors struggle to provide a sliding fee scale to ensure that women have access to services (Kawano, 1990).

Japanese feminist counselors are sometimes trained as social workers and psychologists, but others have received their training primarily within specific feminist therapy centers that provide a yearlong training program for those who desire to become feminist counselors (Kawano, 1990, personal communication, 1999). Through coursework on the psychology of women, group work, and supervision of counseling, women trainees gain the competencies necessary to practice. As a result, feminist counseling is less "professional" than is its counterpart in the United States.

Feminist therapists trained in the West can learn much from Japanese feminist therapists who have retained a strong commitment to social change throughout their twenty-year history. In their now classic statement on therapy for social change, Edna Rawlings and Diane Carter (1977) noted that when feminist therapists are not vigilant about the conflicts of working in powerful social institutions, it is easy to inadvertently serve the status quo rather than meet important social change goals. Rawlings and Carter also noted that psychotherapy for social change is supported by the use of well-trained paraprofessionals and by the creation of counterinstitutions that exist independent of traditional mental health structures. Both of these features are present in Japanese feminist counseling.

Issues women bring to feminist counseling in Japan are often associated with the consequences of inequality that women face within work and home environments. Kiyomi Kawano's (1990) case study described a thirty-nine-year-old married woman and full-time secretary for a labor union who sought counseling initially because of difficulties relating to her eight-year-old daughter. The client, Hideko, had difficulty experiencing and expressing the culturally valued and idealized form of unconditional love for her daughter, who was also experiencing rejection and difficulty in child care and school environments. Second, Hideko was dissatisfied with her relationship with her husband, who participated in a very limited basis in household chores but was highly critical of Hideko for being an inadequate parent and for being "uneducated." He also belittled her commitments to an activist group concerned with environmental goals. Beyond these conflicts, spousal communication was limited. A third problem was Hideko's experience of sex discrimination at work. She was frustrated that she was expected to run personal errands for men, such as buying cigarettes or making tea.

The challenges and issues experienced by Hideko within her home are shared by many other Japanese women. Masami Matsuyuki (1998) noted that in many Japanese households, family members depend on women as mothers and spouses, but women have relatively few options for depending on others for support and nurture. Some Japanese ideals tend to equate maturity in women with three qualities of nurturing (Long, 1996). First, nurturing is associated with a physical relationship. The nurturer shoulders another person's burdens, physically relieves stress, and provides a calm environment for members of a household. One must "be there" physically, which demands a significant quantity of time, not just quality of investment. Second, anger and confrontation are seen as inconsistent with caregiving roles. When the demands of caregiving become extensive or excessive, asking others to compromise is not an option. As a consequence, the nurturer may cope by working even harder to create a calm environment or by "swallowing" her own feelings. Third, nurturing one's children, one's husband, and one's own parents is considered the woman's major role. All other obligations take on lesser importance.

Within feminist therapy, Hideko was able to express her emotional conflicts related to her daughter as well as her anger toward her husband. Hideko recognized that she did not easily practice the type of "motherhood mandate" idealized in Japan. She identified her "musts" and her internalization of the "good girl image," which required that she must be responsive to others' expectations and deny herself. She also began to express her concerns in her marriage and developed greater assertiveness at work. While progress was not always smooth, Hideko developed a new image of herself based on the validation of her own needs and desires.

Kiyomi Kawano (1990) proposed that had Hideko seen a traditional therapist, the therapist would have advised her to quit her job. From a traditional perspective, if Hideko were to quit her job, she would not need to fight about household chores with her spouse. She would give and gain greater love for her daughter if she had more time to spend with her daughter. Her husband would then take greater responsibility as head of household, searching for additional ways to support his family financially.

Kiyomi Kawano (1990) identified the roles of feminist therapy as follows:

1. To "implant the idea" that it is normal for women to explore nontraditional options, particularly those that fall outside the domain of caregiving
2. To search for a new identity based on self-discovery and self-realization
3. To examine and change behavior patterns that induce guilt and are self-defeating

As a part of this process, women learn to examine how their culture contributes to their emotional distress, especially distress marked by guilt, anxiety, and shame. After identifying these messages, women are able to develop a new sense of personal power and skills of self-expression and self-assertiveness. One of the challenges faced by women is giving themselves permission to express their own feelings. Some Japanese women have developed only a limited vocabulary for emotional expression, especially for self-expression. In feminist therapy, women gain permission to care for themselves: "A woman gets accustomed to talking, gains her own vocabulary and gets to know the joy of talking. This joy contains the power to open interpersonal relationships. This learning process requires time and energy directed to the woman herself" (Kawano, 1990, p. 47).

Low self-esteem, a limited sense of self, and lack of personal direction are some of the potential consequences of the realities of caregiving and thus become an important focus in feminist counseling in Japan (Matsuyuki, 1998). A major challenge is to help women transcend confining traditional roles without losing the community and family ties that offer women support and social stability. Japanese women's training in "adaptability" and sensitivity to others are important strengths, and they enhance women's survival skills and endurance over time. However, this adaptability training can limit Japanese women's ability to express their own needs directly, to think independently, or to make deliberate choices and take responsibility for these choices (Iwao, 1993; Kawano, 1990; Matsuyuki, 1998).

Taking self-responsibility is a difficult choice because social rewards for women in Japan are often tied to women's willingness to be compliant *(sunaosa)* or their ability to maintain interpersonal harmony *(ki-kubari)* (Iwao, 1993). As a result of these factors, Kiyomi Kawano (personal communication, 1999) noted that it is often helpful for Japanese women to receive training in assertive communication before they participate in consciousness-raising groups and therapy groups. In addition, a major challenge for Japanese feminist counselors is to identify concepts of independence and self-expression that do not resemble the self-contained individualism of the West but that allow women to develop skills in communication, competence, and responsibility while maintaining the capacity for interdependence (Matsuyuki, 1998). One such concept of independence is referred to in Japan as *jiritsu,* or socially sensitive independence.

Yukari Kamitani's (1993, 1996) studies of the structure of *jiritsu* in Japanese women's lives suggest that it consists of two major components: (1) independence, which involves free decision making and self-assertion, mutual noninterference, as well as self-confidence and self-reliance; and (2) integrated dependence, which includes sympathy and tolerance, mutual reliance, and the capacity for interdependence. The construct of *jiritsu* shares similar themes with relationship differentiation as theorized by relational cultural theory (Jordan, 2000). Although possibilities for integrating relational/cultural therapy and Japanese relationship concepts are promising, it is also important to note that relational-cultural theory (see Chapter 4) is centered primarily in Western concepts of the self and will need to be modified by models of the interdependent self in order to be fully useful in a Japanese context (Kawano, personal communication, 1999).

CONCLUDING COMMENTS

The situations of women around the world are complex and cannot be adequately characterized in a brief commentary. It is my hope that the brief observations in this chapter point to the value of exploring gender-related issues as they are shaped by culture. An encouraging development is the growing interest on the part of American psychologists with global issues. A recent position paper on cultural and gender awareness in international psychology (Rice and Ballou, 2002) calls on psychologists to become more aware of colonialism and global imperialism and the ways in which dominant traditions in psychology can contribute to inadequate and oppressive practices. The position paper identifies five principles, the first of which calls on psychologists to value the history, worldviews, ways of knowing, standpoints, and modes of functioning of diverse people around the world. The exploration of culture-specific and culturally relevant concepts, and an ecological perspective, which focuses on how individuals accommodate themselves to the realities of their circumstances, is important for furthering knowledge about and communication with women throughout the world.

A second theme emphasizes the value of pluralism and difference as the foundation for collaborative work with mental health workers around the world. This principle does not imply that one adopts an uncritical cultural relativistic stance but rather a recognition and appreciation for the multiple methods and points of view and their associated strengths and limitations. A third principle speaks to the importance of acknowledging power differences, reducing power differences, and working toward egalitarian relationships. The fourth principle recommends the critical analysis of dominant psychologies, including the way in which Western methods may be used to inappropriately impose Western individualistic norms on women around the world. The final principle speaks to the profound influence that external macrosystemic factors may have on individuals. Global economic forces, geopolitical forces, and social structural arrangements that privilege some individuals and harm others have a powerful impact on women around the world and must become an important emphasis in a psychology that is to be relevant to people around the world (Rice and Ballou, 2002).

Chapter 7

Feminist Postmodernism, Lesbian/Queer Feminisms, and Third-Wave Feminisms

This chapter summarizes recent contributions to diversity within feminism and feminist therapy. The first approach, feminist postmodernism, emerged as a new force in feminist theory in the 1980s and has continued to be a powerful influence as well as focus of debate throughout the 1990s and the early twenty-first century. In contrast to the second-wave feminisms, which were embedded in social activism, postmodern feminism emerged from within academic disciplines and has become a method for considering the changing nature of knowledge and the limitations of that which is called knowledge. It has become a foundation for questioning existing theory and thinking about the meanings and implications of difference and diversity. As noted by Ann Cacoullos (2001), "the objects or subjects of oppression themselves are seen and acknowledged to be more diverse, such that the phenomena being investigated and theorized are far more complex than they were thirty years ago" (p. 72).

Lesbian and queer theory as well as the third-wave feminisms represent specific ways of approaching diversity, and both approaches have been influenced substantially by postmodern thought. I use the lesbian and queer feminisms to illustrate the way in which second-wave lesbian feminisms (see Chapter 3) have been revised as they have been reexamined through postmodern feminist lenses. The final approach, third-wave feminism, represents feminist thought that has been developed by the daughters of the second-wave generation.

POSTMODERN FEMINISM

To use the following items as a form of self-assessment, please respond to each statement with a "yes" or "no." Agreement with the following items suggests agreement with the principles of postmodern feminist theory.

_____ 1. One of the most important features of feminist theory is the exploration of differences among individuals rather than their commonalities and similarities.

_____ 2. Knowledge and identity, including feminist theory and feminist identity, are unstable and variable; they are influenced by culture, context, time, and life experience.

_____ 3. Feminist theory should challenge dualistic concepts such as masculine/feminine, black/white, objective/subjective, and rational/emotional because these binary constructs distort and oversimplify reality.

_____ 4. One of the major roles of feminist theory is to reveal how power and privilege influence "the canon" and that which we value as knowledge.

_____ 5. The positionalities, or social locations and identities of both clients and therapists, have powerful influences on therapy relationships and should be addressed explicitly.

Patricia Waugh (1998) proposed that the term *postmodernism* is associated with a type of "end-of-millennium consciousness" (p. 177) that has exerted an "enormous grip" on academic disciplines. Postmodernism is linked to a "bewilderingly diverse" array of cultural practices and theories, and "is best thought of as a 'mood' arising out of a sense of the collapse of all those foundations of modern thought that seemed to guarantee a reasonably stable sense of Truth, Knowledge, Self and Value" (p. 178). Janis Bohan's (2002) summary of this "mood" noted that "postmodern thought urges us to doubt our capacity to know anything with certainty and rejects the very possibility of grand theories that are capable of capturing the infinite variety of specific, located experiences" (p. 74). Postmodern perspectives raise metatheoretical questions about the role and function of theory and research in many disciplines, and are "deconstructive" in the sense that "they seek to distance us from and make us skeptical about beliefs concerning truth, knowledge, power, the self, and language that are often taken for granted" (Flax, 1987, p. 624). Postmodern theorists challenge the existence of a stable coherent self that is capable of reason and self-insight, and the belief that reason can provide a reliable and objective basis of knowledge or that knowledge based on reason is "real and unchanging" (p. 624), as well as ahistorical and independent of the context in which it is created. Postmodernists also question the assumption that individuals can escape a predetermined existence and live autonomous, free lives by implementing laws of reason, and the notion that knowledge and truth can be defined in ways that are independent and free of power dynamics. Postmodern theorists argue that claims about truth or knowledge tend "to universalize the particular and the idiosyncratic, to privilege the ethnocentric, and to conflate truth with those prejudices that advantage the knower" (Hawkesworth, 1989, p. 554). In addition, knowledge can be seen as "the imposition of form on the world rather than the result of discovery" (Hawkesworth, 1989, p. 536); the notion of "Truth" should be rejected; it promotes a "destructive illusion" (p. 554).

Since the 1980s, postmodern approaches to feminism have been promoted as ways to transcend the limitations of other feminisms. Feminist postmodern theorists reject the search for a distinctive, universal female standpoint because personal identities are influenced by other individual differences and standpoints, such as race, ethnicity, sexual orientation, class, and disability. Major goals of postmodern feminists are to complicate or problematize the concept of gender as well as to resist any efforts to "homogenize" the experiences of women (Peterson and Runyan, 1999). A postmodern view proposes that reality is embedded within social relationships and historical contexts, is socially created or invented, and is reproduced through power relationships. Rather than searching for *a* truth, the inquirer focuses on how meaning is negotiated and how persons in authority maintain control over these meanings. Feminist postmodernism also emphasizes how truth is shaped by history, the social context, and the views and life experiences of the knower. Knowledge can never be neutral or objective. Feminist postmodernism provides not only a framework for critiquing androcentric biases but also a metatheoretical perspective for evaluating the claims of feminist researchers and theorists (Allen and Baber, 1992; Harding, 1986; Hare-Mustin and Marecek, 1990; Hawkesworth, 1989; Morrow, 2000; Singer, 1992; Wilkinson, 2001).

A major tool of feminist postmodern analysis is deconstruction, which involves challenging bipolar constructs and definitions (e.g., masculine and feminine), showing how reality is created rather than existing in a "natural" or "true" state, and demonstrating how reality is often defined by those with greater power in society. Dualistic concepts are rejected because they reinforce existing power relations. For example, the first term in most bipolar word pairs assumes primacy (e.g., rational versus irrational) over the derivative or "weaker" term (Scott, 1988). Polarized constructs also constrain our ability to see the multiple diversities and positions that exist or to think in nonoppositional categories. For example, when strong is compared to weak, individuals tend to see these words as opposite categories. However, if strong is compared to qualities such as respected, principled, or effective, the bipolar nature of comparisons disappears and it becomes possible to think in nonoppositional or integrative ways (Peterson and Runyan, 1999; Scott, 1988). Deconstructive efforts reveal that constructs such as masculine/feminine, heterosexuality/homosexuality, and white/black are creations that have meaning only when they are contrasted with each other (Morrow, 2000; Wilkinson, 2001).

Postmodern feminist theorists focus primarily on connections between meaning and power, and their inquiries emphasize the power of language as it represents ideas, concepts, and power (Hare-Mustin and Marecek, 1990). When referring to language, postmodern theorists are interested in much more than a system of grammatical rules and methods of expression. Language refers to any method by which "meaning is constructed and cultural practices organized and by which, accordingly, people represent and understand their world, including who they are and how they relate to others" (Scott, 1988, p. 34). The analysis of language reveals how social relationships are understood, institutions are structured, and collective identities are established. Analysis of language also facilitates the examination of how meanings change and how power is communicated. Postmodern feminists often use techniques such as discourse analysis and conversation analysis to consider how language conveys power through mechanisms such as metaphors and dualistic constructs, as well as how "discourses structure both the material conditions of women's lives, and their subjective experiences" (Wilkinson, 2001, p. 25).

Feminist Postmodernism and Other Feminist Epistemologies

In order to understand the contributions of feminist postmodern theory, it is useful to contrast it with two other feminist proposals for understanding "truth": feminist empiricism, which became prominent within feminist psychology in the 1970s; and feminist standpoint theory, which became a significant tool within feminist psychology during the 1980s (Gergen, 2001). Feminist empiricism, which is defined and described in the chapter on liberal feminist theory (see Chapter 2), relies on scientific techniques that are designed to control subjective biases but do not challenge the basic structure of knowledge. Feminist empiricism is based on faith in the "primacy of the senses" (Hawkesworth, 1989, p. 535) and, in contrast to feminist postmodern thought, is built on the assumption that there is a "truth" to be known. Through the elimination of the distorting lenses of biased observers, feminist researchers can presumably arrive at objective knowledge and "unmediated truth about the world" (Hawkesworth, 1989, p. 535). However, such "objective" research methods may also result in context stripping, or the erasure of the specific circumstances and contexts that often modify the "truth" being sought (Morrow, 2000).

A second approach, feminist standpoint theory, has been most closely associated with the belief systems and approaches of cultural feminism, including ecofeminism, and some forms of radical and socialist feminism (see Chapter 4). Feminist standpoint theories, which focus on a unique "women's" point of view and view of reality, have been criticized as being "essentialist" or assuming that there is *one* way of knowing and experiencing that is uniquely female. Elizabeth Spelman (1988) stated,

> Posing an essential "womanness" has the effect of making women inessential in a variety of ways. First of all, if there is an essential womanness that all women have and have always had, then we needn't know anything about any woman in particular. . . . If all women have the same story "as women," we don't need a chorus of voices to tell the story. (p. 158)

If one assumes that women have a distinctive and more complete perspective, then one must also assume that there is some common experience that women share that would lead to a shared vision. Critics propose that standpoint theories put forth universal theories about women and neglect the diverse voices of women of color, working-class women, and lesbians. Jane Flax (1987) contended that feminist standpoint theory "may require the suppression of the important and discomforting voices of persons with experiences unlike our own" (p. 633). A second criticism is that feminist standpoint theories may place men's and women's strengths into dichotomous categories. In their efforts to reject an overemphasis on instrumental reason, standpoint theorists may overemphasize a "unique" female knowledge that is embedded in emotion, care, and intuition (Bohan, 1993; Hawkesworth, 1989). Third, standpoint theories rely on overly optimistic beliefs that women are not substantially damaged by their oppression and are able to retain superior observational and comprehension skills. Unlike men, women are assumed to be "free of determination from their own participation in relations of domination such as those rooted in the social relations of race, class, or homophobia" (Flax, 1987, p. 642). Hawkesworth (1989) noted: "Given the diversity and fallibility of all human knowers, there is no good reason to believe that women are any less prone to error, deception, or distortion than men" (p. 544). Thus, standpoint theories can contain biases that resemble those which have permeated traditional androcentric perspectives.

In contrast to more traditional standpoint theorists, some women-of-color and lesbian theorists have articulated standpoints that are intended to describe the unique experiences of specific groups of women rather than women in general. For example, the standpoints of specific groups of women of color (see Chapter 5) reveal the ways in which complex social interactions of race, gender, class, sexual orientation, nationality, and religion influence and modify the social identity of women.

Strengths and Critiques of Postmodern Feminism

Postmodernism feminism has contributed to heightened awareness of how power and knowledge are interconnected (Butler, 1992). It has encouraged an appreciation of diversity and difference, promoted a new appreciation of pluralism, and reminded theorists and activists that feminist voices cannot be reduced to a common denominator

(Cacoullos, 2001; Hawkesworth, 1989). It has also supported the development of feminist theories of difference and encourages all feminists to question the ways in which their own paradigms "serve to subordinate and erase that which they seek to explain" (Butler, 1992, p. 5). Susan Bordo (1990) cautioned, however, that "attentiveness to difference" may not necessarily lead to the "adequate representation of difference" (p. 140); "attending *too* vigilantly to difference can just as problematically construct an Other who is an exotic alien, a breed apart" (p. 140).

Some feminist critics have suggested that postmodernism can promote a "slide into relativism" because all realities are placed into question, including the notion of women's oppression. If reality and the self are merely constructions, the individual has no real power to reflect on her or his existence, and to resist or challenge ways in which her or his life is constricted (Alcoff, 1988; Allen and Baber, 1992). If this view is taken to its logical conclusion, none of the statuses of race, class, and gender can be used to validate or support one's calls for justice. If all truth is created and relative, no group can legitimately make claims about injustice, and "once again, underneath we are all the same" (Alcoff, 1988, p. 421). Feminist politics, which are based on the perception of the shared needs of a group, become impossible, and feminism exists only as a mode of inquiry (Cacoullos, 2001).

A second criticism is that if there is no "truth," feminism is limited to reaction rather than creation; the only remaining feminism becomes "a wholly negative feminism, deconstructing everything and refusing to construct anything" (Alcoff, 1988, p. 418). Nancy Hartsock (1987) stated, "For those of us who want to understand the world systematically in order to change it, postmodernist theories at their best give little guidance" (pp. 190-191). Alcoff (1988) added, "If gender is simply a social construct, the need and even the possibility of a feminist politics becomes immediately problematical" (p. 420).

A related concern is that postmodern theories are often highly complex and couched in language that is generally inaccessible to those outside of the academic world (Hartsock, 1987). Joanna Russ (1998) characterized postmodern theory as being detached and disconnected to real experience and consisting primarily of "people theorizing from other people's theories about yet more theory" (p. 435). Concerns about the void between theory and real life, the potential for distancing between academic theory and activism, and the limited accessibility of theory represent ongoing challenges that need to be addressed if this approach is to hold significant merit for dealing effectively with women's diversity.

In an effort to propose an approach to postmodernism that transcends these criticisms, Patricia Waugh (1998) has differentiated between "strong" postmodernism and "weak" postmodernism. She argued that a "strong" position, which questions all efforts to discover truth and proposes that the only absolute is uncertainty and shifting and disembodied realities, "threatens the entire identity of feminism as a politics and tries to discredit the emancipatory ideals which have guided it in the past" (p. 190). However, a "weak" position proposes that although our ability to achieve knowledge and objectivity is partial and our models must be open to modification, feminist models can provide an important basis for developing actions based on a shared sense of values, personal significance, and collective consciousness.

In general, feminists have argued that postmodern models should be viewed as fallible but useful. When used flexibly and in conjunction with other feminist theories, they can help feminists create pictures of reality that look more "like a tapestry of many threads and hues than one woven in a single color" (Fraser and Nicholson, 1990, p. 35). Linda Singer (1992) recommended that feminists use postmodern ideas in a strategic fashion in order to increase the strength and viability of feminism in a complicated world. Feminists whose work has been influenced by postmodernism indicate that its most useful purpose is to enhance feminists' abilities to avoid making inappropriate generalizations about men and women and to facilitate the creation of complex theories in which gender is considered one of many relevant categories that include race, class, ethnicity, and sexual orientation (Fraser and Nicholson, 1990).

Postmodernism and Social Constructionism in Feminist Psychology

Janis Bohan (2002) identified social constructionism as one of a variety of approaches to postmodern theorizing, and Mazarin Banaji (1993) called social constructionism "psychology's code word for postmodernism" (p. 261). Mary Gergen (2001) proposed that postmodernism has both deconstructive and reconstructive implications for psychology. While deconstruction entails dissolving meanings, social constructionism offers opportunities for creating models of meaning that emphasize how social influences are integrated within and between persons as well as within communities of persons.

At present, a social constructionistic model is the dominant perspective within the psychology of women as an academic and research discipline (Crawford and Unger, 2004; Gergen, 2001; Matlin, 2004; Morrow, 2000) and is generally consistent with a "weak" feminist postmodern perspective (Waugh, 1998; Wilkinson, 2001). A foundation of social constructionism is the notion that it is not possible to directly apprehend reality, and that the lenses we use to observe behavior actively shape perceptions. That which we see as reality consists of hypotheses, which are also influenced by the contexts in which knowledge or reality are created. Although social constructionism can range from "weak" to "strong" variations (Bohan, 2002), the dominant version of social constructionism in feminist psychology can be summarized as follows: meanings associated with experiences and events vary; the same experience can be observed from a variety of perspectives and can be imbued with divergent meanings.

A feature of social constructionism in feminist psychology is the assumption that "one does not have gender; one does gender" (Allen and Baber, 1992, p. 13; West and Zimmerman, 1987). Stephanie Riger (1992) elaborated, "Gender is something we enact, not an inner core or constellation of traits that we express; it is a pattern of social organization that structures the relations, especially the power relations, between women and men" (p. 737). In keeping with this principle, gender is not merely a static subject variable that exists within the person, but is continuously shaped by multiple levels of interaction. At a social structural level, gender becomes a form of social classification that determines the availability of resources and power to women and men. At the interpersonal level, gender acts as a cue or stimulus that informs individuals how to behave toward men and women. Finally, at an individual level, a person's self-definition as a gendered individual influences the manner in which specific behaviors and traits are attributed to the self (Crawford and Unger, 2000). From a postmodern/social constructionist perspective, important questions about gender include the following: What does gender mean? How is gender created and shaped? Besides difference or similarity, what else is gender? Who benefits from constructions of gender that emphasize similarity or difference (Hare-Mustin and Marecek, 1990; Riger, 1992)?

Feminist psychologists have generally used the word *sex* to refer to biological aspects of being male or female, and the term *gender* to refer to psychological, social, and cultural experiences and characteristics associated with the biological aspects of being female or male. Jeanne Marecek (2002) noted, however, that when gender and sex are conceptualized as distinct and separate categories, "sex stands as some immutable bedrock that remains after gender is stripped away" (p. 14). In reality, biological "facts" are influenced by assumptions and cultural values, and biological sex is much more diverse than previously thought (Golden, 2004). Sex *as well as* gender is influenced by social experience, and for many individuals, neither sex nor gender is fixed and stable. Consistent with the postmodern thinking rejection of two-box categories, Carla Golden (2004) recommended abandoning the sex-gender division and instead stretching our concepts of gender and sex to "diversify and multiply the possibilities" (p. 93).

Mary Gergen (2001) identified the following four themes as major contributions of postmodernism to feminist psychology:

1. The permission it provides to critique narrow ways of conducting "science"
2. Its recognition of the limitations of language and thus the valuing of multiple voices, narrative methods, and creative forms of writing
3. Its invitation to therapists and researchers to practice reflexivity, which encourages continual self-examination and questioning of one's approaches to knowledge
4. Its recognition of the important role of values in knowledge making, which allows one to connect the personal and political

Although it remains important for feminist therapists to carefully consider the strengths and limitations of the various feminist theories, a postmodern perspective does not require the individual to endorse one form of feminism and reject others. Feminist postmodernism or social constructionism provides a framework for organizing the multiple truths of women's lives. It offers much to feminist psychologists because it "embraces complexity and contradiction" and "surpasses theories that offer single-cause deterministic explanations about patriarchy and gender relations" (Gavey, 1989, p. 472).

CONTEMPORARY LESBIAN FEMINISMS AND QUEER THEORY

To use the following items as a form of self-assessment, please respond to each statement with a "yes" or "no." Agreement with the following items suggests agreement with important themes in contemporary lesbian feminist and queer theory.

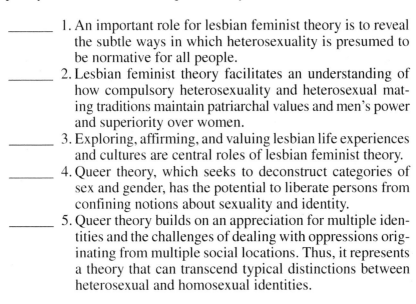

_____ 1. An important role for lesbian feminist theory is to reveal the subtle ways in which heterosexuality is presumed to be normative for all people.

_____ 2. Lesbian feminist theory facilitates an understanding of how compulsory heterosexuality and heterosexual mating traditions maintain patriarchal values and men's power and superiority over women.

_____ 3. Exploring, affirming, and valuing lesbian life experiences and cultures are central roles of lesbian feminist theory.

_____ 4. Queer theory, which seeks to deconstruct categories of sex and gender, has the potential to liberate persons from confining notions about sexuality and identity.

_____ 5. Queer theory builds on an appreciation for multiple identities and the challenges of dealing with oppressions originating from multiple social locations. Thus, it represents a theory that can transcend typical distinctions between heterosexual and homosexual identities.

Lesbian feminist theory has been characterized by a diversity of viewpoints since its earliest years. Some radical feminists viewed lesbian identity as a profoundly political choice that allowed women to achieve complete freedom from patriarchy and male dominance as well as make complete commitments to women and political causes that supported women's liberation (Bunch, [1972] 1987; Gonda, 1998; Radicalesbians, 1973) (see Chapter 3). Radical lesbian feminists embraced the notion that anyone could choose to be lesbian, sometimes implying that "lesbians are the best feminists" (Garber, 2001, p. 20) because they are fully absorbed in women's causes and women's lives. Other lesbian feminists described radical feminists as "de-sexing" lesbian experience, and viewed lesbian sexuality and lesbian erotic expression and sexual practice as crucial to identity (Gonda, 1998). As noted by Kathy Rudy (2001), "definite tensions existed between those who choose lesbian life for reasons of desire and those who choose it for feminist politics; each group imagined the other was inauthentic" (p. 195). These tensions illustrate the variety of assumptions that can emerge within as well as between groups of feminists.

An important theme in lesbian feminism has focused on the nature of lesbian community and the degree to which women-identified women benefit from forming separate women's communities that allow them to develop ethical models embedded in the unique attributes of women who care exclusively for other women (Gonda, 1998; Rudy, 2001). In recent years, lesbians who have been attracted to the social constructionist and postmodern assumptions associated with queer theory have focused on diversity within the lesbian and homosexual experience. At times, they have also labeled lesbians who emphasize the unique, shared features of lesbian experience and community as "essentialist" (Garber, 2001; Rudy, 2001). Many lesbian feminists who have been attracted to queer theory are from a younger generation than radical feminists of the 1970s, and the different philosophies and goals of this younger generation have led to substantial diversity within current lesbian feminist thought.

The following discussion of contemporary lesbian feminism and queer theory is cursory and selective at best. I have chosen to highlight those aspects of lesbian feminism and queer theory that illustrate some of the key principles of postmodern feminism, such as their challenge of bipolar categories and the power dynamics associated with bipolar categories, and their contributions to an understanding of the fluidity and complexity of identity.

Compulsory Heterosexuality, Heterosexism, and Lesbian Experience

Adrienne Rich's ([1980] 1989) classic and frequently reproduced commentary on compulsory heterosexuality is a cornerstone of lesbian feminist critiques of heterosexism. Adrienne Rich proposed that compulsory heterosexuality has been imposed on all women, supports and perpetuates male dominance, and limits women's creative energy and opportunities to form positive bonds with one another. In her efforts to redefine lesbian existence, Rich used the term *lesbian continuum* to represent "a range—through each woman's life and throughout history—of woman-identified experience, not simply the fact that woman has had or consciously desired genital sexual experience with another woman" ([1980] 1989, p. 129). Consistent with postmodern feminist critiques, Rich pointed to the problems of conceptualizing identity through the lens of bipolar constructs such as masculine and feminine, heterosexual and homosexual. In keeping with the notion that identity is complex, Rich noted that lesbian experience includes various forms of "primary intensity between and among women, including the sharing of a rich inner life, the bonding against male tyranny, and the giving and receiving of practical and political support" (p. 129). Rich (1986) warned that the complexities of this continuum and lesbian feminism identity should not be confused with or oversimplified as "lifestyle shopping" (p. 73). She expressed concern that some women would use the continuum as "a safe way to describe their felt connections with women, without having to share in the risks and threats of lesbian existence" (p. 73). An examination of the privilege and power associated with heterosexuality is central to an informed understanding of the lesbian continuum.

Adrienne Rich explored ways in which compulsory heterosexuality becomes the foundation for heterosexism, which can be defined as the assumption that heterosexuality is the only natural form of emotional and sexual expression. Lesbian feminists highlight the necessity of analyzing heterosexuality as an institution rather than merely a sexual preference. More specifically, lesbian feminists examine the manner in which heterosexuality dictates how some members of society, especially heterosexual men, hold greater power than others. Maintaining an almost universal female heterosexuality is an important mechanism of male domination because it guarantees women's sexual availability to men. Women's subordination to men is solidified through various heterosexual norms and traditions, including heterosexual romantic traditions and rites of passage, women's acts of caring for men, prohibitions against cross-dressing, heterosexual pornography and erotica, and heterosexualized humor and dress. Issues such as violence against women and children, sexual harassment, and physical enslavement are also consequences of patriarchal power (Calhoun, 1997).

In addition to analyzing how heterosexuality organizes social and reproductive relationships, lesbian feminism has evaluated heterosexuality as an ideology that subtly erases or prohibits lesbianism and homosexuality. Heterosexism promotes the view that male-female relationships are a fundamental building block of society; in contrast, same-sex intimate relationships are seen as holding no social reality. Lesbian feminists argue that the critical analysis and deconstruction of heterosexist assumptions in society and feminist theory are essential for creating truly liberating feminisms (Calhoun, 1997; Kitzinger, 1996).

Celia Kitzinger (1996) argued that lesbian feminist theorists need not only to deconstruct the assumption of heterosexuality but also to work toward a true inclusion of lesbianism in theory, research, and practice (Kitzinger, 1996; Rose, 1996). The phrase *compulsory heterosexuality* conveys the reality that heterosexuality remains a defining construct and the standard for normalcy for all people. In keeping with their efforts to make lesbian life central to theory, lesbian feminist theorists have emphasized themes that affirm and embrace lesbian life experiences, such as the cultural components of being lesbian. The components include the impact of growing up lesbian in a heterosexual society, the coming-out process, lesbian culture and lesbian lifestyles, lesbian intimate partnership and parenting concerns, differences between lesbian and gay identity, and the life experiences of lesbians who represent diversity in terms of race, ethnicity, and social class (Calhoun, 1997). Choices related to acts of coming out are also important aspects of lesbian feminist theory and social action. The process of coming out and being out requires one to publicly declare one's sexual orientation, which deconstructs heterosexuality. Coming out is an integral component of lesbian feminist theory because it decentralizes heterosexuality, thus makes lesbian experience visible (Stein, 1997).

Diversity Among Lesbians

Linda Garber (2001) noted that in the late 1970s women of color challenged the commonality of "lesbian experience," particularly the notion that independence from men and patriarchy would resolve issues related to classism, racism, and other forms of discrimination. Some radical lesbians believed that "all systems of discrimination derive from sexism, and that therefore racism and sexism are less of a problem for lesbians than for others" (Garber, 2001, p. 20). The works of lesbian feminists of color (e.g., Anzaldúa, 1990; Moraga and Anzaldúa, 1983) challenged this assumption, which resulted in the acknowledgment that "the special attributes we had associated with womanness actually described only the womanness of whites" (Rudy, 2001, p. 202).

Lesbians of color have made important contributions by critiquing white lesbian feminist theory for not attending to the diversity of lesbians and the multiple and intersecting discriminations faced by lesbians of color. Beverly Greene (1997) indicated that the concerns of lesbians of color are often rendered invisible in the scholarly research of both women of color and lesbians. In addition, the "public discourse on the sexuality of particular racial and ethnic groups is shaped by processes that pathologize those [racial and ethnic] groups" (Hammonds, 1997, p. 138). In other words, the sexuality of lesbians of color is often seen as perverse both within racial or ethnic groups and by society in general (Hammonds, 1997). Aída Húrtado (1996) expanded on this problem with the following words: "Many lesbians of Color are not only thought of as traitors to their ethnic/racial communities, but also are often accused of catching 'white women's disease'" (p. 23). Similarly, Audré Lorde (1984) stated that Black lesbian feminists are seen as a threat to "black nationhood" and that "lesbianism" is seen as a white women's problem. Thus, lesbians of color are caught between "the racism of white women and the homophobia of their sisters" (Lorde, 1984, p. 122).

Lesbian feminists of color note that one must understand the specific cultural factors which influence lesbian experience within specific ethnic groups (Greene, 1997; Lorde, 1984). The experiences of lesbians of color have contributed to the growing recognition that identity, including lesbian identity, is not stable but may vary across situations, contexts, and time. For example, lesbians of color often learn to negotiate multiple identities that may sometimes be fragmented. Depending on the issue, context, and demands of a situation, they may identify themselves primarily as persons of color, as females, or as homosexual (Rudy, 2001). In addition, privilege and oppression are not stable and uniform but may vary according to demands of a situation. For example, a white lesbian may experience harassment and discrimination in the workplace but may act in oppressive ways toward women of color within the lesbian community.

Queer Theory

Lesbians of color have offered perspectives that are consistent with postmodern feminism by pointing to the variable and often fragmented nature of identity, privilege, and oppression. Queer theory has offered another approach to conceptualizing diversity. Some lesbian feminists have embraced queer theory, believing a shift from lesbian to queer theory allows for a discussion of sexuality that transcends identity categories and dichotomies associated with constructs such as gender and race. Elizabeth Weed (1997) proposed that queer and feminist theory can be seen as "two branches of the same family tree of knowledge and politics" (p. vii).

Queer theory has been influenced substantially by postmodern perspectives. It seeks to reexamine widespread assumptions about the connections between gender and sexuality, and explores the experiences of people who are marginalized or disparaged because of their sexual orientation and/or gendered experiences. These groups include lesbian, gay, bisexual, transvestite, transsexual, and transgendered persons. Queer theory calls for the elimination of particular identities of sexual orientation, and this shift in orientation allows for an overarching, inclusive umbrella that may incorporate "queer heterosexuals" (Jagdose, 1996). Some queer theorists argue that the categories gay and lesbian create artificial divides between these two groups and that deconstructing these categories will result in a collapse of divisions between other groups as well (e.g., heterosexual/homosexual) (Esterberg, 1997). In general, queer theory emphasizes "challenging that which is perceived as normal" (Rudy, 2001, p. 212), including "the idea that sexuality has any 'normal' parameters at all" (p. 215). Arlene Stein (1997) noted that the term *queer* "signifies the possibility of constructing a nonnormative sexuality that includes all who feel disenfranchised by dominant sexual norms" (p. 192). This definition may include anyone or anything that is not "completely heterosexual" (p. 192) and supports ambiguity or the impossibility of dividing identity into "us and them" categories.

Queer theory allows for a discussion of sexuality that transcends identity categories such as gender and race because it emphasizes the possibility of experiencing a multiplicity of overlapping female sexualities. For example, queer theory increases the visibility of Black women's sexuality by allowing Black women to experience multiple female sexualities. The need to compare Black and white lesbians, or the expectation that Black women need to choose lesbian as a primary identity and race as a secondary identity disappears (Hammonds, 1997). In addition to their openness to racial, class, and ethnic diversity, queer communities expect members to experience multiple or potentially contradictory identities, which allows for strategic coalition-building efforts on a variety of social issues. Furthermore, those who identify themselves as lesbian are less likely to feel confined by rule-based or politically correct versions of how one should act or what one should believe as a lesbian (Rudy, 2001).

Despite these advantages, queer theory is sometimes critiqued for ignoring oppression and experiences that are specific to women (Esterberg, 1997). Efforts to break down divisions between men and women of diverse sexualities can inadvertently contribute to "the valorization of those things associated with the male, public sphere" (Rudy, 2001, p. 216) and decreased attention to the realities of women, especially the relational and caretaking roles that are often central to women's lives. Removing the notion of identity does not change the fact that a lesbian is a woman who negotiates a world that discriminates against her for both her lesbianism and her womanhood. Thus, many lesbian feminists argue that a lesbian feminist theory needs to be attentive to issues of diversity and the multiplicity of identities among lesbians. However, it is premature to remove gender or identity from discussion because oppression due to gender and other identities (e.g., race, ethnicity) is pervasive (Esterberg, 1997; Garber, 2001).

In summary, lesbian and queer feminisms have played significant roles in decentralizing heteronormality, challenging the dichotomous categories of heterosexual and homosexual, and critiquing the notion that identities are fixed and stable. Both lesbian feminism and queer theory emphasize the importance of

- exploring multiple identities and their relationships to oppression;
- deconstructing and decentering assumptions about normative heterosexuality as well as the subtle and not-to-subtle ways in

which heterosexism permeates psychological theory and notions about normality;
- emphasizing social action; and
- identifying and appreciating the diversity among those with marginalized sexualities with regard to age, social class, race, culture, and ethnicity.

THIRD-WAVE FEMINISMS

To use the following items as a form of self-assessment, please respond to each statement with a "yes" or "no." Agreement with these items suggests agreement with important themes in third-wave feminist theory.

_____ 1. To be relevant to new generations of women and men, feminists must become less politically correct, more flexible, and more tolerant of apparent contradictions.

_____ 2. Conveying feminist ideas and messages can often best be accomplished by using contemporary methods such as music, media, and the Internet. These tools are also useful assets for feminist therapy.

_____ 3. Helping women overcome the limiting effects of internalized cultural messages about beauty and body ideals is one of the most important targets of feminist activism and therapy.

_____ 4. Successful activism requires the building of coalitions across boundaries of gender, race, culture, and sexual orientation.

_____ 5. Autobiographical accounts are especially valuable learning tools because of their accessibility, appeal to a wide audience, and ability to demonstrate tangibly how individuals deal with contradictions and paradoxes in their lives.

During the 1990s, a group of primarily young adult women (Generation Xers) identified themselves as third-wave feminists (e.g., Walker, 1995). Third-wave-feminist Barbara Findlen (1995) stated, "We are the first generation for whom feminism has been entwined in the fabric of our lives; it is natural that many of us are feminists"

(p. xii). Third-wave feminists have been critical of some second-wave feminists, sometimes characterizing second-wave feminists as being somewhat inflexible and dogmatic, too concerned with political correctness, and as promoting unspoken but influential "rules" about what one must believe and do to be a "real" feminist (Walker, 1995). Some young feminists identify their efforts to live by these "rules" as impinging on their creativity and as contributing to a lack of spontaneity, artificial efforts to "measure up," and misguided efforts to gain the approval of second-wave feminists. As a result, a major goal of young feminists has been to reclaim feminism on their own terms, to correct some of the inflexibilities and mistakes of the previous generation, and to challenge distortions of feminism that have permeated American culture in recent years. Consistent with postmodern themes, third-wave feminists have both deconstructed previous feminisms and have contributed to reconstructed ways of conceptualizing feminism (Dicker and Piepmeier, 2003; Hernández and Rehman, 2002).

As daughters of the second wave, third-wave feminists recognize the major economic opportunities available to them as well as the significant social change brought about by the previous generation's contributions to activist causes associated with such issues as sexual harassment, reproductive freedom, and affirmative action. However, they have been critical of the previous generation's limited progress combating major social issues such as the AIDS epidemic, violence against women, economic crises, and ecological concerns. In keeping with their desire to endorse a feminism of action, Generation X third-wave women have been involved in a wide variety of activist causes, such as voter registration, affordable health care, parental laws related to abortion, sex education, violence against women, and the combating of subtle forms of racism. In addition to major concerns addressed by second-wave feminists, third-wave feminists have been concerned with issues such as HIV infection, equal/gendered access to the Internet, global issues in feminism, child sexual abuse, eating disorders and body image, self-mutilation, and sexual health (Baumgardner and Richards, 2000; Hernández and Rehman, 2002). An emphasis on activism and organizing across categories can be seen in the mission statement of Third Wave, which reads, "Third Wave is a member-driven multiracial, multicultural, multisexuality national nonprofit organization devoted to feminist and youth activism for change" (cited in Heywood and Drake, 1997, p. 7).

Deborah Siegel (1997) suggested that a major task of third-wave feminists is consciousness changing rather than consciousness raising. While feminists of the second wave needed to raise awareness of sexism and other oppressions, third-wave feminists face the challenge of changing the perceptions of those whose education about feminism has consisted of hearing pejorative descriptions of feminists (e.g., as hating men or as refusing to shave their legs) or being exposed to backlash rhetoric (e.g., the use of the phrase *victim feminism* to characterize feminist activism) (Baumgardner and Richards, 2000; Walker, 1995). Young feminists have sought to fight a feminist backlash by proposing a feminism that is flexible, expands on what it means to be feminist, and allows individuals to express their individuality and uniqueness. Reflecting this flexibility, Jennifer Baumgardner and Amy Richards (2000) proposed that "feminism wants you to be whoever you are—but with a political consciousness" (pp. 56-57).

Leslie Heywood and Jennifer Drake (1997) also characterized third-wave feminists as persons who have learned to deal with the contentious climate surrounding feminism by developing "modes of thinking that can come to terms with multiple, constantly shifting bases of oppression in relation to the multiple, interpenetrating axes of identity, and the creation of a coalition politics based on these understandings" (p. 3). Heywood and Drake see third-wave feminisms as drawing "strategically" (p. 3) from a variety of feminisms, including postmodern feminisms, second-wave feminisms, women-of-color feminisms, working-class feminisms, and prosex feminism. Furthermore, they have noted the variable nature of oppression, and the fact that the experiences deemed oppressive by one individual or group of women may be experienced as benign or nonoppressive by others. They propose that whereas "different strains of feminisms directly contradict each other" (p. 3), it is possible to transcend these contradictions and create a hybrid feminism that is meaningful to contemporary women and men.

As a component of their efforts to engage in consciousness changing, third-wave feminists have often emphasized the "personal" dimension of "the personal is political." Their writings have often been highly personal, and several anthologies consist primarily of accounts of encountering feminism in a personal way (Findlen, 1995;

Walker, 1995). Some young feminists have argued that academic writings on feminist theory have been of limited help to those attempting to live their lives as feminists, and they believe that the political implications of feminism are often most clearly revealed in personal writings. Furthermore, personal writings are more accessible to a wide audience, and they truly show a respect and appreciation for the diversity of experience and identity (Dicker and Piepmeier, 2003; Hernández and Rehman, 2002). The Internet and "zines" have become important methods for sharing these ideas and theories as well as for building activist coalitions (Baumgardner and Richards, 2000; Orr, 1997; Siegel, 1997; Findlen, 1995; Walker, 1995).

Lisa Rubin and Carol Nemeroff (2001) proposed that younger women sometimes feel intimidated by the erudite writings of academic feminists, and that it is important for young feminists to have a variety of spaces in which to formulate their own feminisms. The spaces that allow young women to explore their views and approaches to activism include informal discussion groups, focus groups, Internet chat rooms, and local zines. In contrast to the consciousness-raising groups of second-wave feminists, which focused on shared aspects of oppression, these discussion opportunities are likely to be facilitated by an emphasis on the diversity of meanings and activities of feminism.

The wide-ranging interests and emphases of third-wave feminists are visible in the Thirteen-Point Manifesta of Jennifer Baumgardner and Amy Richards (2000), which listed some of the following as important to their generation:

1. Outing and energizing unacknowledged feminists
2. Preserving abortion rights
3. Challenging double standards of sexual expression and health
4. Increasing awareness of feminist history
5. Increasing the visibility of lesbian, bisexual, and women-of-color feminists
6. Liberating adolescents from violence, sexual harassment, "slut bashing," disengaged educators, and bullying
7. Practicing "autokeonony," which involves viewing activism as arising from a close connection between the self and community, which can foster personal balance and motivation for action

This younger generation of feminists has also focused substantial energy on women's experiences with their bodies and physical appearance, highlighting the ubiquitous and often subtle media images that blanket the culture with unrealistic physical images of women. As noted by Amelia Richards (1998), "body image may be the pivotal third wave issue—the common struggle that mobilizes the current feminist generation" (p. 196). Lisa Rubin and Carol Nemeroff (2001) argued that although many external barriers to women's success have been eliminated or at least substantially reduced by the past generations' efforts, "the truest, biggest, and most crippling obstacles are internal" (p. 97) and often center on the body and its relationship to identity. They also added that the personal implications of body self-acceptance are "indeed political" (p. 98). This perspective lends itself to an expanded view of the political implications of personal change. In addition, when young feminists choose unconventional forms of physical appearance (e.g., body piercing, tattoos, alternative dress), they may be symbolically resisting narrow images of physical perfection and are engaging in social change (Baumgardner and Richards, 2000; Rubin and Nemeroff, 2001).

In summary, third-wave feminists have highlighted the importance of recognizing multiple identities and rejecting polarities or convenient dichotomies such as male versus female or good versus evil. Thus, they tend to express appreciation for such feminisms as global feminism and women-of-color feminisms (Hernández and Rehman, 2002). In addition, these third-wave feminists have aspired to be honest about the daily ambiguities, contradictions, and messy dilemmas that confront them. For example, Nomy Lamm (1995) stated, "My contradictions can coexist, cuz they exist inside of me, and I'm not gonna simplify them so that they fit into the linear, analytical pattern that I know they're supposed to" (p. 85). Consistent with this point of view, many published personal narratives embrace seemingly contradictory identities such as being feminist and Christian, a spiritual tradition which often endorses patriarchal values; being male and feminist; desiring to be "treated as a lady" and being feminist; wanting to be married and devoting oneself to the care of children while also being a feminist; working as a model and participating in the beauty culture while also being feminist; or enjoying hip-hop music, which is often identified as antifeminist, and being feminist (Findlen, 1995; Walker, 1995).

COMMONALITIES OF POSTMODERN, LESBIAN/QUEER, AND THIRD-WAVE FEMINISMS

The feminisms discussed in this chapter are characterized by many similarities, including a focus on power and privilege, and an emphasis on valuing difference and flexibility. Postmodern feminism provides principles for thinking about diversity and power, and lesbian/queer feminisms and third-wave feminisms provide insights about how these principles can be applied to specific groups and within specific contexts. Each of these feminisms is attentive to the socially constructed nature of knowledge and indicates that it is important for feminists to engage in ongoing self-conscious recognition of their own positions of power, privilege, and oppression; and to be cognizant of how these social experiences influence their everyday and social action activities.

Postmodern feminism has been described by some as providing a useful framework for questioning assumptions but an inadequate foundation for activism (Alcoff, 1988; Allen and Baber, 1992; Cacoullos, 2001). If no reality is certain, what is the basis for activism? Despite these concerns, postmodern influences in lesbian/queer theory and third-wave feminisms have not limited activist efforts but appear to support a variety of activist causes. The lesbian/queer and third-wave feminisms have supported coalition building among groups that may share many but not all of the same goals. Recognition of the impermanence, partial, and fluid nature of reality has supported pragmatic, time-limited approaches to social action projects.

IMPLICATIONS OF POSTMODERN, LESBIAN/QUEER, AND THIRD-WAVE FEMINISMS FOR PRACTICE

Although the implications of the feminisms described in this chapter are multiple, I will focus on two major themes that are relevant to feminist therapy practice: (1) implications for conceptualizing identity, identity development, and gender/social identity analysis and (2) the use of constructivism and narrative therapy to help women create meaningful but unique social narratives of their lives.

Issues Related to Identity

The Nature of Identity

Each of the theoretical perspectives described in this chapter challenges traditional boundaries or understandings of identity. Postmodern feminists indicate that identity is socially constructed, fluid, and varies across contexts. Identity may be contradictory, partial, and strategic. Postmodern feminism also challenges the notion that we can accurately conceptualize identity in bipolar categories such as masculine and feminine, homosexual and heterosexual, and feminist and nonfeminist. Queer theory deconstructs binary categories of sexuality and sexual orientation, and both queer and lesbian theories reveal how power is expressed through language associated with heterosexual behavior patterns. Third-wave feminists seek to define feminism and feminist identity more flexibly, noting the problems with feminisms that are rule-bound or based on political correctness. Third-wave feminists also suggest that "real world" living may require one to live with imperfection, inconsistency, paradox, and time-bound or place-bound realities.

Identity Development

Since the 1970s, psychology witnessed the proliferation of identity development models that conceptualize how individuals integrate new aspects of awareness within a core sense of self. These identity development models typically focus on how aspects of identity associated with privilege (e.g., whiteness) or minority status, marginalization, or oppression (e.g., lesbian identity, feminist identity, Black identity) are integrated within the self. Most of these models propose that individuals move through phases that are initially characterized by internalized prejudice or privilege, a lack of recognition or salience with regard to a particular identity, or satisfaction with things as they are. Over time, individuals become increasingly aware of societal prejudices and privilege and often experience periods of upheaval and questioning. Later phases are generally marked by cognitive flexibility, and internal standards of self-definition (Cross and Vandiver, 2001; Downing and Roush, 1985; Helms, 1995).

In their original forms, most models of identity development proposed a relatively linear path that focused on one aspect of identity, such as feminist identity (e.g., Downing and Roush, 1985), racial identity (e.g., Cross, 1991), or gay identity (e.g., Cass, 1979). Over time, however, theorists and researchers have recognized that identity development may not follow an orderly pathway, particularly when individuals are negotiating multiple aspects of identity that may be associated with different levels of privilege (e.g., being white, holding middle-class status) and/or oppression (e.g., being a person of color or lesbian). For example, even when persons occupy only one "minority" status, such as being lesbian, they negotiate varied aspects of identity such as sexual attraction and desire, patterns of intimacy, generational status, community support or prejudice, and political commitments (Fassinger, 2000).

It is important for therapists to recognize that multiple identities may be negotiated in a variety of ways, including primary identification with one or several aspects of identity, identification with multiple aspects of self in a segmented fashion (specific aspects of identity become more salient in specific contexts), and identification with multiple aspects of self as they intersect with one another in an integrated manner (Reynolds and Pope, 1991). Recent models have focused on interrelationships among aspects of identity, with various aspects postulated to take on different levels of salience depending on life events, family and cultural background, experiences of privilege and oppression, and numerous other variables. Furthermore, once a specific aspect of identity is negotiated, it may remain fluid and changing over time (Anthias, 1999; Jones and McEwen, 2000).

In light of these features of identity, feminist therapists seek to be attentive to the narrative and meaning of clients' multiple identities, recognizing that a person's priorities and self-definitions may shift significantly in different contexts. The identities that are relevant personally to clients may be associated with, but not limited to, gender, race, culture, ethnicity, geographic location, intellectual ability, sexual orientation, class, age, body size, religious affiliation, acculturation status, and other sociodemographic variables. The interaction of these group identities and statuses are reflected in multidimensional concepts of identity that are influenced by visibility (the degree to which they are easily discernable to others), situational salience or relevance, and experiences of oppression or privilege (Deaux and Stewart, 2001; Suyemoto, 2002; Worell and Remer, 2003).

Social Identity Analysis

Gender-role analysis has been identified as a hallmark of feminist assessment therapy since the early years of feminist therapy practice (Kaschak, 1981). Gender-role analysis was originally defined as the exploration of the impact of gender and gender socialization on identity and psychological well-being. With greater knowledge about the multidimensionality of identity and the way in which gender is modified by many other social locations such as age, race/ethnicity, and sexual orientation, gender-role analysis was increasingly seen as encompassing assessment about the intersections of gender as well as other relevant identity statuses (e.g., race, ethnicity, culture, lesbian identity). For example, Laura Brown (1990b) indicated that comprehensive gender-role analysis is needed to focus on the exploration of gender in light of personal values, family dynamics, life stage, cultural/ethnic background, experiences of trauma, and current environment. Postmodern perspectives, which indicate that perceptions of identity may vary significantly across contexts, imply that our assessment of gender and intersecting social identities should be modified further.

Given the complexity, variability, and different levels of salience of various social identities, it may be difficult for the feminist therapist to ask a standardized set of orderly assessment questions to understand the role that gender and intersecting identities play in a client's life. To conduct an individualized and comprehensive social identity analysis, the feminist therapist is attentive to what a client does and does not communicate about important experiences and activities in her or his life, and asks follow-up questions that are relevant to aspects of identity the client views as important or unimportant. Open-ended questions about identity, roles, and the contexts in which an individual interacts with others are likely to be important points of entry for assessing social identity. These questions are based on the assumptions that identity can be situational, variable, and contextualized. Some of these questions may include the following: What roles, identities, and social memberships are most important and least important at this point in your life? What roles and/or identities are most frequently noticed and appreciated (or underappreciated) by others? When do you feel powerful (or weak, or discriminated against), and what roles and identities are you most aware of when you feel powerful or a lack of power? When are you most aware of/least aware of being female/male, lesbian, a person of color, feminist? What does lesbian identity, spiritual/religious identity, feminist identity, or ethnic identity mean to you? How do you see yourself as similar to and/or different from other women or men you know? How does your sense of "who am I" vary in different circumstances?

Feminist narrative therapists Anne Prouty and Maria Bermúdez (1999) use the metaphor of "parts" to examine multiple aspects of identity. During an initial session, they encourage clients to draw and define the different parts, or roles, and identities that are relevant to their self-definitions. Following the identification of different parts, clients are encouraged to explore how each role emerged, evolved, was nurtured, reinforced, empowered and disempowered, and/or shamed and shunned. "Deconstructing" questions are posed in order to question dominant stories about their parts, and "reconstructing" questions are designed to explore new possibilities. Examples of deconstructing questions include the following: How did each role or part develop, and how do they interact? Who or what promoted or discouraged various arts? How or when are different parts of the self at war with one another? What sources of power are available to the different parts? Examples of reconstructing questions include the following: What parts work together effectively? What parts can you use to increase your self-confidence, flexibility, or your sense of control? How can you increase the satisfaction associated with each part? These questions are designed to help clients become more aware of their multiple identities, to promote collaboration between the therapist and client, and to increase clients' awareness of options and choices.

Within family therapy circles, various clinicians have modified the genogram, a major family assessment tool, in ways that are consistent with the assumption that multiple social identities may influence the self and the family. These specialized genograms focus on gender issues in the family (e.g., the gendergram in White and Tyson-Rawson, 1995), spiritual issues and resources (e.g., Dunn and Dawes, 1999; Frame, 2001), and multicultural themes (Thomas, 1998). The multicultural genogram (Thomas, 1998) can be structured to take into account the following factors: ethnicity, race, immigration/acculturation, social class, gender, and spirituality. Finally, the socially constructed genogram (Milewski-Hertlein, 2001) is built on the client's personal perceptions of what a family is, and depicts how the person sees himself or herself in this social context.

In summary, the goal of social identity analysis and gender-role analysis is to gain a clear sense of how an individual views herself or himself so that she or he can begin to become an active agent in constructing new and satisfying (although potentially partial) identities. As suggested by the feminist theories described in this chapter, seeking a permanent and coherent identity may be less important than living effectively with a range of overlapping identities and, at times, apparently contradictory identities.

Constructivism and Narrative Therapies

Constructivism, which can be seen as a form of postmodern thought, highlights "the personal and collective processes by which people organize their experience and coordinate their relationships with one another" (Neimeyer and Stewart, 2000, p. 338). Constructivism has become an important framework for psychotherapy and is based on the assumption that people are active agents as interpreters of their lives and creators of meaning. Common themes underlying the variety of constructivist psychotherapies include recognition of the unique and distinctive qualities of meaning making for each individual, the valuing of assessments and techniques that are specific to each individual, and resistance to diagnostic systems that magnify clients' deficits and pathologize clients. These approaches are also critical of systems that rely on universal diagnostic categories, which "fail to capture the richness and subtlety of any given individual's way of interpreting the social world and constructing relationships with others" (p. 341).

The phrase *narrative therapy* has become an important metaphor for conceptualizing constructivist and postmodern themes in counseling. The metaphor of narrative makes salient the notion that people are the authors and main characters of their lives and actively create meaning by weaving the past, present, and future together in a coherent life story. Loss of meaning often occurs when individuals lose a sense of continuity and order in their lives; thus, the use of narratives and life sketches represents an important therapeutic means for helping individuals gain or regain a sense of meaning. Extensions of the narrative metaphor can be seen in narrative models of the self, narrative diagnoses or ways of organizing problems in living, and narrative reconstructions of the self and world (Neimeyer and Stewart, 2000; White, 1995; Zimmerman and Dickerson, 1994).

Many of the more recent family therapies have incorporated constructionistic and narrative methods as foundations of treatment. As noted in Chapter 2, the family therapies have been critiqued by feminists for their implicit endorsement of the white, middle-class, two-parent, nuclear family as the standard for normalcy in family life (Bograd, 1999). However, family therapy concepts and practices have evolved substantially since the 1980s as practitioners have become increasingly aware of diversity within the family and society. The most significant shifts in family therapy theory include increased recognition of the diversity of family structures, and the inseparable and complex intersections of race, class, sexual orientation, and gender in shaping personal and family identity. Consistent with this recognition, recent articles on family therapy focus on integrating multicultural and feminist perspectives (e.g., Bryan, 2001) and attend to issues of poverty in the family (e.g., Ziemba, 2001).

Important concepts within the narrative therapies include the concepts of co-authoring, shared subjectivity (or honoring the subjectivity of clients' problem definitions), and externalizing (as opposed to internalizing) questions. The concept of co-authoring challenges the view of the therapist as expert and emphasizes achieving shared meaning within the counseling relationship (Winslade, Crocket, and Monk, 1997). Shared subjectivity refers to the creation of conceptual understandings of problems that avoid "objectifying modes of thinking and behaving" (p. 56). Narrative therapists avoid terms such as *diagnosis, assessment,* and *treatment* "which grant precedence to 'regimes of truth' over clients' knowledge about their own lives" (p. 56). Finally, externalizing questions or interventions reflect narrative therapists' resistance to lodging problems within the client, which may merely place clients into professional molds. Thus, they tend to avoid using internalizing terms such as *resistance* and *denial,* which tend to place blame on individuals. Externalizing questions, which can be defined as a form of deconstruction, are problem-focused. According to Wendy Drewery and John Winslade (1997), the externalizing conversation "focuses on the problem rather than on the person and then mobilizes the client's resources against the problem" (p. 45). This way of thinking about issues allows individuals to see themselves as capable of solving problems and reverses psychological trends that support seeing problems as the consequences of personal deficits. The concepts of externalizing, co-authoring, and shared subjectivity reflect the postmodern assumption that language conveys power and that *"what we say, and how we say it, matter"* (p. 34). The language we use affects our thinking about problems and clients. According to this narrative view, the language of professional psychology merely reinforces traditional authority rather than freeing clients to create stories that allow them to construct their own meanings and engage in productive change. These concepts are highly compatible with basic assumptions of feminist therapy.

Janet Lee (1997) identified narrative approaches as offering positive alternatives to women who are "re-authoring" their lives. Narrative therapy eschews diagnoses that may encourage victim blaming, places value on relational themes that are important to many women, empowers women by validating their own stories and meaning, and thus supports self-sufficiency and competency. Through their emphasis on uniqueness and flexibility, narrative approaches also allow for conceptualizations of gender and other social identities that are flexible. In other words, gender is not unitary or static, and women construct their lives and meanings within the multiple social locations they inhabit, including locations influenced by gender, race, class, age, and sexual orientation.

CONCLUDING COMMENTS

Postmodern, lesbian/queer, and third-wave feminisms have challenged the adequacy of traditional feminisms. A major implication of each of the three feminisms presented in this chapter is that feminist therapists need to be consistently aware of power dynamics and how language and meaning are produced and reproduced in psychotherapy. Of particular importance is the need for feminist therapists to practice flexibly and to scrutinize continuously their own practices, assumptions, and beliefs about power, oppression, empowerment, and social change.

Attentiveness to difference and power is crucial, as is the need for feminist therapists to recognize their own "positionality" vis-à-vis their clients. Positionality refers to awareness of how the social positioning of individuals and the power relationships in which they participate inform their knowledge base and experience, and how social and political forces affect this process. Both therapists and clients juggle "polyrhythmic realities" (Sheared, 1994) associated with their roles as raced and gendered beings and in their roles as workers, partners, therapists, and clients. The differences and complex identities that individuals bring to psychotherapy (e.g., learning style, cultural background, class status, religion, sexual orientation, age, race, and gender) and the borders and boundaries between these identities can become important aspects of discussion as clients and therapists seek to create complex but potentially incomplete or partial models of oppression, reality, and empowerment (Maher and Tetreault, 2001).

Chapter 8

Developing a Personal Approach to Feminist Therapy

INTRODUCTION

A major rationale for this book is the assumption that feminist therapists benefit from examining their personal assumptions and considering the compatibility of these assumptions with various feminist theoretical perspectives. The goal of this activity is to encourage counselors and therapists to create personal models of feminist therapy that reflect clarity and consistency of theory and practice. Feminist therapy can be best described as a conceptual framework or philosophical perspective for organizing one's assumptions about psychotherapy, and the theories described in this book are useful for clarifying this metaframework. Theory provides a foundation that can be used to guide practice, allow an overarching overview of one's work and goals, and create a base from which to engage in self-reflective practice.

Theoretical notions about human problems and psychotherapy often represent deeply held complex convictions about the nature of human functioning (Mark, 1990). A recent study found that clinical psychologists' theory-based assumptions about psychological problems had a more significant impact on their explanations of problems than did atheoretical descriptive checklists. Theoretical frameworks rather than atheoretical criteria represented in the DSM-IV (American Psychiatric Association, 1994) were found to be the most influential contributors to clinical psychologists' organization and conceptualizations of symptom patterns (Kim and Ahn, 2002). Personal ties to a theory are powerful influences on one's assessment of issues as well as one's practices and interventions in therapy. To avoid practicing in inconsistent ways or unconsciously imposing theoretical biases on clients, it is important for feminist psychotherapists and counselors to explore the intricacies of theory and to make self-reflective choices about their theoretical orientations. Ongoing reflection about the core components and evolving aspects of one's theoretical worldview lends authenticity and coherence to one's interventions.

Laura Brown's (1994) thoughts about the importance of theory and feminist therapy are especially informative. She posed and responded to the following question:

> Why is it important to understand the various models of feminism and the therapy theories that they reflect? It is, I would argue, because the models and theories by which any psychotherapy is practiced inform reality for the therapist and the client. Those constructs that a particular model names and defines become real, present, and observable in the psychotherapy process of practitioners who use that model. (p. 48)

The feminist therapist's personal orientation to feminist theory may have a profound impact on the nature of feminist therapy that one practices. If feminist therapists mistakenly assume that feminist philosophy is a monolithic entity, they are likely to draw erroneous conclusions or overgeneralizations about the nature of feminist psychotherapy. Alternatively, if therapists do not systematically explore the intersection between feminist theory, psychotherapy theory, and feminist therapy, they risk the possibility of putting together a collection of ideas that are subjectively appealing but have no clear rationale. Mismatches between interventions and assumptions may result in blank spots and diminished effectiveness on the part of the feminist therapist. The unsystematic combination of approaches and theories may also result in confusion on the part of the therapist or client or, at worst, unethical behavior. For example, if the feminist therapist does not have a clear theoretical understanding of the principle of egalitarianism or the skill of self-disclosure, she or he may engage in inappropriate boundary violations.

Participants in the 1993 National Conference on Education and Training in Feminist Practice (Brabeck and Brown, 1997) identified feminist theory as an essential foundation for sound feminist therapy and practice. These participants reached consensus about nine features of a feminist theory of psychological practice, and these principles are paraphrased or directly quoted in the following list:

1. Feminist theory is a political enterprise and is associated with the goal of social transformation.
2. "A goal of feminist practice is the creation of a feminist consciousness that becomes as unconscious as patriarchal consciousness is currently" (p. 32).
3. Theory creation is embedded in or can be derived from human connections and experience, written materials, group solidarity, and activism. These sources inform how the personal is political and how experiences become the foundation for social transformation goals.
4. Gender is an important aspect of women's oppression and interacts with other forms of oppression that include but are not limited to culture, class, age, race, ethnicity, sexual orientation, ability, and linguistic status. Feminist practitioners make efforts to become aware of how their experiences with regard to these hierarchies influence their work.
5. An appreciation of diversity is an essential foundation for practice. Diversity (e.g., religion, sexual orientation, ethnicity) "is a goal in its own right but also is necessary for feminist theory to be complete and reflective of the total range of human experience" (p. 32).
6. "Feminist theory affirms, attends to, and authorizes the experience of the oppressed in their own voices" (p. 32). Feminist practitioners are attentive to the ways they may play oppressive roles in their relationship to others.
7. Feminist practitioners seek and rely on models of the self and development that are expansive. These models appreciate the varied ways in which individuals view identity, and honor the multiple subjectivities that individuals may hold.
8. Feminist theory recognizes complex and multifaceted causes of distress, placing special emphasis on sociocultural contexts. Each person is also viewed as competent and responsible for participating in change.
9. Feminist theory is not static but continually evolving.

More recently, a task force of feminist psychologists met to articulate assumptions and guidelines for psychological practice with girls and women. This project was initiated in 2000 and sponsored by the American Psychological Association's Societies of Counseling Psychology and Psychology of Women. Along with psychologists Roberta Nutt and Joy Rice, I am one of three co-chairs of this task force.

Following a variety of group meetings and electronic communications efforts, our twenty-five-member task force met for a weekend retreat in April 2002. The deliberations of the task force were informed by the products of many previous documents that articulated practices for working effectively with women (e.g., American Psychological Association, 1975, 1978, 1979; Worell and Johnson, 1997) as well as the Guidelines for Psychotherapy with Lesbian, Gay, and Bisexual Clients (American Psychological Association, 2000) and Guidelines on Multicultural Education, Training, Research, Practice, and Organizational Change for Psychologists (American Psychological Association, 2002b). Following a highly productive retreat that culminated in the articulation of basic guidelines, members then developed literature reviews to support the basic guideline statements (Enns, 2002; Worell, 2002).

The resulting draft (Nutt, Rice, and Enns, 2003) was reviewed by the executive boards of the sponsoring societies at their January 2003 mid-year meetings and approved for submission to the APA's Council of Representatives. The Board of Professional Affairs (BPA) of the American Psychological Association and its Committee on Professional Practice and Standards (COPPS) have since reviewed the document and provided feedback for revisions, which are now in progress (Nutt, Rice, and Enns, 2003).

The guidelines are informed by a feminist and multicultural framework, intended to be aspirational statements rather than to imply mandated practices, and designed to clarify optimal practices for a broad range of psychological practice with girls and women. Although they are written primarily for psychologists, they are also relevant to members of a wide range of other mental health professionals. Because the guidelines remain under review at the time of this writing, I will not reproduce the guidelines but instead summarize main points associated with the three main sections of the document: (1) diversity, social context, and power; (2) professional responsibility; and (3) best practices (see also Enns, 2004, for additional discussion of themes).

The first section of the guidelines describes assumptions and foundations for working with girls and women, including the recognition that girls and women are socialized into multiple social group memberships, and that girls and women have both shared and unique identities. Psychologists seek to gain information about the various privileges and oppressions associated with social group memberships and strive to understand power imbalances that exist among themselves and those with whom they work. Attentiveness to power imbalances includes efforts to understand institutional and social relationships that facilitate and detract from women's and girls' physical and mental health (Nutt et al., 2003).

Proposed guidelines relevant to professional responsibility encourage psychologists to engage in continuous self-reflection, education, and consultation, and to develop awareness of their own socialization, social identities, values, attitudes, privileges, and oppressions that may affect their practice with girls and women. The guidelines also call for psychologists to be mindful of the potentially oppressive values and biases that are embedded in psychological research, theory, and practice and to create and use gender and culturally sensitive practices (Nutt et al., 2003).

A final section on best practices encourages practitioners to create and implement approaches that foster empowering alliances and practices; make use of affirming assessments and conceptual frameworks; conceptualize issues within the sociopolitical framework that recognizes the importance of gender, culture, and power dynamics; incorporate a wide range of mental health, educational, and community resources; and challenge unhealthy power structures at interpersonal, institutional, and systemic levels (Nutt et al., 2003).

This section has outlined two sets of consensus statements, one that articulates common understandings about the role of feminist theory in feminist practice (Brabeck and Brown, 1997) and one that seeks to articulate consensus values related to psychological practice with girls and women (Nutt et al., 2003). Both sets of statements may be useful to readers who are working toward developing personal approaches to feminist therapy. I encourage readers to consider the degree to which their frameworks and practices are consistent with these consensus statements.

CREATING A PERSONAL THEORETICAL APPROACH

Questions to Facilitate the Creation of a Personal Theoretical Approach

The feminist theories described in this book speak to four inter-related themes: description, analysis, vision, and strategy. First, feminist theory is useful for defining the interlocking influences of racism, sexism, ageism, heterosexism, colonialism, and other "isms" that affect personal experience. This descriptive component contributes to consciousness raising and a feminist therapist's sense of purpose. A second facet of theory is analysis, or explanations regarding why reality exists as it does. Analysis is central to considering why oppression exists, who benefits from it, how oppression changes over time, and how it varies across contexts. A third feature of theory is vision, or the values, principles, and goals that support feminist practice. Finally, strategy focuses on action or the specific tools for overcoming oppression and supporting the positive growth of clients and society (Bunch, 1987).

I encourage readers to reflect on these four overlapping themes as they consider and clarify their feminist theoretical approaches. Many of these questions are adapted from reflection questions proposed by Judith Worell and Pam Remer (2003) and Gwyn Kirk and Margo Okazawa-Rey (1998). If applied to each of the theories discussed in this book, these questions are likely to contribute to comprehensive knowledge of feminist foundations as well as clarity about one's personal preferences.

1. What historical and cultural events are associated with the emergence of this theory?
2. What are the main arguments and assumptions underlying the theory?
3. What major theorists, writers, and activists were influential in the creation of this theory? What were or are their views regarding oppressions related to race, gender, class, nationality, and sexual orientation? Which of these social statuses are descriptive of the theorists as individuals, and how do the social locations of the theorists influence the theory? To what degree

do you share similar or different social locations with these theorists?

4. How does this theory conceptualize women's problems and the way in which these problems are influenced by various "isms"? How, according to this perspective, can these problems be eradicated?

5. What are the primary goals or social change implications associated with this theory? What methods and strategies are recommended for achieving these goals? What is the role of the individual in effecting change?

6. Who are the critics of this theory? What concerns of critics do you find compelling or not compelling?

7. What issues received the greatest attention in this theory? Are some issues overemphasized? Are some issues left out? What gaps between theory and practice exist?

8. To what degree does this theory attend to diversity and the multiple realities of women?

9. What theory or theories can be used to fill in gaps or to clarify issues not addressed by this theory? Is it possible to combine the strengths of these theories and eliminate limitations?

10. What are the consistencies and inconsistencies between this theory and the psychological personality and counseling theories that inform your work with clients?

11. To what degree are psychological concepts such as assessment, diagnosis, pathology, and mental illness consistent with this theory?

12. To what degree does this theory reflect the nine attributes of a feminist theory of practice? (See previous section, Brabeck and Brown, 1997.)

13. Based on the answers to your questions, what theory or combination of theories is most useful to you as a feminist therapist? Write a statement that describes your approach, making sure that you address each of the following: description, analysis, vision, and strategy or interventions.

14. What aspects of your own theory are still evolving? What information will you need to seek to round out your theoretical foundation?

Challenges in Developing a Personal Approach

Since the 1990s, feminist therapy has gained visibility and recognition, and is now featured as a major theoretical approach in introductory counseling texts (e.g., Corey, 2004; Murdock, 2004; Sharf, 2004; Sommers-Flanagan and Sommers-Flanagan, 2004). Feminist therapists have achieved consensus about many principles and practices of feminist therapy, and these consensus values are summarized in a variety of sources (e.g., Brabeck and Brown, 1997; Nutt et al., 2003; Worell and Remer, 2003; Wyche and Rice, 1997). However, two areas of practice, the role of social change and the role of assessment in feminist therapy, remain particularly complex. As a result, I summarize current issues and encourage readers to consider carefully the relevance of these issues to their personal approaches to feminist therapy.

Social Change: Essential Activity for the Feminist Therapist?

A recent survey of 140 Australian feminist counselors (Chester and Bretherton, 2001) found that roughly 95 percent shared the views that women should be viewed positively and as capable of reaching their potential, and that their concerns should be seen as influenced by gender-role stereotyping and sociocultural experiences. These views are most consistent with liberal and cultural feminist perspectives and are generally compatible with the professional culture of counseling and mainstream practices and theory in psychology (Marecek and Kravetz, 1998).

Only 40 percent of respondents in Andrea Chester and Diane Bretherton's (2001) study described themselves as involved in social action, and only 26 percent viewed social activism as an essential quality of a feminist counselor. Similarly, Jeanne Marecek and Diane Kravetz's (1998) qualitative study of twenty-five American feminist therapists found that these therapists emphasized concepts which were compatible with individual empowerment and the professional practice of psychology. Although holding opinions about the value of social and political change, "they worked within existing gender arrangements and social institutions and did not overly challenge systems of power operating in society" (p. 26). The findings of Rebecca Beardsley and colleagues (1998), which were based on the responses of 170 individuals, also found that the use of political analysis and encouraging clients to be involved in social change were uncommon practices of experienced, self-identified feminist therapists.

In contrast to these realities, initial formulations (e.g., Rawlings and Carter, 1977) viewed social action as central to feminist therapy. More recently, the Feminist Therapy Institute (FTI) (2000) code of ethics stated that the feminist therapist "seeks multiple avenues" for implementing social change such as helping clients negotiate the criminal justice system; questioning community practices that may be harmful to clients or therapists; and participating in public education, advocacy, and legislative lobbying. Likewise, actions directed toward achieving social justice are identified by Mary Brabeck and Kathleen Ting (2000) as important feminist ethical commitments. Within the field of psychology in general, social activism has been identified as an important component of self-care and well functioning (Coster and Schwebel, 1997), and recent ethical codes (e.g., American Psychological Association, 2002a) speak to the importance of social justice as an ethical commitment.

Given increased recognition of social change as an important activity within the larger field of psychology, it is surprising that social change is not more frequently seen as essential by practicing feminist therapists. Several influences may help account for relatively low levels of commitment of social action, including limited or no training for participating in social change, fear of a backlash if one identifies oneself publicly as feminist, and the social isolation of feminist therapists who may often practice in climates that provide limited opportunity for ongoing interaction with feminist colleagues (Beardsley et al., 1998; Marecek and Kravetz, 1998).

For feminist therapists who are most attracted to liberal and cultural feminist theoretical foundations, social change may not be a defining feature of feminist therapy. Alternatively, some feminist therapists may view social change as synonymous with treating the client respectfully and equally (liberal feminism) or highlighting the growth-supporting relational qualities of the counseling relationship (cultural feminism). In these cases, social change is defined as individual transformation. However, all other feminisms discussed in this book speak to the importance of social transformation both within and without counseling. In light of the diversity of thought and practice about social change and social activism, I encourage readers to consider the following questions:

1. How do you define social change, activism, and/or transformation? How does your definition compare to the definitions of social change associated with various feminist theories?
2. How do you gain information about human rights and social justice issues? How do you maintain connections with other feminists with whom you might cooperate in fighting injustice?
3. What are the social change activities in which you are willing to become involved at the individual level? Local community level? Within the work setting? Within professional organizations? At the legislative level? Within criminal justice and education systems?
4. Do you believe it is empowering for clients to be involved in social change issues? If so, what types of social change activities may be most appropriate and at what stages of counseling might these activities be most appropriate?

Assessment, Diagnosis, and Conceptualization

A second major area that merits further consideration is the conceptualization of clients' difficulties. Feminist therapy has often been described primarily as a framework or conceptual model for thinking about problems in living. This conceptual framework may be integrated with a wide range of specific techniques that are consistent with this framework. One of the ways in which one's theoretical orientation is most evident is through one's assessment of clients' problems and thus careful attention to this aspect of feminist therapy is crucial. Assessment and diagnosis are also particularly complex issues because conceptualization according to an external validating structure is often necessary for gaining necessary monetary support for services.

Counselors with liberal feminist orientations are likely to endorse the view that women's difficulties or diminished accomplishments are the consequences of learned behaviors and socialization. Furthermore, the symptoms of disorders such as agoraphobia, depression, and eating disorders are linked to the stereotyping of women and/or women's overly rigid adherence to traditional gender roles (Franks and Rothblum, 1983). Liberal feminist therapists are likely to use traditional diagnostic categories but make efforts to apply diagnoses fairly by applying a single standard of mental health to men and women. Thus, they may experience little or no conflict about practicing in most professional psychology contexts.

Therapists influenced by cultural feminist perspectives are most likely to question diagnostic categories if they are based on androcentric or culturally biased models, or devalue women's traditional strengths (Jordan and Hartling, 2002; Stiver, 1991). They are likely to view woman-centered explanations of women's distress as an "antidote to the effect of patriarchal oppression" (Radden, 2001, p. 73). For example, the relational/cultural model of depression indicates that a woman's core self is built on relational strengths. Because society denigrates a woman's capacity to be attuned to others, she may be defined as dependent or immature, and she becomes vulnerable to depression and low self-esteem (Jack, 1987, 1991, 1999; Kaplan, 1986). Feminist therapists influenced by cultural feminist theory tend to view disconnections from others as a major contributor to distress and mutual empowerment and reconnection as central to health (Jordan and Hartling, 2002). Recent assessment trends referred to as "relational diagnosis" (Kaslow, 1996), which views problems as rooted in relationships, may also be attractive to some cultural feminist therapists. Jennifer Radden (2001) cautions that despite its criticism of androcentric models, cultural feminist approaches only infrequently challenge basic psychological assumptions about the individual self; they do not place significant emphasis on social-contextual relationships that move beyond the confines of nuclear family relationships or microsystemic relationships. Thus, Radden (2001) refers to this feminist therapy approach as "relational individualism" (p. 71) or "autonomous relationality" (p. 72).

Radical, socialist, woman-of-color, lesbian/queer, postmodern, and global feminists often operate from "transformation" or "social change" frameworks that question the basic tenets and foundation of mental health systems. Many social change feminists avoid using diagnostic labels, except in rare circumstances, because they are seen as embedded in oppressive, culturally circumscribed beliefs that exaggerate power differentials, label the person rather than the social circumstances as the cause of problems, and lead to an overemphasis on individual change efforts (Rawlings and Carter, 1977). Those who adopt a transformation framework generally view the DSM-IV (American Psychiatric Association, 1994, 2000) as a political and economic document that controls who can provide and receive remuneration for services and often reinforces current hierarchical power structures within society. Although many social change feminist therapists prefer to use descriptive phrases or culturally appropriate terms in order to avoid the mystification of standard diagnostic terminology, they may use traditional categories on behalf of clients if the denial of service is at stake (e.g., for health insurance reimbursement).

Many social change feminist therapists are attentive to specific ways in which diagnostic or conceptual criteria are associated with subtle forms of racism, ethnocentrism, classism, cultural bias, or heterosexism (e.g., Brown, 1994; Espín and Gawelek, 1992; Jackson and Greene, 2000; Kaschak, 1992). For example, women-of-color feminists are especially attentive to the manner in which diagnostic categories equate white, middle-class values with normalcy; lesbian and queer feminists are concerned about the ways in which heterosexism permeates standards of normalcy; and global feminists are sensitive to the ways in which Western standards of the self and mental health influence conceptual frameworks. These feminist therapists are also attentive to how the intersections of race, sex, culture, and class influence the type of psychological distress that clients display, as well as how specific biases (e.g., racism, heterosexism) influence the manner in which diagnostic frameworks are applied. These feminist therapists are also cognizant of omission bias, or the ways in which conceptual frameworks do not include the realities and experiences of persons who are often marginalized within society and thus contribute to their invisibility. Connotation bias, which involves using phrases with negative meanings or implications when referring to nondominant groups in society, is also a major concern of social transformation therapists (Chernin, Holden, and Chandler, 1997). An example of connotation bias is that lesbian relationships are sometimes characterized as fused or enmeshed when more appropriate language would refer to "the ability for empathic relating" or "self-boundary flexibility" (Morton, 1998).

Postmodern feminists seek to deconstruct the language of diagnostic labeling and the manner in which labeling conveys power and dominant cultural values. Consistent with its critique of dualistic categories, postmodern feminists are likely to be concerned with the ways in which diagnostic language places "abnormal" and "normal" behavior into discrete categories rather than conceptualizing behavior along a more flexible continuum. Psychotherapies influenced by postmodern ideas eschew traditional diagnostic categories that place problems into arbitrary categories rather than individualized under- standings, reinforce traditional bases of power (e.g., psychiatry), grant "third-person object status" to clients and limit their sense of agency (Winslade, Crocket, and Monk, 1997, p. 55), and give greater credence to "professional 'regimes of truth' over clients' knowledge about their own lives" (p. 56). "Coconstructive" models, such as those that are based on mutual decision making between therapist and client and are consciously attentive to power dynamics, represent op- tions that are attractive to feminist therapists operating from a post- modern framework. Such coconstructive models do not view prob- lems as lodged within the person but as embedded in a complex web of interactions and cultural systems (Rigazio-DiGilio, 2000).

The Complexities of Assessment: The Example of PTSD

The complexities of conceptualizing women's problems within a feminist framework can be illustrated through the examination of the diagnostic category of post-traumatic stress disorder. PTSD has been endorsed by many feminist therapists as a diagnostic category that serves as "a rhetorical resource for voicing their objections, as femi- nists, to conventional diagnoses and the medical model" (Marecek, 1999, p. 162). The label of PTSD has been viewed by many feminist therapists as conceptualizing the impact of the external environment and social/situational origins on individual distress, "normalizing" and destigmatizing women's reactions to traumatic events in their lives, and avoiding victim-blaming and scapegoating attitudes (Becker, 2000; Marecek, 1999). During the 1980s, feminist therapists began to use PTSD to organize knowledge about the aftermath of trauma, but they expressed concern about the DSM-III-R definition of trauma as "outside the range of usual human experience" (American Psychiat- ric Association, 1987, p. 480), and as categorizing symptoms too nar- rowly to account for the range of posttrauma stress reactions of women (Lerman, 1989). To increase the adequacy of this diagnosis for women, several feminist therapists explored possibilities for ex- panding on or redefining PTSD by referring to these patterns as abuse/oppression artifact disorders (Brown, 1992a) and complex post- traumatic stress disorder (Herman, 1992).

When the DSM-IV (American Psychiatric Association, 1994) redefined trauma to include exposure to "an event or events that involved actual or threatened death or serious injury, or a threat to the physical integrity of self or others" (p. 427), this diagnostic category became even more attractive to many feminist therapists. The new definition included the very types of stress and trauma associated with various forms of interpersonal trauma. Despite these positive changes, Dana Becker (2000) argued that the DSM-IV redefinition "increased by millions the number of those eligible for a PTSD diagnosis and has identified those women who qualify for it as a mental disorder" (p. 425). She noted that it is not possible to normalize a pattern of behavior while also calling it a disorder. If the use of this label proliferates, large groups of women may be placed in a new "catchall" category, which may be associated with decreased attention to the individualized patterns of response experienced by victims. An additional issue is that although PTSD originally highlighted the environmental contributors to posttrauma distress, research has increasingly focused on biological factors associated with PTSD, including the possibility that sex differences associated with PTSD may be related to hormonal differences between men and women (Wolfe and Kimerling, 1997). Thus, even a diagnostic category designed to be attentive to external causal factors can be used to support biological and intrapsychic hypotheses and treatment. Finally, racism, sexism, heterosexism, classism, and ageism also interact with the ways in which trauma is experienced, and the current conceptualization of PTSD does not provide insight about these complicated intersections (Sanchez-Hucles and Hudgins, 2001). In summary, the social change implications associated with the forms of violence that lead to PTSD-like symptoms might be ignored or minimized as more specialized treatments for individuals are developed.

Susan Berg (2002) proposed that feminist therapists' use of PTSD as a diagnostic category varies according to their feminist theoretical orientations. Those with liberal feminist views will see PTSD as a compensatory reaction to violence and view it as honoring "the subjective experience of the victim-patient by validating and substantiating her claims of violence and pain" (p. 58). She also predicted that although many radical feminist therapists are likely to resist the PTSD label because it emphasizes the "dysfunction" of individuals and depoliticizes problems related to violence (e.g., Burstow, 2003) those with socialist feminist orientations are likely to see PTSD as an accurate depiction of the individual impact of abuse in a classist, racist, capitalistic society. For those working from a socialist feminist framework, a PTSD label can provide relief to the client because the symptoms can be meaningfully named, and can also provide a basis for political action by those who share this diagnosis and can speak to the profound individual effects of the social problem of violence (Berg, 2002).

It is likely that feminist therapists who are especially cognizant of diversity issues (e.g., heterosexism, racism) will be concerned that the PTSD diagnosis does not address how insidious and sometimes indirect forms of daily psychological violence associated with racism, anti-Semitism, homophobia, and other "isms" may also result in symptom patterns that may resemble but not be identical to classic PTSD symptoms (Brown, 1992a; Root, 1992). Finally, postmodern feminists are likely to be aware of the ways in which popular diagnoses such as PTSD can be used in unintended ways. For example, Dana Becker (2000) argued that PTSD has become associated with "good girl" responses to trauma, while borderline personality disorder is often used to label "bad girl" responses to trauma. Postmodern feminist counselors are likely to make efforts to deconstruct these binary categories and reconstruct or coconstruct more meaningful ways of conceptualizing the aftermath of abuse and violence.

Options for Expanding Conceptual Frameworks

This brief overview of PTSD-related strengths and limitations reveals that even those diagnostic categories that have been endorsed by prominent feminist therapists (e.g., Walker, 1994) remain controversial. In response to the individually focused DSM, some feminist therapists have proposed models that expand the frameworks of traditional diagnosis. Hannah Lerman (1996) suggested that the person-in-environment (PIE) system (Karls and Wandrei, 1994) may hold promise for feminist therapists who believe that the DSM is adequate for conceptualizing the individual aspect of problems but desire a more complete model for assessing roles and social systems in which persons are embedded. The PIE model organizes problems in living into four categories. One factor focuses on clinical syndromes as represented by the DSM and a second on physical health issues. A third category consists of social functioning issues, which focuses functioning within roles related to the family, occupation, life situation, and other interpersonal contexts. A fourth category represents environmental problems associated with economic, education, legal, health, and social/affectional institutions. The model is designed to facilitate assessment of individual, interpersonal, and environmental problems.

A second promising model that may help feminist therapists integrate individual assessment with social-systemic conceptual frameworks is feminist ecological theory (Ballou, Matsumoto, and Wagner, 2002). Based on the assumption that human experience consists of multiple spheres of influence, this model seeks to integrate themes from the following social justice traditions: feminism, multiculturalism, liberation and critical psychology, and ecopsychology. The core of the circle consists of individual dimensions of the self. A series of rings radiate from this core and represent increasingly wider social systems. The first circle represents the microsystem, which includes daily interpersonal interactions and systems such as friends, the local neighborhood and church, work, school, and family. The second circle is the exosystem, which is used to conceptualize the impact of regional or national systems such as ethnicity, culture, religion, legal and economic systems, educational and political systems, and other social institutions. The macrosystem refers to global environmental issues, worldviews and ideologies, and political and economic issues. In addition to these circles of influence, one is encouraged to consider the intersecting lines of age, race, class, sex, and gender. Even when feminist therapists are compelled by practical demands or institutional expectations to offer formal diagnoses that conform with the DSM-IV (American Psychiatric Association, 1994, 2000), they may expand their own conceptualizations by exploring the specific impact of these larger systems on their clients and developing more complete and rich frameworks of understanding that take social-systemic issues into account.

To conclude this section, I list a series of questions to help readers clarify their thinking about assessment issues.

1. What aspects of human experience are important in arriving at a complete conceptual framework?
2. To what degree do you endorse traditional models of diagnosis (e.g., DSM-IV-TR)? Why? Is it possible to integrate aspects of

traditional diagnosis within a more complete framework? If so, what micro- and macrosystems need to be considered in developing a complete framework?

3. Challenging incomplete, androcentric, racist, heterosexist diagnostic practices has been a major focus of feminist psychologists' activism since the mid-1980s. To what degree is the ongoing challenge of diagnostic practices an important social justice issue? What current practices need to be challenged?

TOWARD INTEGRATION
AND ONGOING EXPLORATION

As we enter the twenty-first century, it is clear that single-cause theories of oppression and liberation represent an inadequate foundation for feminist therapy. In order to create integrated, flexible models that are open to modification, feminist therapists recognize that experiences have multiple meanings. Feminist therapists benefit from asking, "What are the *various* meanings of this event or experience to or about this person? What can be understood from *all* of them rather than from choosing one correct insight?" (Kaschak, 1992, p. 35). In contrast, efforts to identify *the* right meaning of women's experience lead to narrow thinking. All experience is organized by the meaning that individuals attribute to events. Personal meanings are influenced by various agents of socialization, including the family, peer groups, institutions, the media, and other social institutions. The messages conveyed through these agents do not have uniform meanings but are organized and elaborated in unique ways by the individual who is influenced variously by diverse social locations such as sexual orientation, race, ethnicity, culture, and class. A major task of the feminist therapist is to "maintain the tension between women as a category and each individual woman, between micro details and broad strokes, similarities and differences" (Kaschak, 1992, p. 224).

To connect feminist political theories with feminist therapy, I have proposed relatively clear distinctions between and among feminisms. In reality, the boundaries among feminisms are often flexible and overlapping. Furthermore, feminist theory is not static but continually evolving. In similar fashion, feminist therapists cannot be categorized neatly; they hold diverse views of feminism and the practice of psychotherapy. The purpose of this book has not been to pigeonhole specific forms of feminist therapy but to encourage psychologists to reflect on how their therapeutic approaches may or may not be consistent with certain forms of feminist philosophy.

Feminist therapy has grown and expanded dramatically since the mid-1970s. As feminist therapy becomes more diverse and complex, it is especially important for feminist therapists to examine how their philosophical and theoretical perspectives influence practice. Students in clinical, counseling, and social work training programs, learn that their assumptions about the nature of humanity have wide-ranging influences on practices. Therapists spend time examining the assumptions underlying systems of psychotherapy in order to develop personal theories that are internally consistent. As a logical extension of this process, it is important to clarify the nature of personal feminist visions and how they are informed by the various feminist theories.

References

Abramowitz, C. V. and Dockeki, P. R. (1977). The politics of clinical judgment: Early empirical returns. *Psychological Bulletin, 84,* 460-476.

Adams, D. (1988). Treatment models of men who batter: A profeminist analysis. In K. Yllo and M. Bograd (Eds.), *Feminist perspectives on wife abuse* (pp. 176-199). Newbury Park, CA: Sage.

Adams, J. M. (2000). Individual and group psychotherapy with African American women: Understanding the identity and context of the therapist and patient. In L. C. Jackson and B. Greene (Eds.), *Psychotherapy with African American women: Innovations in psychodynamic perspectives and practice* (pp. 33-61). New York: Guilford Press.

Adams, M. (2001). Core processes of racial identity development. In C. L. Wijeyesinghe and B. W. Jackson III (Eds.), *New perspectives on racial identity development: A theoretical and practical anthology* (pp. 209-242). New York: New York University Press.

Addams, J. ([1913] 1960). If men were seeking the franchise. In E. C. Johnson (Ed.), *Jane Addams: A centennial reader* (pp. 107-113). New York: Macmillan.

Adleman, J. and Barrett, S. E. (1990). Overlapping relationships: The importance of the feminist ethical perspective. In H. Lerman and N. Porter (Eds.), *Feminist ethics in psychotherapy* (pp. 87-91). New York: Springer.

Adleman, J. and Enguídanos, G. (Eds.) (1995). *Racism in the lives of women: Testimony, theory and guides to antiracist practice.* Binghamton, NY: The Haworth Press.

Agel, J. (Ed.) (1971). *The radical therapist.* New York: Ballantine Books.

Agras, W. S., Walsh, B. T., Fairburn, C. G., Wilson, G. T., and Kraemer, H. C. (2000). A multicenter comparison of cognitive-behavioral therapy and interpersonal psychotherapy for bulimia nervosa. *Archives of General Psychiatry, 57,* 459-466.

Alcoff, L. (1988). Cultural feminism versus post-structuralism: The identity crisis in feminist theory. *Signs: Journal of Women in Culture and Society, 13,* 405-436.

Allen, K. R. and Baber, K. M. (1992). Ethical and epistemological tensions in applying a postmodern perspective to feminist research. *Psychology of Women Quarterly, 16,* 1-15.

Allen, P. (1971). Free space. In A. Koedt, S. Firestone, A. Rapone, and E. Levine (Eds.), *Notes from the third year* (pp. 93-98). New York: Notes from the Third Year.

Allen, P. G. (Ed.) (1989). *Spider woman's granddaughters.* New York: Fawcett Press.

Alpert, J. (1973). Mother right: A new feminist theory. *Ms., 2*(2), 52-55, 88-94.

American Psychiatric Association (1980). *Diagnostic and statistical manual of mental disorders* (Third edition). Washington, DC: American Psychiatric Association.

American Psychiatric Association (1987). *Diagnostic and statistical manual of mental disorders* (Third edition, Revised). Washington, DC: American Psychiatric Association.

American Psychiatric Association (1994). *Diagnostic and statistical manual of mental disorders* (Fourth edition). Washington, DC: American Psychiatric Association.

American Psychiatric Association (2000). *Diagnostic and statistical manual of mental disorders* (Fourth edition, Text revision). Washington, DC: American Psychiatric Association.

American Psychological Association (1975). Report of the Task Force on Sex Bias and Sex-Role Stereotyping in Psychotherapeutic Practice. *American Psychologist, 30,* 1169-1175.

American Psychological Association (1978). Guidelines for therapy with women: Task Force on Sex Bias and Sex-Role Stereotyping in Psychotherapeutic Practice. *American Psychologist, 33,* 1122-1123.

American Psychological Association (1979). Principles concerning the counseling and psychotherapy of women. *Counseling Psychologist, 8,* 21.

American Psychological Association (2000). Guidelines for psychotherapy with lesbian, gay, and bisexual clients. *American Psychologist, 55,* 1440-1451.

American Psychological Association (2002a). *Ethical principles and code of conduct.* Washington, DC: Author.

American Psychological Association (2002b). *Guidelines on Multicultural Education and Training, Research, Practice, and Organizational Change for Psychologists.* Washington, DC: Author.

Anderson, A. (1999). Feminist psychology and global issues: An action agenda. *Women and Therapy, 22*(1), 7-21.

Anonymous (1971). Manifesto. In J. Agel (Ed.), *The radical therapist* (pp. xv-xxiii). New York: Ballantine Books.

Anthias, F. (1999). Beyond unities of identity in high modernity. *Identities, 6*(1), 121-144.

Anthias, F. and Yuval-Davis, N. (1990). Contextualizing feminism—Gender, ethnic and class divisions. In T. Lovell (Ed.), *British feminist thought: A reader* (pp. 103-118). Cambridge, MA: Basil Blackwell Ltd.

Anthony, S. B. ([1871] 1981a). Suffrage and the working woman. In E. C. DuBois (Ed.), *Elizabeth Cady Stanton/Susan B. Anthony: Correspondence, writings, speeches* (pp. 139-145). New York: Schocken Books.

Anthony, S. B. ([1872] 1981b). Constitutional argument. In E. C. DuBois (Ed.), *Elizabeth Cady Stanton/Susan B. Anthony: Correspondence, writings, speeches* (pp. 152-165). New York: Schocken Books.

Anthony, S. B. ([1877] 1981c). Homes of single women. In E. C. DuBois (Ed.), *Elizabeth Cady Stanton/Susan B. Anthony: Correspondence, writings, speeches* (pp. 146-151). New York: Schocken Books.

Anzaldúa, G. (1983). La Prieta. In C. Moraga and G. Anzaldúa (Eds.), *This bridge called my back* (pp. 198-209). New York: Kitchen Table/Women of Color Press.

Anzaldúa, G. (1987). *Borderlands, la frontera: The new mestiza.* San Francisco: Aunt Lute Books.

Anzaldúa, G. (Ed.) (1990). *Making face, making soul: Creative and critical perspectives of women of color.* San Francisco: Aunt Lute Books.

Anzaldúa, G. E. and Keating, A. (Eds.) (2002). *This bridge we call home: Radical visions for transformation.* New York: Routledge.

Aoki, Y. (1997). Feminism and imperialism [interview]. In S. Buckley (Ed.), *Broken silence: Voices of Japanese feminism* (pp. 1-31). Berkeley: University of California Press.

Asian Women United of California (Eds.) (1989). *Making waves: An anthology of writings by and about Asian American women.* Boston: Beacon.

Asian Women United of California (Eds.) (1997). *Making more waves: New writings by Asian American women.* Boston: Beacon.

Associated Press Worldstream (2000a). *Majority of female public servants say they face sex harassment at work.* December 27.

Associated Press Worldstream (2000b). *More Japanese women reporting sexual harassment: Government report.* May 2.

Atkinson, T.-G. (1974). *Amazon odyssey.* New York: Links.

Ault-Riché, M. (Ed.) (1986). *Women and family therapy.* Rockville, MD: Aspen.

Avis, J. M. (1988). Deepening awareness: A private study guide to feminism and family therapy. In L. Braverman (Ed.), *Women, feminism, and family therapy* (pp. 15-46). Binghamton, NY: The Haworth Press.

Baber, K. M. and Allen, K. R. (1992). *Women and families: Feminist reconstructions.* New York: Guilford Press.

Ballou, M. and Brown, L. S. (Eds.) (2002). *Rethinking mental health and disorder: Feminist perspectives.* New York: Guilford Press.

Ballou, M. and Gabalac, N. W. (1985). *A feminist position on mental health.* Springfield, IL: Charles C Thomas.

Ballou, M., Matsumoto, A., and Wagner, M. (2002). Toward a feminist ecological theory of human nature: Theory building in response to real-world dynamics. In M. Ballou and L. S. Brown (Eds.), *Rethinking mental health and disorder: Feminist perspectives* (pp. 99-141). New York: Guilford Press.

Ballou, M., Reuter, J., and Dinero, T. (1979). An audio-taped consciousness-raising group for women: Evaluation of the process dimension. *Psychology of Women Quarterly, 4,* 185-193.

Ballou, M. and West, C. (2000). Feminist therapy approaches. In M. Biaggio and M. Hersen (Eds.), *Issues in the psychology of women* (pp. 273-297). New York: Kluwer Academic/Plenum.

Banaji, M. R. (1993). The psychology of gender: A perspective on perspectives. In A. E. Beall and R. J. Sternberg (Eds.), *The psychology of gender* (pp. 251-273). New York: Guilford Press.

Banks, O. (1981). *Faces of feminism.* New York: St. Martin's Press.

Banner, L. W. (1980). *Elizabeth Cady Stanton: A radical for woman's rights.* Boston: Little, Brown and Co.

Barlow, D. H. and Durand, V. M. (2002). *Abnormal psychology: An integrative approach* (Third edition). Belmont, CA: Wadsworth.

Barnett, R. C. and Hyde, J. S. (2001). Women, men, work, and family: An expansionist theory. *American Psychologist, 56,* 781-796.

Barrett, C. J., Berg, P. I., Eaton, E. M., and Pomeroy, E. L. (1974). Implications of women's liberation and the future of psychotherapy. *Psychotherapy: Theory, Research and Practice, 11,* 11-15.

Bartlett, E. A. (Ed.) (1988). *Sarah Grimké: Letters on the equality of the sexes and other essays.* New Haven, CT: Yale University Press.

Bartlett, E. A. (1992). Beyond either/or: Justice and care in the ethics of Albert Camus. In E. B. Cole and C. S. Coultrap-McQuin (Eds.), *Explorations in feminist ethics* (pp. 82-88). Bloomington: Indiana University Press.

Basu, A. (Ed.) (1995). *The challenge of local feminisms: Women's movements in global perspective.* Boulder, CO: Westview Press.

Basu, A. (2000). Globalization of the local/localization of the global: Mapping transnational women's movements. *Meridians, 1*(1), 68-84.

Baumgardner, J. and Richards, A. (2000). *Manifesta: Young women, feminism, and the future.* New York: Farrar, Straus, and Giroux.

Beale, F. M. (1970). Double jeopardy: To be Black and female. In R. Morgan (Ed.), *Sisterhood is powerful* (pp. 340-353). New York: Random House.

Beardsley, B., Morrow, S. L., Castillo, L., and Weitzman, L. (1998). Perceptions and behaviors of practicing feminist therapists: Development of the feminist multicultural practice instrument. Paper presented at the twenty-third annual conference of the Association for Women in Psychology, Baltimore. March.

Becker, D. (2000). When she was bad: Borderline personality disorder in a post-traumatic age. *American Journal of Orthopsychiatry, 70,* 422-431.

Becker, D. (2001). Diagnosis of psychological disorders: DSM and gender. In J. Worell (Ed.), *Encyclopedia of women and gender* (pp. 333-343). San Diego: Academic Press.

Becker, D. and Lamb, S. (1994). Sex bias in the diagnosis of borderline personality disorder and posttraumatic stress disorder. *Professional Psychology, 25,* 55-61.

Belenky, M. J., Clinchy, B. M., Goldberger, N. R., and Tarule, J. M. (1986). *Women's ways of knowing.* New York: Basic Books.

Bem, S. L. (1976). Probing the promise of androgyny. In A. G. Kaplan and J. P. Bean (Eds.), *Beyond sex-role stereotypes: Readings toward a psychology of androgyny* (pp. 47-62). Boston: Little, Brown and Co.

Bem, S. L. (1983). Gender schema theory and its implications for child development: Raising gender-aschematic children in a gender-schematic society. *Signs: Journal of Women in Culture and Society, 8,* 598-616.

Bem, S. L. (1987). Gender schema theory and the romantic tradition. In P. Shaver and C. Hendrick (Eds.), *Sex and gender* (pp. 251-271). Newbury Park, CA: Sage.

Bem, S. L. (1993). *The lenses of gender: Transforming the debate on sexual inequality.* New Haven, CT: Yale University Press.

Berg, S. H. (2002). The PTSD diagnosis: Is it good for women? *Affilia, 17*(1), 55-68.

Berger, R. J., Searles, P., and Cottle, C. E. (1991). *Feminism and pornography.* Westport, CT: Praeger.

Berkeley, K. C. (1999). *The women's liberation movement in America.* Westport, CT: Greenwood.

Bernal, D. D. (1998). Using a Chicana feminist epistemology in educational research. *Harvard Educational Review, 68,* 555-579.

Bernstein, J., Morton, P., Seese, L., and Wood, M. (1969). Sisters, brothers, lovers . . . listen . . . In B. Roszak and T. Roszak (Eds.), *Masculine/feminine: Readings in sexual mythology and the liberation of women* (pp. 251-254). New York: Harper Colophon Books.

Betz, N. E. (1994). Basic issues and concepts in career counseling for women. In W. B. Walsh and S. H. Osipow (Eds.), *Career counseling for women* (pp. 1-41). Hillsdale, NJ: Erlbaum.

Betz, N. E. (2002). Women's career development: Weaving personal themes and theoretical constructs. *The Counseling Psychologist, 30,* 467-481.

Betz, N. E. and Hackett, G. (1981). The relationship of career-related self-efficacy expectations to perceived career options in college women and men. *Journal of Counseling Psychology, 28,* 399-410.

Betz, N. E. and Hackett, G. (1997). Applications of self-efficacy to the career assessment of women. *Journal of Career Assessment, 5,* 382-402.

Black, N. (1989). *Social feminism.* Ithaca, NY: Cornell University Press.

Blazina, C. and Marks, L. I. (2001). College men's affective reactions to individual therapy, psychoeducational workshops, and men's support group brochures: The influence of gender-role conflict and power dynamics upon help-seeking attitudes. *Psychotherapy: Theory, Research, Practice, Training, 38,* 297-305.

Bograd, M. (1988). Power, gender and the family: Feminist perspectives on family systems theory. In M. A. Dutton-Douglas and L. E. Walker (Eds.), *Feminist psychotherapies: Integration of therapeutic and feminist systems* (pp. 118-133). Norwood, NJ: Ablex.

Bograd, M. (1999). Strengthening domestic violence theories: Intersections of race, class, sexual orientation, and gender. *Journal of Marital and Family Therapy, 25,* 275-289.

Bohan, J. S. (1993). Regarding gender: Essentialism, constructionism, and feminist psychology. *Psychology of Women Quarterly, 17,* 5-21.

Bohan, J. S. (2002). Sex differences and/in the self: Classic themes, feminist variations, postmodern challenges. *Psychology of Women Quarterly, 26,* 74-88.

Bolen, J. S. (1984). *Goddesses in every woman.* San Francisco, CA: Harper and Row.

Bordo, S. (1990). Feminism, postmodernism, and gender-skepticism. In L. J. Nicholson (Ed.), *Feminism/postmodernism* (pp. 133-156). New York: Routledge.

Boston Lesbian Psychologies Collective (Eds.) (1987). *Lesbian psychologies.* Urbana: University of Illinois Press.

Boyd, J. A. (1990). Ethnic and cultural diversity: Keys to power. *Women and Therapy, 9(1/2),* 151-167.

Brabeck, M. (Ed.) (2000). *Practicing feminist ethics in psychology.* Washington, DC: American Psychological Association.

Brabeck, M. and Brown, L. (1997). Feminist theory and psychological practice. In J. Worell and N. G. Johnson (Eds.), *Shaping the future of feminist psychology* (pp. 15-35). Washington, DC: American Psychological Association.

Brabeck, M. and Ting, K. (2000). Feminist ethics: Lenses for examining ethical psychological practice. In M. Brabeck (Ed.), *Practicing feminist ethics in psychology* (pp. 17-35). Washington, DC: American Psychological Association.

Bradshaw, C. K. (1990). A Japanese view of dependency: What can amae psychology contribute to feminist theory and therapy? *Women and Therapy, 9(1/2),* 67-86.

Braverman, L. (Ed.) (1988). *Women, feminism, and family therapy.* Binghamton, NY: The Haworth Press.

Brien, L. and Sheldon, C. (1977). Gestalt therapy and women. In E. I. Rawlings and D. K. Carter (Eds.), *Psychotherapy for women* (pp. 120-127). Springfield, IL: Charles C Thomas.

Brodsky, A. (1976). The consciousness-raising group as a model for therapy with women. In S. Cox (Ed.), *Female psychology: The emerging self* (pp. 372-377). Chicago: Science Research Associates.

Brodsky, A. (1977). Therapeutic aspects of consciousness-raising groups. In E. I. Rawlings and D. K. Carter (Eds.), *Psychotherapy for women* (pp. 300-309). Springfield, IL: Charles C Thomas.

Brodsky, A. (1980). A decade of feminist influence on psychotherapy. *Psychology of Women Quarterly, 4,* 331-343.

Brooke (1975). The retreat to cultural feminism. In Redstockings (Eds.), *Feminist revolution* (pp. 79-83). New York: Redstockings Inc.

Brooks, G. R. (1998). *A new psychotherapy for traditional men.* San Francisco: Jossey-Bass.

Brooks, G. R. and Good, G. E. (Eds.) (2001). *The new handbook of psychotherapy and counseling with men: A comprehensive guide to settings, problems, and treatment approaches* (Volumes 1 and 2). San Francisco: Jossey-Bass.

Brooks, G. R. and Silverstein, L. B. (1995). Understanding the dark side of masculinity: An interactive systems model. In R. F. Levant and W. S. Pollack (Eds.), *A new psychology of men* (pp. 280-333). New York: Basic Books.

Brooks, L. and Forrest, L. (1994). Feminism and career counseling. In W. B. Walsh and S. H. Osipow (Eds.), *Career counseling for women* (pp. 87-134). Hillsdale, NJ: Erlbaum.

Broverman, I. K., Broverman, D. M., Clarkson, F., Rosenkrantz, P., and Vogel, S. (1970). Sex-role stereotyping and clinical judgments of mental health. *Journal of Consulting and Clinical Psychology, 45,* 250-256.

Brown, J. (1971). Mothers of the millennium. In J. Agel (Ed.), *The radical therapist* (pp. 164-168). New York: Ballantine.

Brown, L. M. and Gilligan, C. (1992). *Meeting at the crossroads: Women's psychology and girls' development.* Cambridge, MA: Harvard University Press.

Brown, L. S. (1986). Gender-role analysis: A neglected component of psychological assessment. *Psychotherapy: Theory, Research, and Practice, 23,* 243-248.

Brown, L. S. (1990a). The meaning of a multicultural perspective for theory-building in feminist therapy. *Women and Therapy, 9*(1/2), 1-22.

Brown, L. S. (1990b). Taking account of gender in the clinical assessment interview. *Professional Psychology: Research and Practice, 21,* 12-17.

Brown, L. S. (1991a). Antiracism as an ethical imperative: An example from feminist therapy. *Ethics and Behavior, 1*(2), 113-127.

Brown, L. S. (1991b). Ethical issues in feminist therapy: Selected topics. *Psychology of Women Quarterly, 15,* 323-336.

Brown, L. S. (1992a). A feminist critique of the personality disorders. In L. S. Brown and M. Ballou (Eds.), *Personality and psychopathology: Feminist reappraisals* (pp. 206-228). New York: Guilford Press.

Brown, L. S. (1992b). While waiting for the revolution: The case for a lesbian feminist psychotherapy. *Feminism and Psychology, 2*(2), 239-253.

Brown, L. S. (1993). Antidomination training as a central component of diversity in clinical psychology education. *The Clinical Psychologist, 46,* 83-87.

Brown, L. S. (1994). *Subversive dialogues: Theory in feminist therapy.* New York: Basic Books.

Brown, L. S. (1995). Anti-racism as an ethical norm in feminist therapy practice. In J. Adleman and G. Engudíanos (Eds.), *Racism in the lives of women: Testimony, theory, and guides to antiracist practice* (pp. 137-148). Binghamton, NY: The Haworth Press.

Brown, L. S. (1997). The private practice of subversion: Psychology as Tikkun Olam. *American Psychologist, 52,* 449-462.

Brown, L. S. (2000a). Feminist ethical considerations in forensic practice. In M. M. Brabeck (Ed.), *Practicing feminist ethics in psychology* (pp. 75-100). Washington, DC: American Psychological Association.

Brown, L. S. (2000b). Feminist therapy. In C. R. Snyder and R. E. Ingram (Eds.), *Handbook of psychological change: Psychotherapy processes and practices for the 21st century* (pp. 358-380). New York: Wiley.

Brown, L. S. and Ballou, M. (Eds.) (1992). *Personality and psychopathology: Feminist reappraisals.* New York: Guilford Press.

Brown, L. S. and Brodsky, A. M. (1992). The future of feminist therapy. *Psychotherapy: Theory, Research, and Practice, 29,* 51-57.

Brown, L. S. and Walker, L. E. A. (1990). Feminist therapy perspectives on self-disclosure. In G. Stricker and M. Fisher (Eds.), *Self-disclosure in the therapeutic relationship* (pp. 135-154). New York: Plenum.

Brown, R. M. (1975). The shape of things to come. In M. Myron and C. Bunch (Eds.), *Lesbianism and the women's movement* (pp. 69-77). Baltimore, MD: Diane Press.

Brownmiller, S. (1975). *Against our will: Men, women, and rape.* New York: Simon & Schuster.

Brownmiller, S. (1999). *In our time: Memoir of a revolution.* New York: Dial Press.

Bryan, L. A. (2001). Neither mask nor mirror: One therapist's journey to ethically integrate feminist family therapy and multiculturalism. *Journal of Feminist Family Therapy, 12*(2/3), 105-121.

Bunch, C. ([1972] 1987). Lesbians in revolt. In C. Bunch (Ed.), *Passionate politics: Feminist theory in action* (pp. 161-181). New York: St. Martin's Press.

Bunch, C. ([1976] 1987). Learning from lesbian separatism. In C. Bunch (Ed.), *Passionate politics* (pp. 182-191). New York: St. Martin's Press.

Bunch, C. ([1978] 1987). Lesbian-feminist theory. In C. Bunch (Ed.), *Passionate politics* (pp. 196-202). New York: St. Martin's Press.

Bunch, C. (1987). Not by degrees: Feminist theory and education. In C. Bunch (Ed.), *Passionate politics* (pp. 240-253). New York: St. Martin's Press.

Burden, D. S. and Gottlieb, N. (1987). Women's socialization and feminist groups. In C. Brody (Ed.), *Women's therapy groups: Paradigms of feminist treatment* (pp. 24-39). New York: Springer.

Burgess, A. W. and Holmstrom, L. L. (1974). Rape trauma syndrome. *American Journal of Psychiatry, 131,* 981-986.

Burn, S. M. (2000). *Women across cultures: A global perspective.* Mountain View, CA: Mayfield.

Burris, B. (1973). The fourth world manifesto. In A. Koedt, E. Levine, and A. Rapone (Eds.), *Radical feminism* (pp. 322-357). New York: Quadrangle Books.

Burstow, B. (1992). *Radical feminist therapy: Working in the context of violence.* Newbury Park, CA: Sage.

Burstow, B. (2002). Adult basic education for psychiatric survivors: Survival skills. *Adult Basic Education, 12*(2), 99-110.

Burstow, B. (2003). Toward a radical understanding of trauma and trauma work. *Violence Against Women, 9,* 1293-1317.

Butler, J. (1992). Contingent foundations: Feminism and the question of "postmodernism." In J. Butler and J. Scott (Eds.), *Feminists theorize the political* (pp. 3-21). New York: Routledge.

Butler, K. (2001). Revolution on the horizon: DBT challenges the borderline diagnosis. *Psychotherapy Networker,* May/June, 26-39.

Butler, M. (1985). Guidelines for feminist therapy. In L. B. Rosewater and L. E. A. Walter (Eds.), *Handbook of feminist therapy* (pp. 32-38). New York: Springer.

Butler, S. and Wintram, C. (1991). *Feminist groupwork.* Newbury Park, CA: Sage.

Byars, A. M. and Hackett, G. (1998). Applications of social cognitive theory to the career development of women of color. *Applied and Preventive Psychology, 7,* 255-267.

Cacoullos, A. R. (2001). American feminist theory. *American Studies International, 39*(1), 72-117.

Calhoun, C. (1997). Separating lesbian theory from feminist theory. In D. T. Meyers (Ed.), *Feminist social thought: A reader* (pp. 200-218). New York: Routledge.

Campbell, B., Schellenberg, E. G., and Senn, C. Y. (1997). Evaluating measures of contemporary sexism. *Psychology of Women Quarterly, 21,* 89-102.

Caplan, P. J. (1984). The myth of women's masochism. *American Psychologist, 39,* 130-139.

Caplan, P. J. (1989). *Don't blame mother: Mending the mother-daughter relationship.* New York: Harper and Row.

Caplan, P. J. (1991). Delusional dominating personality disorder (DDPD). *Feminism and Psychology, 1,* 171-174.

Caplan, P. J. (1995). *They say you're crazy.* Reading, MA: Addison-Wesley.

Carden, M. L. (1974). *The new feminist movement.* New York: Russell Sage Foundation.

Cass, V. (1979). Homosexual identity formation: A theoretical model. *Journal of Homosexuality, 4,* 219-235.

Castillo, A. (1995). *Massacre of the dreamers: Essays on Xicanisma.* New York: Plume.

Chadwick, B. A. and Heaton, T. B. (1999). *Statistical handbook on the American family.* Phoenix, AZ: Orynx Press.

Charlotte Perkins Gilman Chapter of the New American Movement (1984). In A. M. Jaggar and P. S. Rothenberg (Eds.), *Feminist frameworks* (pp. 152-154). New York: McGraw-Hill.

Chase, K. (1977). Seeing sexism: A look at feminist therapy. *State and Mind,* March/April, 12-22.

Chernin, J., Holden, J. M., and Chandler, C. (1997). Bias in psychological assessment: Heterosexism. *Measurement and Evaluation in Counseling and Development, 30,* 68-76.

Chesler, P. (1971). Patient and patriarch: Women in the psychotherapeutic relationship. In V. Gornick and B. Moran (Eds.), *Woman in sexist society* (pp. 362-392). New York: Mentor.

Chesler, P. (1972). *Women and madness.* New York: Doubleday.

Chesler, P. (1997). Women and madness: A feminist diagnosis. *Ms., 8*(3), 36-41.

Chester, A. and Bretherton, D. (2001). What makes feminist counseling feminist? *Feminism and Psychology, 11,* 527-545.

Chin, J. L. (Ed.) (2000). *Relationships among Asian American women.* Washington, DC: American Psychological Association.

Chodorow, N. J. (1978). *The reproduction of mothering.* Berkeley: University of California Press.

Chodorow, N. J. (1999). *The power of feeling: Personal meaning in psychoanalysis, gender, and culture.* New Haven, CT: Yale University Press.

Chow, E. N. (1996). The development of feminist consciousness among Asian American women. In E. N. Chow, D. Wildinson, and M. B. Zinn (Eds.), *Race, class, and gender: Common bonds, difference voices* (pp. 251-264). Thousand Oaks, CA: Sage.

Clopton, N. A. and Sorell, G. T. (1993). Gender differences in moral reasoning: Stable or situational? *Psychology of Women Quarterly, 17,* 85-101.

Collard, A. (1989). *Rape of the wild: Man's violence against animals and the earth.* Bloomington: Indiana University Press.

Collier, H. V. (1982). *Counseling women.* New York: Free Press.

Collins, P. H. (1986). Learning from the outsider within: The sociological significance of Black feminist thought. *Social Problems, 33*(6), S14-S32.

Collins, P. H. (1991). The meaning of motherhood in Black culture and Black mother-daughter relationships. In P. Bell-Scott, B. Guy-Sheftall, J. J. Royster, J. Sims-Wood, M. DeCosta-Willis, and L. P. Fultz (Eds.), *Double stitch: Black women write about mothers and daughters* (pp. 42-60). New York: Harper Collins.

Collins, P. H. (2000). *Black feminist thought: Knowledge, consciousness, and the politics of empowerment* (Second edition). New York: Routledge.

Comas-Díaz, L. (1987). Feminist therapy with mainland Puerto Rican women. *Psychology of Women Quarterly, 11,* 461-474.

Comas-Díaz, L. (1988). Feminist therapy with Hispanic/Latina women: Myth or reality? In L. Fulani (Ed.), *The psychopathology of everyday racism and sexism* (pp. 39-61). Binghamton, NY: The Haworth Press.

Comas-Díaz, L. (1991). Feminism and diversity in psychology: The case of women of color. *Psychology of Women Quarterly, 15,* 597-609.

Comas-Díaz, L. (1994). An integrative approach. In L. Comas-Díaz and B. Greene (Eds.), *Women of color: Integrating ethnic and gender identities in psychotherapy* (pp. 287-318). New York: Guilford Press.

Comas-Díaz, L. (2000). An ethnopolitical approach to working with people of color. *American Psychologist, 55,* 1319-1325.

Comas-Díaz, L. and Duncan, J. W. (1985). The cultural context: A factor in assertiveness training with mainland Puerto Rican women. *Psychology of Women Quarterly, 9,* 463-476.

Comas-Díaz, L. and Greene, B. (Eds.) (1994a). *Women of Color: Integrating ethnic and gender identities in psychotherapy.* New York: Guilford Press.

Comas-Díaz, L. and Greene, B. (1994b). Women of color with professional status. In L. Comas-Díaz and B. Greene (Eds.), *Women of color: Integrating ethnic and gender identities in psychotherapy* (pp. 347-388). New York: Guilford Press.

Combahee River Collective (1982). A Black feminist statement. In G. T. Hull, P. B. Scott, and B. Smith (Eds.), *All the women are white, all the Blacks are men, but some of us are brave* (pp. 13-22). Old Westbury, NY: The Feminist Press.

Cook, E. P. (1985). Androgyny: A goal for counseling? *Journal of Counseling and Development, 63,* 567-571.

Cooper-White, P. (1989). Peer and clinical counseling—Is there a place for both in the battered women's movement? Paper presented at the Third National Nursing Conference on Violence Against Women. Concord, California. May.

Corey, G. (2004). *Theory and practice of counseling and psychotherapy* (Seventh edition). Belmont, CA: Wadsworth.

Costello, C. B. and Stone, A. J. (Eds.) (2001). *The American woman: 2001-2002.* New York: Norton.

Coster, J. S. and Schwebel, M. (1997). Well-functioning in professional psychologists. *Professional Psychology: Research and Practice, 28,* 5-13.

Craighead, W. E., Craighead, L. W., and Ilardi, S. S. (1998). Psychosocial treatments for major depressive disorder. In P. E. Nathan and J. M. Gorman (Eds.), *A guide to treatments that work* (pp. 226-239). New York: Oxford University Press.

Crawford, M. and Marecek, J. (1989). Psychology reconstructs the female: 1968-1988. *Psychology of Women Quarterly, 13,* 147-165.

Crawford, M. and Unger, R. (2004). *Women and gender: A feminist psychology* (Fourth edition). Boston: McGraw-Hill.

Cross, T., Klein, F., Smith, B., and Smith, B. (1982). Face-to-face, day-to-day—Racism CR. In G. T. Hull, P. B. Scott, and B. Smith (Eds.), *All the women are white, all the Blacks are men, but some of us are brave* (pp. 52-56). Old Westbury, NY: The Feminist Press.

Cross, W. (1991). *Shades of Black: Diversity in African-American identity.* Philadelphia: Temple University Press.

Cross, W. E. Jr. and Vandiver, B. J. (2001). Nigrescence theory and measurement: Introducing the Cross Racial Identity Scale (CRIS). In J. G. Ponterotto, J. M. Casas, L. M. Suzuki, and C. M. Alexander (Eds.), *Handbook of multicultural counseling* (Second edition) (pp. 371-393). Thousand Oaks, CA: Sage.

Crowley-Long, K. (1998). Making room for many feminisms: The dominance of the liberal political perspective in the psychology of women course. *Psychology of Women Quarterly, 22,* 113-130.

Daly, M. (1978). *Gyn/ecology: The metaethics of radical feminism.* Boston: Beacon Press.

Davis, A. Y. (1981). *Women, race, and class.* New York: Vintage Books.

de Beauvior, S. (1952). *The second sex.* New York: Knopf.

Deaux, K. and Major, B. (1987). Putting gender into context: An interactive model of gender-related behavior. *Psychological Review, 94,* 369-389.

Deaux, K. and Stewart, A. (2001). Framing gendered identities. In R. K. Unger (Ed.), *Handbook of the psychology of women and gender* (pp. 84-97). New York: Wiley.

Deckard, B. S. (1979). *The women's movement.* New York: Harper and Row.

Diamond, I. and Orenstein, G. F. (Eds.) (1990). *Reweaving the world: The emergence of ecofeminism.* San Francisco: Sierra Club Books.

Dickensheets, T. (1996). The role of the education mama. *Japan Quarterly, 43*(3), 73-78.

Dicker, R. and Piepmeier, A. (Eds.) (2003). *Catching the wave: Reclaiming feminism for the 21st century.* Boston: Northeastern University Press.

DiQuinzio, P. and Young, I. M. (Eds.) (1997). *Feminist ethics and social policy.* Bloomington: Indiana University Press.

Doherty, M. A. (1973). Sexual bias in personality theory. *The Counseling Psychologist, 4,* 67-74.

Donovan, J. (2000). *Feminist theory: Intellectual traditions* (Third edition). New York: Continuum Publishing Co.

Douglas, E. T. (1970). *Margaret Sanger: Pioneer of the future.* New York: Holt, Rinehart and Winston.

Douglas, M. A. (1985). The role of power in feminist therapy: A reformulation. In L. B. Rosewater and L. E. A. Walker (Eds.), *Handbook of feminist therapy* (pp. 241-249). New York: Springer.

Downing, N. E. and Roush, K. L. (1985). From passive acceptance to active commitment: A model of feminist identity development for women. *Counseling Psychologist, 13,* 695-709.

Drewery, W. and Winslade, J. (1997). The theoretical story of narrative therapy. In G. Monk, J. Winslade, K. Crocket, and D. Epston (Eds.), *Narrative therapy in practice: The archaeology of hope* (pp. 32-52). San Francisco: Jossey-Bass.

DuBois, E. C. (Ed.) (1981). *Elizabeth Cady Stanton/Susan B. Anthony: Correspondence, writings, speeches.* New York: Schocken Books.

Dunn, A. B. and Dawes, S. J. (1999). Spirituality-focused genograms: Keys to uncovering spiritual resources in African American families. *Journal of Multicultural Counseling and Development, 27,* 240-254.

Dunn, K. F. and Cowan, G. (1993). Social influence strategies among Japanese and American college women. *Psychology of Women Quarterly, 17,* 39-52.

DuPlessis, R. B. and Snitow, A. (1998). *The feminist memoir project: Voices from women's liberation.* New York: Three Rivers Press.

Dutton-Douglas, M. A. and Walker, L. E. (Eds.) (1988). *Feminist psychotherapies: Integration of therapeutic and feminist systems.* Norwood, NJ: Ablex.

Dworkin, A. (1980). Why so-called radical men love and need pornography. In L. Lederer (Ed.), *Take back the night: Women on pornography* (pp. 148-154). New York: William Morrow.

Dworkin, A. (1981). *Pornography: Men possessing women.* New York: Perigee.

Eccles, J. S. (1994). Understanding women's educational and occupational choices: Applying the Eccles et al. model of achievement-related choices. *Psychology of Women Quarterly, 18,* 585-610.

Echols, A. (1989). *Daring to be bad: Radical feminism in America.* Minneapolis: University of Minnesota Press.

Ehara, Y. (2000). Feminism's growing pains. *Japan Quarterly, 47*(3), 41-48.

Eichenbaum, L. and Orbach, S. (1983). *Understanding women: A feminist psycho-analytic approach.* New York: Basic Books.

Eisenstein, Z. (1979). Developing a theory of capitalist patriarchy and socialist feminism. In Z. Eisenstein (Ed.), *Capitalist patriarchy and the case for socialist feminism* (pp. 5-40). New York: Monthly Review Press.

Eisenstein, Z. (1981). *The radical future of liberal feminism.* Boston: Northeastern University Press.

Eisler, R. (1988). *The chalice and the blade.* San Francisco: Harper.

Eisler, R. (1990). The Gaia tradition and the partnership future: An ecofeminist manifesto. In I. Diamond and G. F. Orenstein (Eds.), *Reweaving the world: The emergence of ecofeminism* (pp. 23-34). San Francisco: Sierra Club Books.

Elias, M. (1975). Sisterhood therapy. *Human Behavior,* April, pp. 56-61.

Elkin, I., Shea, M. T., Watkins, J. T., Imber, S. D., Sotsky, S. M., Collins, J. F., Glass, D. R., Pilkonis, P. E., Leber, W. R., Docherty, J. P., et al. (1989). National Institute of Mental Health Treatment of Depression Collaborative Research Program: General effectiveness of treatments. *Archives of General Psychiatry, 46,* 971-982.

Enns, C. Z. (1987). Gestalt therapy and feminist therapy: A proposed integration. *Journal of Counseling and Development, 66,* 93-95.

Enns, C. Z. (1988). Dilemmas of power and quality in marital and family counseling: Proposals for a feminist perspective. *Journal of Counseling and Development, 67,* 242-248.

Enns, C. Z. (1991). The "new" relationship models of women's identity: A review and critique for counselors. *Journal of Counseling and Development, 69,* 209-217.

Enns, C. Z. (1992a). Self-esteem groups: A synthesis of consciousness-raising and assertiveness training. *Journal of Counseling and Development, 71,* 7-13.

Enns, C. Z. (1992b). Toward integrating feminist psychotherapy and feminist philosophy. *Professional Psychology: Research and Practice, 23,* 453-466.

Enns, C. Z. (1993). Twenty years of feminist counseling and therapy: From naming biases to implementing multifaceted practice. *The Counseling Psychologist, 21,* 3-87.

Enns, C. Z. (1994). Archetypes and gender: Goddesses, warriors, and psychological health. *Journal of Counseling and Development, 73,* 127-133.

Enns, C. Z. (2000). Gender issues in counseling. In S. D. Brown and R. W. Lent (Eds.), *Handbook of counseling psychology* (Third edition) (pp. 601-638). New York: Wiley.

Enns, C. Z. (2002). A summary of task force activities. Unpublished manuscript.

Enns, C. Z. (2004). Counseling girls and women: Attitudes, knowledge, and skills. In D. R. Atkinson and G. Hackett (Eds.), *Counseling diverse populations* (Third edition) (pp. 285-306). Boston: McGraw-Hill.

Enns, C. Z., Campbell, J., Courtois, C., Gottlieb, M., Lese, K., Gilbert, M., and Forrest, L. (1998). Working with clients who may have experienced childhood abuse: Recommendations for assessment and practice. *Professional Psychology: Research and Practice, 29,* 245-256.

Enns, C. Z. and Hackett, G. (1990). Comparisons of feminist and nonfeminist women's reactions to variants of nonsexist and feminist counseling. *Journal of Counseling Psychology, 37,* 33-40.

Enns, C. Z. and Hackett, G. (1993). A comparison of feminist and nonfeminist women's and men's reactions to nonsexist and feminist counseling: A replication and extension. *Journal of Counseling and Development, 71,* 499-509.

Erikson, E. H. (1968). *Identity: Youth and crisis.* New York: Norton.

Espín, O. M. (1986). Cultural and historical influences on sexuality in Hispanic/Latina women. In J. Cole (Ed.), *All American women* (pp. 272-284). New York: Free Press.

Espín, O. M. (1987). Psychological impact of migration on Latinas: Implications for psychotherapeutic practice. *Psychology of Women Quarterly, 11,* 489-503.

Espín, O. M. (1990). How inclusive is feminist psychology? *Association for Women in Psychology Newsletter,* fall, 1-2.

Espín, O. M. (1994). Feminist approaches. In L. Comas-Díaz and B. Greene (Eds.), *Women of color: Integrating ethnic and gender identities in psychotherapy* (pp. 265-286). New York: Guilford Press.

Espín, O. M. (1995). On knowing you are the unknown: Women of color constructing psychology. In J. Adleman and G. Enguídanos (Eds.), *Racism in the lives of women: Testimony, theory, and guides to antiracist practice* (pp. 127-136). Binghamton, NY: The Haworth Press.

Espín, O. M. and Gawelek, M. A. (1992). Women's diversity: Ethnicity, race, class, and gender in theories of feminist psychology. In L. S. Brown and M. Ballou (Eds.), *Personality and psychopathology: Feminist reappraisals* (pp. 88-107). New York: Norton.

Essed, P. (1991). *Understanding everyday racism: An interdisciplinary theory.* Newbury Park, CA: Sage.

Esterberg, K. G. (1997). *Lesbian and bisexual identities: Constructing communities, constructing selves.* Philadelphia, PA: Temple University Press.

Estes, C. P. (1992). *Women who run with the wolves: Myths and stories of the wild woman archetype.* New York: Ballantine.

Eugene, T. M. (1995). There is a balm in Gilead: Black women and the black church as agents of a therapeutic community. *Women and Therapy, 16*(2/3), 55-71.

Evans, M. D., Hollon, S. D., DeRubeis, R. J., Piascki, J. M., Grove, W. M., Garvey, M. J., and Tuason, V. B. (1992). Differential rates of relapse following cognitive therapy and pharmacotherapy for depression. *Archives of General Psychiatry, 49,* 802-808.

Farmer, H. S. (1997). *Diversity and women's career development: From adolescence to adulthood.* Thousand Oaks, CA: Sage.

Fassinger, R. E. (1990). Causal models of career choice in two samples of college women. *Journal of Vocational Behavior, 36,* 225-248.

Fassinger, R. E. (1996). Notes from the margins: Integrating lesbian experience into the vocational psychology of women. *Journal of Vocational Behavior, 48,* 160-175.

Fassinger, R. E. (2000). Gender and sexuality in human development: Implications for prevention and advocacy in counseling psychology. In S. D. Brown and R. W. Lent (Eds.), *Handbook of counseling psychology* (Third edition) (pp. 346-378). New York: Wiley.

Fassinger, R. E. and O'Brien, K. M. (2000). Career counseling with college women: A scientist-practitioner-advocate model of intervention. In D. A. Luzzo (Ed.), *Career counseling of college students: An empirical guide to strategies that work* (pp. 253-266). Washington, DC: American Psychological Association.

Feminist Therapy Institute (1990). Feminist Therapy Institute code of ethics. In H. Lerman and N. Porter (Eds.), *Feminist ethics in psychotherapy* (pp. 37-40). New York: Springer.

Feminist Therapy Institute (2000). *Feminist therapy code of ethics* [revised 1999]. San Francisco: Feminist Therapy Institute.

The Feminists (1973). The Feminists: A political organization to annihilate sex roles. In A. Koedt, E. Levine, and A. Rapone (Eds.), *Radical feminism* (pp. 368-378). New York: Quadrangle Books.

Ferree, M. M. and Hess, B. B. (1985). *Controversy and coalition: The new feminist movement.* Boston: Twayne.

Ferree, M. M. and Hess, B. B. (1995). *Controversy and coalition: The new feminist movement across four decades of change* (Third edition). New York: Routledge.

Findlen, B. (Ed.) (1995). *Listen up: Voices from the next feminist generation.* Seattle, WA: Seal Press.

Firestone, S. (1970). *The dialectic of sex.* New York: Morrow.

Fischer, A. R. and Good, G. E. (1997). Men and psychotherapy: An investigation of alexithymia, intimacy, and masculine gender roles. *Psychotherapy: Theory, Research, Practice, Training, 34,* 160-170.

Fitzgerald, L. F. and Rounds, J. (1994). Women and work: Theory encounters reality. In W. B. Walsh and S. H. Osipow (Eds.), *Career counseling for women* (pp. 327-353). Hillsdale, NJ: Erlbaum.

Flax, J. (1987). Postmodernism and gender relations in feminist theory. *Signs: Journal of Women in Culture and Society, 12,* 621-643.

Flores, L. Y. and O'Brien, K. M. (2002). The career development of Mexican American adolescent women: A test of social cognitive career theory. *Journal of Counseling Psychology, 49,* 14-27.

Flores-Ortiz, Y. G. (1995). Psychotherapy with Chicanas at midlife: Cultural/clinical considerations. In J. Adleman and G. Enguídanos (Eds.), *Racism in the lives of women: Testimony, theory, and guides to antiracist practice* (pp. 251-259). Binghamton, NY: The Haworth Press.

Foa, E. B., Dancu, C. B., Hembree, E. A., Jaycox, L. H., Meadows, E. A., and Street, G. P. (1999). A comparison of exposure therapy, stress inoculation training, and their combination for reducing posttraumatic stress disorder in female assault victims. *Journal of Consulting and Clinical Psychology, 67*(2), 194-200.

Foa, E. B. and Rothbaum, B. O. (1998). *Treating the trauma of rape: Cognitive-behavioral therapy for PTSD.* New York: Guilford Press.

Foa, E. B. and Street, G. P. (2001). Women and traumatic events. *Journal of Clinical Psychiatry, 62* (Suppl. 17), 29-34.

Foa, E. B. and Zoellner, L. A. (1998). Posttraumatic stress disorder in female victims of assault: Theory and treatment. In E. Sanavio (Ed.), *Behavior and cognitive therapy today: Essays in honor of Hans J. Eysenck* (pp. 87-101). Oxford: Pergamon.

Fodor, I. G. (1988). Cognitive behavior therapy: Evaluation of theory and practice for addressing women's issues. In M. A. Dutton-Douglas and L. E. Walker (Eds.), *Feminist psychotherapies: Integration of therapeutic and feminist systems* (pp. 91-117). Norwood, NJ: Ablex.

Fodor, I. and Rothblum, E. D. (1984). Strategies for dealing with sex-role stereotypes. In C. Brody (Ed.), *Women therapists working with women* (pp. 86-95). New York: Springer.

Foreman, A. (1977). *Femininity as alienation: Women and the family in Marxism and psychoanalysis.* London: Pluto Press.

Frame, M. W. (2001). The spiritual genogram in training and supervision. *The Family Journal: Counseling and Therapy for Couples and Families, 9,* 109-115.

Frankenberg, R. (1993). *The social construction of whiteness: White women, race matters.* Minneapolis: University of Minnesota Press.

Franks, V. and Rothblum, E. D. (Eds.) (1983). *The stereotyping of women.* New York: Springer.

Fraser, N. and Nicholson, L. (1990). Social criticism without philosophy: An encounter between feminism and postmodernism. In L. J. Nicholson (Ed.), *Feminism/postmodernism* (pp. 19-38). New York: Routledge.

Fredrickson, B. L. and Roberts, T. A. (1997). Objectification theory: Toward understanding women's lived experiences and mental health risks. *Psychology of Women Quarterly, 21,* 173-206.

Freedman, E. B. (2002). *No turning back: The history of feminism and the future of women.* New York: Ballantine Books.

Freeman, J. (1995). From seed to harvest: Transformations of feminist organizations and scholarship. In M. M. Ferree and P. Y. Martin (Eds.), *Feminist organizations: Harvest of the new women's movement* (pp. 397-408). Philadelphia, PA: Temple University Press.

Freire, P. (1970). *Pedagogy of the oppressed.* New York: Seabury Press.

Friedan, B. ([1963] 1983). *The feminine mystique* (Twentieth anniversary edition). New York: Norton.

Friedman, M. (2000). Feminism in ethics: Conceptions of autonomy. In M. Fricker and J. Hornsby (Eds.), *The Cambridge companion to feminism in philosophy* (pp. 205-224). New York: Cambridge University Press.

Frye, M. (1983). *The politics of reality: Essays in feminist theory*. Trumansburg, NY: Crossing Press.

Fujieda, M. and Fujimura-Fanselow, K. (1995). Women's studies: An overview. In K. Fujimura Fanselow and A. Kameda (Eds.), *Japanese women: New feminist perspectives on the past, present and future* (pp. 155-180). New York: The Feminist Press.

Fukuzawa, K. (1995). Women's hiring woes. *Japan Quarterly, 42*(2), 155-161.

Fulani, L. (1988). Poor women of color do great therapy. In L. Fulani (Ed.), *The psychopathology of everyday racism and sexism* (pp. 111-120). Binghamton, NY: The Haworth Press.

Fulcher, J. A. (2002). Domestic violence and the rights of women in Japan and the United States. *Human Rights,* summer, 16-17.

Fuller, M. ([1845] 1976). Woman in the nineteenth century. In B. G. Chevigny (Ed.), *The woman and the myth: Margaret Fuller's life and writings* (pp. 239-279). Old Westbury, NY: The Feminist Press.

Gage, J. J. ([1884] 1968). Address at a convention. In A. S. Kraditor (Ed.), *Up from the pedestal* (pp. 137-140). Chicago: Quadrangle Books.

Ganley, A. L. (1988). Feminist therapy with male clients. In M. A. Dutton-Douglas and L. E. Walker (Eds.), *Feminist psychotherapies: Integration of therapeutic and feminist systems* (pp. 186-205). Norwood, NJ: Ablex.

Gannon, L. (1982). The role of power in psychotherapy. *Women and Therapy, 1*(2), 3-11.

Garb, H. N. (1997). Race bias, social class bias, and gender bias in clinical judgment. *Clinical Psychology: Science and Practice, 4,* 99-120.

Garber, L. (2001). *Identity poetics: Race, class, and the lesbian-feminist roots of queer theory*. New York: Columbia University Press.

García, A. M. (Ed.) (1997). *Chicana feminist thought: The basic historical writings*. New York: Routledge.

Garrison, D. (1981). Karen Horney and feminism. *Signs: Journal of Women in Culture and Society, 6,* 672-691.

Gavey, N. (1989). Feminist poststructuralism and discourse analysis. *Psychology of Women Quarterly, 13,* 459-475.

Gergen, M. (2001). *Feminist reconstructions in psychology*. Thousand Oaks, CA: Sage.

Gervasio, A. H. and Crawford, M. (1989). Social evaluations of assertiveness: A critique and speech act reformulation. *Psychology of Women Quarterly, 13,* 1-25.

Giddings, P. (1984). *When and where I enter: The impact of Black women on race and sex in America*. New York: Wm. Morrow and Co.

Gilbert, L. A. (1980). Feminist therapy. In A. Brodsky and R. T. Hare-Mustin (Eds.), *Women and psychotherapy* (pp. 245-265). New York: Guilford Press.

Gilbert, L. A. (1981). Toward mental health: The benefits of psychological androgyny. *Professional Psychology: Research and Practice, 12,* 29-38.

Gilbert, L. A. (1993). *Two careers/one family: The promise of gender equality.* Beverly Hills, CA: Sage.

Gilbert, L. A. and Rader, J. (2001). Current perspectives on women's adult roles: Work, family, and life. In R. K. Unger (Ed.), *Handbook of the psychology of women and gender* (pp. 156-169). New York: Wiley.

Gilbert, L. A. and Sher, M. (1999). *Gender and sex in counseling and psychotherapy.* Boston: Allyn & Bacon.

Gilbert, S. and Thompson, J. K. (1996). Feminist explanations of the development of eating disorders: Common themes, research findings, and methodological issues. *Clinical Psychology: Science and Practice, 3,* 183-202.

Gilligan, C. (1977). In a different voice: Women's conception of self and morality. *Harvard Educational Review, 47,* 481-517.

Gilligan, C. (1982). *In a different voice.* Cambridge, MA: Harvard University Press.

Gilligan, C., Lyons, N. P., and Hanmer, T. J. (1990). *Making connections.* Cambridge, MA: Harvard University Press.

Gilman, C. P. S. (1898). *Women and economics.* Boston: Small, Maynard, and Co.

Gilman, C. P. ([1915] 1979). *Herland.* New York: Pantheon Books.

Gilman, C. P. (1923). *His religion and hers: A study in the faith of our fathers and the work of our mothers.* New York: The Century Company.

Glaser, K. (1976). Women's self-help groups as an alternative to therapy. *Psychotherapy: Theory, Research, and Practice, 13,* 77-81.

Glenn, M. (1971). Introduction. In J. Agel (Ed.), *The radical therapist* (pp. ix-xxiii). New York: Ballantine.

Glick, P. and Fiske, S. T. (1997). Hostile and benevolent sexism: Measuring ambivalent sexist attitudes toward women. *Psychology of Women Quarterly, 21,* 119-136.

Goldberger, N. R. (1996). Cultural imperatives and diversity in ways of knowing. In N. R. Goldberger and J. M. Tarule (Eds.), *Knowledge, difference, and power: Essays inspired by "Women's Ways of Knowing"* (pp. 335-371). New York: Basic Books.

Golden, C. (2004). The intersexed and the transgendered: Rethinking sex/gender. In J. C. Chrisler, C. Golden, and P. D. Rozee (Eds.), *Lectures on the psychology of women* (Third edition) (pp. 81-95). Boston: McGraw-Hill.

Goldenberg, N. R. (1976). A feminist critique of Jung. *Signs: Journal of Women in Culture and Society, 2,* 443-449.

Goldman, E. ([1917] 1969a). Marriage and love. In E. Goldman (Ed.), *Anarchism and other essays* (pp. 227-239). New York: Dover Publications, Inc.

Goldman, E. ([1917] 1969b). The tragedy of woman's emancipation. In E. Goldman (Ed.), *Anarchism and other essays* (pp. 213-225). New York: Dover Publications, Inc.

Goldman, E. ([1917] 1969c). Woman suffrage. In E. Goldman (Ed.), *Anarchism and other essays* (pp. 195-211). New York: Dover Publications, Inc.

Gomberg, L. E. (2001). What women in groups can learn from the goddess: The maiden-mother-crone trinity. *Women and Therapy, 23*(4), 55-70.

Gonda, C. (1998). Lesbian theory. In S. Jackson and J. Jones (Eds.), *Contemporary feminist theories* (pp. 113-130). New York: New York University Press.

Gondolf, E. (1988). *Battered women as survivors.* Lexington, MA: D.C. Heath and Company.

Good, G., Gilbert, L., and Scher, M. (1990). Gender aware therapy: A synthesis of feminist therapy and knowledge about gender. *Journal of Counseling and Development, 68,* 376-380.

Good, G. and Mintz, L. M. (1990). Gender role conflict and depression in college: Evidence for compounded risk. *Journal of Counseling and Development, 69,* 17-21.

Good, G. E., Robertson, J. M., Fitzgerald, L. F., and Stevens, M. (1996). The relation between masculine role conflict and psychological distress in male university counseling center clients. *Journal of Counseling and Development, 75,* 44-49.

Good, G. E., Robertson, J. M., O'Neil, J. M., and Fitzgerald, L. F. (1995). Male gender role conflict: Psychometric issues and relations to psychological distress. *Journal of Counseling Psychology, 42,* 3-10.

Goodman, L. A., Koss, M. P., and Russo, N. R. (1993). Violence against women: Mental health effects. Part II. Conceptualizations of posttraumatic stress. *Applied and Preventive Psychology, 2,* 23-130.

Goodrich, T. J., Rampage, C., Ellman, B., and Halstead, K. (1988). *Feminist family therapy.* New York: Norton.

Gordon, E. W., Miller, F., and Rollock, D. (1990). Coping with communicentric bias in knowledge production in the social sciences. *Educational Researcher, 19,* 4-19.

Gordon, S. (1991). *Prisoners of men's dreams.* Boston: Little, Brown and Co.

Greene, B. (1986). When the therapist is white and the patient is Black: Considerations for psychotherapy in the feminist heterosexual and lesbian communities. In D. Howard (Ed.), *The dynamics of feminist therapy* (pp. 41-65). Binghamton, NY: The Haworth Press.

Greene, B. (1990). What has gone before: The legacy of racism and sexism in the lives of Black mothers and daughters. In L. Brown and M. P. Root (Eds.), *Diversity and complexity in feminist therapy* (pp. 207-230). Binghamton, NY: The Haworth Press.

Greene, B. (1992). Still here: A perspective on psychotherapy with African-American women. In J. C. Chrisler and D. Howard (Eds.), *New directions in feminist psychology: Practice, theory, and research* (pp. 13-25). New York: Springer.

Greene, B. (1994). African American women. In L. Comas-Díaz and B. Greene (Eds.), *Women of color: Integrating ethnic and gender identities in psychotherapy* (pp. 10-29). New York: Guilford Press.

Greene, B. (1995). An African American perspective on racism and anti-Semitism within feminist organizations. In J. Adleman and G. Enguídanos (Eds.), *Racism in the lives of women: Testimony, theory, and guides to antiracist practice* (pp. 303-313). Binghamton, NY: The Haworth Press.

Greene, B. (1997). Lesbian women of color: Triple jeopardy. *Journal of Lesbian Studies, 1*(1), 109-147.

Greene, B. and Sanchez-Hucles, J. (1997). Diversity: Advancing an inclusive feminist psychology. In J. Worell and N. G. Johnson (Eds.), *Shaping the future of feminist psychology: Education, research, and practice* (pp. 173-202). Washington, DC: American Psychological Association.

Greenspan, M. (1986). Should therapists be personal? Self-disclosure and therapeutic distance in feminist therapy. In D. Howard (Ed.), *The dynamics of feminist therapy* (pp. 5-17). Binghamton, NY: The Haworth Press.

Greenspan, M. (1993). *A new approach to women and therapy.* New York: Wiley.

Greenspan, M. (1995). On being a feminist and a psychotherapist. *Women and Therapy, 17*(1/2), 229-241.

Grice, H. (2000). Asian American women's prose narratives: Genre and identity. In E. M. Ghymn (Ed.), *Asian American studies: Identity, images, issues past and present* (pp. 179-204). New York: Peter Lang.

Grimké, S. ([1838] 1972). Letters on the equality of the sexes and the condition of woman. In M. Schneir (Ed.), *Feminism: The essential historical writings* (pp. 35-48). New York: Vantage Books.

Gulanick, N. A., Howard, G. S., and Moreland, J. (1979). Evaluation of a group program designed to increase androgyny in feminine women. *Sex Roles, 5,* 811-827.

Gurko, M. (1976). *The ladies of Seneca Falls: The birth of the women's rights movement.* New York: Schocken Books.

Gutek, B. A. (2001). Women and paid work. *Psychology of Women Quarterly, 25,* 379-393.

Guy-Sheftall, B. (Ed.) (1995). *Words of fire: An anthology of African-American feminist thought.* New York: The New Press.

Hackett, G. and Lonborg, S. D. (1994). Career assessment and counseling for women. In W. B. Walsh and S. H. Osipow (Eds.), *Career counseling for women* (pp. 43-85). Hillsdale, NJ: Erlbaum.

Halifax, N. V. D. (1997). Feminist art psychotherapy: Contributions from feminist theory and contemporary art practice. *American Journal of Art Therapy, 36,* 49-55.

Halleck, S. L. (1971). *The politics of therapy.* New York: Science House Inc.

Hammond, V. W. (1987). "Conscious subjectivity" or use of one's self in therapeutic process. *Women and Therapy, 6*(4), 75-82.

Hammonds, E. (1997). Black (w)holes and the geometry of Black female sexuality. In E. Weed and N. Schor (Eds.), *Feminism meets queer theory* (pp. 136-156). Bloomington: Indiana University Press.

Hanisch, C. (1971). The personal is political. In J. Agel (Ed.), *The radical therapist* (pp. 152-157). New York: Ballantine.

Hardiman, R. (2001). Reflections on white identity development theory. In C. L. Wijeyesinghe and B. W. Jackson III (Eds.), *New perspectives on racial identity development: A theoretical and practical anthology* (pp. 108-128). New York: New York University Press.

Harding, S. (1986). *The science question in feminism.* Ithaca, NY: Cornell University Press.

Harding, S. (1990). Feminism, science, and the anti-enlightenment critiques. In L. J. Nicholson (Ed.), *Feminism/postmodernism* (pp. 83-106). New York: Routledge.

Hare-Mustin, R. T. (1978). A feminist approach to family therapy. *Family Process, 17,* 181-194.

Hare-Mustin, R. T. and Marecek, J. (1986). Autonomy and gender: Some questions for therapists. *Psychotherapy: Theory, Research, and Practice, 23,* 205-212.

Hare-Mustin, R. T. and Marecek, J. (Eds.) (1990). *Making a difference: Psychology and the construction of gender.* New Haven, CT: Yale University Press.

Hare-Mustin, R. T., Marecek, J., Kaplan, A. G., and Liss-Levinson, N. (1979). Rights of clients, responsibilities of therapists. *American Psychologist, 34,* 3-16.

Hartmann, H. (1981). The unhappy marriage of Marxism and feminism: Toward a more progressive union. In L. Sargent (Ed.), *Women and revolution: A discussion of the unhappy marriage of Marxism and feminism* (pp. 1-41). Boston: South End Press.

Hartsock, N. (1983). The feminist standpoint: Developing the ground for a specifically feminist historical materialism. In S. Harding and M. B. Hintikka (Eds.), *Discovering reality* (pp. 283-310). Dordrecht, The Netherlands: D. Reidel Publishing Co.

Hartsock, N. (1984). Staying alive. In A. M. Jaggar and P. S. Rothenberg (Eds.), *Feminist frameworks* (pp. 266-276). New York: McGraw-Hill.

Hartsock, N. (1987). Rethinking modernism: Minority vs. majority theories. *Cultural Critique, 7,* 187-206.

Hartung, C. M. and Widiger, T. A. (1998). Gender differences in the diagnosis of mental disorders: Conclusions and controversies of the DSM-IV. *Psychological Bulletin, 123,* 260-278.

Hawkesworth, M. E. (1989). Knowers, knowing, known: Feminist theory and claims of truth. *Signs: Journal of Women in Culture and Society, 14,* 533-557.

Hawxhurst, D. M. and Morrow, S. L. (1984). *Living our visions: Building feminist community.* Tempe, AZ: Fourth World.

Hayes, J. A. and Mahalik, J. R. (2000). Gender role conflict and psychological distress in male counseling center clients. *Psychology of Men and Masculinity, 1,* 116-125.

Held, V. (1998). Feminist reconceptualizations in ethics. In J. A. Kournany (Ed.), *Philosophy in a feminist voice: Critiques and reconstructions* (pp. 92-115). Princeton, NJ: Princeton University Press.

Helms, J. E. (1990). "Womanist" identity attitudes: An alternative to feminism in counseling theory and research. Unpublished manuscript.

Helms, J. E. (1995). An update of Helms's white and people of color model racial identity models. In J. G. Ponterotto, J. M. Casas, L. A. Suzuki, and C. M. Alexander (Eds.), *Handbook of multicultural counseling* (pp. 181-198). Thousand Oaks, CA: Sage.

Heppner, M. J., Davidson, M. M., and Scott, A. B. (2003). The ecology of women's career barriers: Creating social justice through systemwide intervention. In M. Kopala and M. A. Keitel (Eds.), *Handbook of counseling women* (pp. 173-184). Thousand Oaks, CA: Sage.

Herman, J. (1981). *Father-daughter incest.* Cambridge, MA: Harvard University Press.

Herman, J. L. (1992). *Trauma and recovery: The aftermath of violence.* New York: Basic Books.

Herman, J. L. and Ojerholm, A. J. (1995). Judy Herman: Cleaning house. *Women and Therapy, 17*(1/2), 243-250.

Hernández, D. and Rehman, B. (Eds.) (2002). *Colonize this! Young women of color on today's feminism.* New York: Seal Press.

Hewlett, S. A. (1986). *A lesser life: The myth of women's liberation in America.* New York: Wm. Morrow and Co., Inc.

Heywood, L. and Drake, J. (Eds.) (1997). *Third wave agenda: Being feminist, doing feminism.* Minneapolis: University of Minnesota Press.

Higgenbotham, E. B. (1992). African American women's history and the meta-language of race. *Signs: Journal of Women in Culture and Society, 17,* 251-274.

Hill, M. (1980). *Charlotte Perkins Gilman: The making of a radical feminist 1860-1896.* Philadelphia: Temple University Press.

Hill, M. and Ballou, M. (1998). Making therapy feminist: A practice survey. *Women and Therapy, 21*(2), 1-16.

Hochschild, A. (1989). *The second shift.* New York: Viking.

Hoffman, L. (1981). *Foundations of family therapy.* New York: Basic Books.

Hole, J. and Levine, E. (1971). The first feminists. In A. Koedt, S. Firestone, A. Rapone, and E. Levine (Eds.), *Notes from the third year* (pp. 5-10). New York: Quadrangle Books.

Holroyd, J. (1976). Psychotherapy and women's liberation. *The Counseling Psychologist, 6,* 22-32.

hooks, b. (1981). *Ain't I a woman?* Boston: South End Press.

hooks, b. (1984). *Feminist theory: From margin to center.* Boston: South End Press.

hooks, b. (1989). *Talking back: Thinking feminist, thinking Black.* Boston: South End Press.

hooks, b. (2000). *Feminism is for everybody.* Cambridge, MA: South End Press.

hooks, b., Steinem, G., Vaid, U., and Wolf, N. (1993). Get real about feminism—The myths, the backlash, the movement. *Ms., 4*(2), 34-43.

Horney, K. ([1926] 1967). The flight from womanhood: The masculinity complex in women as viewed by men and women. In H. Kelman (Ed.), *Feminine psychology* (pp. 54-70). New York: Norton.

Horney, K. ([1932] 1967). The dread of woman. In H. Kelman (Ed.), *Feminine psychology* (pp. 133-146). New York: Norton.

Horney, K. ([1933] 1967). The denial of the vagina. In H. Kelman (Ed.), *Feminine psychology* (pp. 147-161). New York: Norton.

Horney, K. ([1934] 1967). The overvaluation of love. In H. Kelman (Ed.), *Feminine psychology* (pp. 182-213). New York: Norton.

Horney, K. (1939). *New ways in psychoanalysis*. New York: Norton.

Horney, K. (1945). *Our inner conflicts*. New York: Norton.

Húrtado, A. (1989). Relating to privilege: Seduction and rejection in the subordination of white women and women of color. *Signs: Journal of Women in Culture and Society, 14,* 833-855.

Húrtado, A. (1996). *The color of privilege: Three blasphemies on race and feminism*. Ann Arbor: University of Michigan Press.

Hurvitz, N. (1973). Psychotherapy as a means of social control. *Journal of Consulting and Clinical Psychology, 40,* 232-239.

Iwao, S. (1993). *The Japanese woman: Traditional image and changing reality*. New York: Free Press.

Jack, D. (1987). Self-in-relation theory. In R. Formanik and A. Gurian (Eds.), *Women and depression: A lifespan perspective* (pp. 41-45). New York: Springer.

Jack, D. (1991). *Silencing the self: Women and depression*. Cambridge, MA: Harvard University Press.

Jack, D. C. (1999). Silencing the self: Inner dialogues and outer realities. In T. Joiner and J. C. Coyne (Eds.), *The interactional nature of depression: Advances in interpersonal approaches* (pp. 221-246). Washington, DC: American Psychological Association.

Jackson, A. P. and Sears, S. J. (1992). Implications of an Africentric worldview in reducing stress for African American women. *Journal of Counseling and Development, 71,* 184-190.

Jackson, L. C. and Greene, B. (Eds.) (2002). *Psychotherapy with African American women: Innovations in psychodynamic perspectives and practice*. New York: Guilford Press.

Jaffee, S. and Hyde, J. S. (2000). Gender differences in moral orientation: A meta-analysis. *Psychological Bulletin, 126,* 703-726.

Jagdose, A. (1996). *Queer theory: An introduction*. New York: New York University Press.

Jaggar, A. M. (1983). *Feminist politics and human nature*. Totowa, NJ: Rowman and Allenheld.

Jaggar, A. M. and Rothenberg, P. S. (Eds.) (1984). *Feminist frameworks*. New York: McGraw-Hill.

Jakubowski, P. A. (1977). Assertion training for women. In E. I. Rawlings and D. K. Carter (Eds.), *Psychotherapy for women* (pp. 147-190). Springfield, IL: Charles C. Thomas.

Jenkins, Y. M. (2000). The Stone Center theoretical approach revisited: Applications for African American women. In L. C. Jackson and B. Greene (Eds.), *Psychotherapy with African American women* (pp. 62-81). New York: Guilford Press.

Jitsukawa, M. (1997). In accordance with nature: What Japanese women mean by being in control. *Anthropology and Medicine, 4,* 177-201.

Johnson, M. (1976). An approach to feminist therapy. *Psychotherapy: Theory, Research, and Practice, 13,* 72-76.

Johnson, M. (1987). Feminist therapy in groups: A decade of change. In C. Brody (Ed.), *Women's therapy groups: Paradigms of feminist treatment* (pp. 13-23). New York: Springer.

Jones, S. R. and McEwen, M. K. (2000). A conceptual model of multiple dimensions of identity. *Journal of College Student Development, 41,* 405-414.

Jordan, J. V. (1991). The meaning of mutuality. In J. V. Jordan, A. G. Kaplan, J. B. Miller, I. P. Stiver, and J. L. Surrey (Eds.), *Women's growth in connection* (pp. 81-96). New York: Guilford Press.

Jordan, J. V. (2000). The role of mutual empathy in relational/cultural therapy. *Journal of Clinical Psychology, 56,* 1005-1016.

Jordan, J. V. (2001). A relational-cultural model: Healing through mutual empathy. *Bulletin of the Menninger Clinic, 65I*(1), 92-103.

Jordan, J. V. and Hartling, L. M. (2002). New developments in relational-cultural theory. In M. Ballou and L. S. Brown (Eds.), *Rethinking mental health and disorder: Feminist perspectives* (pp. 48-70). New York: Guilford Press.

Jordan, J. V., Kaplan, A. G., Miller, J. B., Stiver, I. P., and Surrey, J. L. (Eds.) (1991). *Women's growth in connection.* New York: Guilford Press.

Jordan, J. V. and Surrey, J. L. (1986). The self-in-relation: Empathy and the mother-daughter relationship. In. T. Bernay and D. W. Cantor (Eds.), *The psychology of today's woman: New psychoanalytic visions* (pp. 81-104). Hillsdale, NJ: Analytic Press.

Joseph, G. (1981). The incompatible ménage a trois: Marxism, feminism, and racism. In L. Sargent (Ed.), *Women and revolution* (pp. 91-107). Boston: South End Press.

Josselson, R. (1987). *Finding herself: Pathways to identity development in women.* San Francisco: Jossey-Bass.

Josselson, R. (1996). *Revising herself: The story of women's identity from college to midlife.* New York: Oxford University Press.

Jung, C. G. ([1954] 1959). Psychological aspects of the mother archetype. In S. H. Read, M. Fordham, and G. Adler (Eds.), and R. F. C. Hull (Trans.), *The collected works of C. G. Jung,* Volume 9, part 1 (pp. 75-110). New York: Pantheon Books.

Juntunen, C. (1996). Relationship between a feminist approach to career counseling and career self-efficacy beliefs. *Journal of Employment Counseling, 33,* 130-143.

Kafka, P. (2000). *(Out)classed women: Contemporary Chicana writers on inequitable gendered power relations*. Westport, CT: Greenwood Press.

Kamitani, Y. (1993). The structure of jiritsu (socially sensitive independence) in young Japanese women. *Psychological Reports, 72*, 855-866.

Kamitani, Y. (1996). The structure of jiritsu (socially sensitive independence) in middle-aged Japanese women. *Psychological Reports, 78*, 1355-1362.

Kantrowitz, R. E. and Ballou, M. (1992). A feminist critique of cognitive-behavioral therapy. In L. S. Brown and M. Ballou (Eds.), *Personality and psychopathology: Feminist reappraisals* (pp. 70-87). New York: Guilford Press.

Kanuha, V. (1990). The need for an integrated analysis of oppression in feminist therapy ethics. In H. Lerman and N. Porter (Eds.), *Feminist ethics in psychotherapy* (pp. 24-35). New York: Springer.

Kaplan, A. G. (1976). Androgyny as a model of mental health for women: From theory to therapy. In A. G. Kaplan and J. P. Bean (Eds.), *Beyond sex-role stereotypes: Reading toward a psychology of androgyny* (pp. 353-362). Boston: Little, Brown and Co.

Kaplan, A. G. (1979). Clarifying the concept of androgyny: Implications for therapy. *Psychology of Women Quarterly, 3*, 223-230.

Kaplan, A. G. (1986). The "self-in relation": Implications for depression in women. *Psychotherapy: Theory, Research, and Practice, 23*, 234-242.

Kaplan, A. G. and Surrey, J. L. (1984). The relational self in women: Developmental theory and public policy. In L. E. Walker (Ed.), *Women and mental health policy* (pp. 79-94). Beverly Hils, CA: Sage.

Kaplan, M. (1983). A woman's view of DSM-III. *American Psychologist, 38*, 786-792.

Kappeler, S. (1986). *The pornography of representation*. Minneapolis: University of Minnesota Press.

Karls, J. M. and Wandrei, K. E. (1994). *PIE manual: Person-in-environment system*. Washington, DC: NASW Press.

Kaschak, E. (1981). Feminist psychotherapy: The first decade. In S. Cox (Ed.), *Female psychology: The emerging self* (pp. 387-400). New York: St. Martin's Press.

Kaschak, E. (1992). *Engendered lives: A new psychology of women's experience*. New York: Basic Books.

Kaschak, E. (1998). Growing pains. *Women's Review of Books, 15*(6), 17-18.

Kashima, Y., Yamaguchi, S., Kim, U., San-Chin, C., Gelfand, M., and Yuki, M. (1995). Culture, gender, and self: A perspective from individualism-collectivism research. *Journal of Personality and Social Psychology, 69*, 925-937.

Kasl, C. D. (1992). *Many roads, one journey: Moving beyond the 12 Steps*. New York: HarperCollins.

Kaslow, F. (Ed.) (1996). *Handbook of relational diagnosis and dysfunctional family patterns*. New York: Wiley.

Kawano, K. (1990). Feminist therapy with Japanese women. *Journal of Social Work Practice, 4*(3/4), 44-55.

Kaysen, S. (1994). *Girl, interrupted.* New York: Vintage Books.

Kerber, L. K. (1986). Some cautionary words for historians. *Signs: Journal of Women in Culture and Society, 11*, 304-310.

Khor, D. (1999). Organizing for change: Women's grassroots activism in Japan. *Feminist Studies, 25*, 633-661.

Kihara, M. O., Kramer, J. S., Bain, D., Kihara, M., and Mandel, J. (2001). Knowledge of and attitudes toward the pill: Results of a national survey in Japan. *Family Planning Perspectives, 33*(3), 123-127.

Kim, N. S. and Ahn, W. (2002). Clinical psychologists' theory-based representations of mental disorders predict their diagnostic reasoning and memory. *Journal of Experimental Psychology: General, 131*, 451-476.

King, D. K. (1988). Multiple jeopardy, multiple consciousness: The context of a Black feminist ideology. *Signs: Journal of Women in Culture and Society, 14*, 42-72.

King, Y. (1990). Healing the wounds: Feminism, ecology, and the nature/culture dualism. In I. Diamond and G. F. Orenstein (Eds.), *Reweaving the world: The emergence of ecofeminism* (pp. 106-121). San Francisco: Sierra Club Books.

Kingston, M. A. (1976). *The woman warrior.* New York: Knopf.

Kirk, G. and Okazawa-Rey, M. (Eds.) (1998). *Women's lives: Multicultural perspectives.* Mountain View, CA: Mayfield Publishing Company.

Kirk, S. (1983). The role of politics in feminist counseling. In J. H. Robbins and R. J. Siegel (Eds.), *Women changing therapy* (pp. 179-189). Binghamton, NY: The Haworth Press.

Kirsch, B. (1974). Consciousness-raising groups as therapy for women. In V. Franks and V. Burtle (Eds.), *Women in therapy* (pp. 326-354). New York: Brunner/Mazel.

Kirsch, B. (1987). Evolution of consciousness-raising groups. In C. Brody (Ed.), *Women's therapy groups* (pp. 43-54). New York: Springer.

Kitzinger, C. (1996). The token lesbian chapter. In S. Wilkinson (Ed.), *Feminist social psychologies: International perspectives* (pp. 119-144). Philadelphia, PA: Open University Press.

Kitzinger, C. and Perkins, R. (1993). *Changing our minds: Lesbian feminism and psychology.* New York: New York University Press.

Klein, M. H. (1976). Feminist concepts of therapy outcome. *Psychotherapy: Theory, Research and Practice, 13*, 89-95.

Klonoff, E. A., Landrine, H., and Campbell, R. (2000). Sexist discrimination may account for well-known gender differences in psychiatric symptoms. *Psychology of Women Quarterly, 24*, 93-99.

Koedt, A. (1973). Lesbianism and feminism. In A. Koedt, E. Levine, and A. Rapone (Eds.), *Radical feminism* (pp. 246-258). New York: Quadrangle Books.

Kohlberg, L. (1981). *The philosophy of moral development.* San Francisco: Harper and Row.

Koss, M. and Harvey, M. (1991). *The rape victim: Clinical and community interventions.* Newbury Park, CA: Sage.

Kozu, J. (1999). Domestic violence in Japan. *American Psychologist, 54,* 50-54.

Kravetz, D. (1976). Consciousness-raising groups and group psychotherapy: Alternative mental health resources for women. *Psychotherapy: Theory, Research, and Practice, 13,* 66-71.

Kravetz, D. (1978). Consciousness-raising groups in the 1970s. *Psychology of Women Quarterly, 3,* 168-186.

Kravetz, D. (1980). Consciousness-raising and self-help. In A. Brodsky and R. T. Hare-Mustin (Eds.), *Women and psychotherapy* (pp. 267-284). New York: Guilford Press.

Kravetz, D. (1987). Benefits of consciousness-rasing groups for women. In C. Brody (Ed.), *Women's therapy groups: Paradigms of feminist treatment* (pp. 55-66). New York: Springer.

Kravetz, D. and Jones, L. E. (1991). Supporting practice in feminist service agencies. In M. Bricker-Jenkins, N. R. Hooyman, and N. Gottlieb (Eds.), *Feminist social work practice in clinical settings* (pp. 233-249). Newbury Park, CA: Sage.

Kreps, B. (1973). Radical feminism 1. In A. Koedt, E. Levine, and A. Rapone (Eds.), *Radical feminism* (pp. 234-239). New York: Quadrangle Books.

Kumagai, F. (1995). Families in Japan: Beliefs and realities. *Journal of Comparative Family Studies, 26*(1), 135-163.

Kumagai, F. (1996). *Unmasking Japan today.* Westport, CT: Praeger.

Kupers, T. A. (1997). The politics of psychiatry: Gender and sexual preference in DSM-IV. In M. R. Walsh (Ed.), *Women, men, and gender: Ongoing debates* (pp. 240-347). New Haven, CT: Yale University Press.

Kurdek, L. (1998). Relationship outcomes and their predictors: Longitudinal evidence from heterosexual married, gay cohabitating, and lesbian cohabitating couples. *Journal of Marriage and the Family, 60,* 553-568.

LaFromboise, T. D., Berman, J. S., and Sohi, B. K. (1994). In L. Comas-Díaz and B. Greene (Eds.), *Women of color: Integrating ethnic and gender identities in therapy* (pp. 30-71). New York: Guilford Press.

LaFromboise, T. D., Heyle, A. M., and Ozer, E. J. (1990). Changing and diverse roles of women in American Indian cultures. *Sex Roles, 22,* 455-476.

Laidlaw, T. A. and Malmo, C. (Eds.) (1990). *Healing voices.* San Francisco: Jossey-Bass.

Lamm, N. (1995). It's a big fat revolution. In B. Findlen (Ed.), *Listen up: Voices from the next feminist generation* (pp. 85-94). Seattle, WA: Seal Press.

Landrine, H. (1989). The politics of personality disorder. *Psychology of Women Quarterly, 13,* 325-339.

Larrington, C. (Ed.) (1992). *The feminist companion to mythology.* San Francisco: HarperCollins.

LaRue, L. J. M. (1970). Black liberation and women's lib. *Trans-Action*, November/December, p. 61.

Lauter, E. and Rupprecht, C. S. (Eds.) (1985). *Feminist archetypal theory*. Knoxville: University of Tennessee Press.

Layton, M. (1995). Emerging from the shadows. *Family Therapy Networker, 19*(3), 35-41.

LeBlanc, R. M. (1999). *Bicycle citizens: The political world of the Japanese housewife*. Berkeley: University of California Press.

Lee, J. (1997). Women re-authoring their lives through feminist narrative therapy. *Women and Therapy, 20*(3), 1-22.

Leidig, M. W. (1977). Feminist therapy. Unpublished manuscript.

Lent, R. W., Brown, S. D., and Hackett, G. (2000). Contextual supports and barriers to career choice: A social cognitive analysis. *Journal of Counseling Psychology, 47*, 36-49.

Lerman, H. (1976). What happens in feminist therapy? In S. Cox (Ed.), *Female psychology: The emerging self* (pp. 378-384). Chicago: Science Research Associates.

Lerman, H. (1986). *A mote in Freud's eye*. New York: Springer.

Lerman, H. (1987). Introduction. In C. Brody (Ed.), *Women's therapy groups* (pp. xxiii-xxviii). New York: Springer.

Lerman, H. (1989). Theoretical and practical implications of the post-traumatic stress disorder diagnosis for women. Paper presented at the annual convention of the American Psychological Association, New Orleans, Louisiana. August.

Lerman, H. (1992). The limits of phenomenology: A feminist critique of the humanistic personality theories. In L. S. Brown and M. Ballou (Eds.), *Personality and psychopathology: Feminist reappraisals* (pp. 8-19). New York: Guilford Press.

Lerman, H. (1996). *Pigeonholing women's misery*. New York: Basic Books.

Lerman, H. and Rigby, D. N. (1990). Boundary violations: Misuse of the power of the therapist. In H. Lerman and N. Porter (Eds.), *Feminist ethics in psychotherapy* (pp. 51-59). New York: Springer.

Lerner, G. (1971). *The Grimké sisters from South Carolina: Pioneers for women's rights and abolition*. New York: Schocken Books.

Lerner, G. (1979). *The majority finds its past: Placing women in history*. New York: Oxford Press.

Lerner, H. G. (1983). Female dependency in context: Some theoretical and technical considerations. *American Journal of Orthopsychiatry, 53*, 697-705.

Lerner, H. G. (1988). *Women in therapy*. Northvale, NJ: Aronson.

Leupnitz, D. A. (1988). *The family interpreted*. New York: Basic Books.

Levinson, D. (1978). *The seasons of a man's life*. New York: Knopf.

Lieberman, M. A. and Bond, G. R. (1976). The problem of being a woman: A survey of 1,700 women in consciousness-raising groups. *Journal of Applied Behavior Science, 12*, 363-379.

Lieberman, M. A., Solow, N., Bond, G. R., and Reibstein, J. (1979). The psycho-therapeutic impact of women's consciousness-raising groups. *Archives of General Psychiatry, 36,* 161-168.

Lim, S. G., Tsutakawa, M., and Donnelly, M. (Eds.) (1989). *The forbidden stitch: An Asian American women's anthology.* Corvallis, OR: Calyx.

Lim-Hing, S. (Ed.) (1994). *The very inside: Anthology of writing by Asian and Pacific Islander lesbian and bisexual women.* Toronto: Sister Vision.

Lindsey, K. (1974). On the need to develop a feminist therapy. *Rough Times: A Journal of Radical Therapy, 4,* 2-3.

Linehan, M. (1993). *Cognitive-behavioral treatment of borderline personality disorder.* New York: Guilford Press.

Linehan, M. M., Armstrong, H. E., Saurez, A., Allmon, D., and Heard, H. L. (1991). Cognitive behavioral treatment of chronically parasuicidal borderline patients. *Archives of General Psychiatry, 48,* 1060-1064.

Lips, H. J. (2003). *A new psychology of women: Gender, culture, and ethnicity* (Second edition). Mountain View, CA: Mayfield.

Little, L. F. (1990). Gestalt therapy with females involved in intimate violence. In S. M. Stith and M. B. Williams (Eds.), *Comprehensive treatment approaches to domestic violence* (pp. 47-65). New York: Springer.

Liu, D. and Boyle, E. H. (2001). Making the case: The women's convention and equal employment opportunity in Japan. *International Journal of Comparative Sociology, 42*(4), 389-404.

Long, S. O. (1996). Nurturing and femininity: The ideal of caregiving in postwar Japan. In A. E. Imamura (Ed.), *Re-imaging Japanese women* (pp. 156-176). Berkeley: University of California Press.

Longres, J. and McLeod, E. (1980). Consciousness raising and social work practice. *Social Casework, 61,* 267-277.

Lopez, S. R. (1989). Patient variable biases in clinical judgment: Conceptual overview and methodological considerations. *Psychological Bulletin, 106,* 184-203.

Lorde, A. (1983). An open letter to Mary Daly. In C. Moraga and G. Anzaldúa (Eds.), *This bridge called my back* (p. 97). New York: Women of Color Press.

Lorde, A. (1984). *Sister outsider.* Trumansburg, NY: The Crossing Press.

Louie, S. C. (2000). Interpersonal relationships: Independence versus interdependence. In J. L. Chin (Ed.), *Relationships among Asian American women* (pp. 211-222). Washington, DC: American Psychological Association.

Lyons, N. (1983). Two perspectives: On self, relationships and morality. *Harvard Educational Review, 53,* 125-145.

MacKinnon, C. A. ([1982] 1993). Feminism, Marxism, method, and the state: Toward a feminist jurisprudence. In P. B. Bart and E. G. Moran (Eds.), *Violence against women: The bloody footprints* (pp. 201-227). Newbury Park, CA: Sage.

MacKinnon, C. A. (1989). *Toward a feminist theory of the state.* Cambridge, MA: Harvard University Press.

Mahalik, J. R. (1999). Interpersonal psychotherapy with men who experience gender role conflict. *Professional Psychology, 30,* 5-13.

Mahalik, J. R. and Cournoyer, R. J. (2000). Identifying gender role conflict messages that distinguish mildly depressed from depressed men. *Psychology of Men and Masculinity, 1,* 109-115.

Mahalik, J. R., Cournoyer, R. J., DeFranc, W., Cherry, M., and Napolitano, J. M. (1998). Men's gender role conflict and use of psychological defenses. *Journal of Counseling Psychology, 45,* 247-255.

Mahalik, J. R., Ormer, A. V., and Simi, N. L. (2000). Ethical issues in using self-disclosure in feminist therapy. In M. M. Brabeck (Ed.), *Practicing feminist ethics in psychology* (pp. 189-201). Washington, DC: American Psychological Association.

Maher, F. A. and Tetreault, M. K. T. (2001). *The feminist classroom: Dynamics of gender, race, and privilege* (Expanded edition). Lanham, MD: Rowman and Littlefield Publishers.

Major, B. (1993). Gender, entitlement, and distribution of family labor. *Journal of Social Issues, 49,* 141-159.

Mander, A. V. and Rush, A. K. (1974). *Feminism as therapy.* New York: Random House.

Mardorossian, C. M. (2002). Toward a new feminist theory of rape. *Signs: Journal of Women in Culture and Society, 27,* 743-775.

Marecek, J. (1999). Trauma talk in feminist clinical practice. In S. Lamb (Ed.), *New versions of victims: Feminist struggle with the concept* (pp. 158-182). New York: New York University Press.

Marecek, J. (2001). Disorderly constructs: Feminist frameworks for clinical psychology. In R. K. Unger (Ed.), *Handbook of the psychology of women and gender* (pp. 303-316). New York: Wiley.

Marecek, J. (2002). Unfinished business: Postmodern feminism in personality theory. In M. Ballou and L. S. Brown (Eds.), *Rethinking mental health and disorder: Feminist perspectives* (pp. 3-28). New York: Guilford Press.

Marecek, J. and Kravetz, D. (1977). Women and mental health: A review of feminist change efforts. *Psychiatry, 40,* 323-329.

Marecek, J. and Kravetz, D. (1998). Power and agency in feminist therapy. In I. B. Seu and C. Heenan (Eds.), *Feminism and psychotherapy* (pp. 13-29). London: Sage.

Marecek, J., Kravetz, D., and Finn, S. (1979). Comparison of women who enter feminist therapy and women who enter traditional therapy. *Journal of Consulting and Clinical Psychology, 4,* 734-742.

Mark, C. G. (1990). The personal relationship between therapists and their theoretical orientation. In D. W. Cantor (Ed.), *Women as therapists: A multitheoretical casebook* (pp. 33-55). New York: Springer.

Markus, H. and Kitayama, S. (1991). Culture and the self: Implications for cognition, emotion, and motivation. *Psychological Review, 98,* 224-253.

Markus, H. and Oyserman, D. (1989). Gender and thought: The role of the self-concept. In M. Crawford and M. Gentry (Eds.), *Gender and thought: Psychological perspectives* (pp. 100-127). New York: Springer.

Maslow, A. H. (1956). Self-actualizing people: A study of psychological health. In C. E. Moustakas (Ed.), *The self* (pp. 160-194). New York: Harper Colophon.

Matlin, M. W. (2004). *The psychology of women* (Fifth edition). Belmont, CA: Wadsworth.

Matsui, Y. (1995). The plight of Asian migrant women working in Japan's sex industry. In K. Fujimura-Fanselow and A. Kameda (Eds.), *Japanese women* (pp. 309-319). New York: The Feminist Press.

Matsui, Y. (1996). *Women in the new Asia: From pain to power.* New York: Zed Books.

Matsuyuki, M. (1998). Japanese feminist counseling as a political act. *Women and Therapy, 21*(2), 65-77.

Matthews, N. A. (1994). *Confronting rape: The feminist anti-rape movement and the state.* New York: Routledge.

Mattis, J. S. (2002). Religion and spirituality in the meaning-making and coping experiences of African American women: A qualitative analysis. *Psychology of Women Quarterly, 26,* 309-321.

Mazure, C. M., Keita, G. P., and Blehar, M. C. (2002). *Summit on women and depression: Proceedings and recommendations.* Washington, DC: American Psychological Association. (Available online at <www.apa.org/pi/wpo/womenanddepression.pdf>.)

McCarn, S. R. and Fassinger, R. E. (1996). Revisioning sexual minority identity formation: A new model of lesbian identity and its implications for counseling and research. *The Counseling Psychologist, 24,* 508-534.

McGrath, E., Keita, G. P., Strickland, B. R., and Russo, N. F. (Eds.) (1990). *Women and depression.* Washington, DC: American Psychological Association.

McIntosh, P. (1989). White privilege: Unpacking the invisible knapsack. *Peace and Freedom,* July/August, 10-12.

McNair, L. D. (1992). African American women in therapy: An Afrocentric and feminist synthesis. *Women and Therapy, 12*(1/2), 5-19.

McWhirter, E. H. (1991). Empowerment in counseling. *Journal of Counseling and Development, 69,* 222-227.

McWhirter, E. H., Hackett, G., and Bandalos, D. L. (1998). A causal model of the educational plans and career expectations of Mexican American high school girls. *Journal of Counseling Psychology, 45,* 166-181.

Mednick, M. T. (1989). On the politics of psychological constructs: Stop the bandwagon, I want to get off. *American Psychologist, 44,* 1118-1123.

Mehrhof, B. and Kearon, P. (1971). Rape: An act of terror. In A. Koedt, A. Rapone, and E. Levine (Eds.), *Notes from the third year: Women's liberation* (pp. 79-81). New York: Radical Feminists.

Messner, M. A. (1998). The limits of "the male sex role": An analysis of the men's liberation and men's rights movements' discourse. *Gender and Society, 12,* 255-276.

Milewski-Hertlein, K. A. (2001). The use of a socially constructed genogram in clinical practice. *The American Journal of Family Therapy, 29,* 23-38.

Miller, D. (1995). *Women who hurt themselves: A book of hope and understanding.* New York: Basic Books.

Miller, J.B. (1976). *Toward a new psychology of women.* Boston: Beacon Press.

Miller, J. B. (1991). The development of women's sense of self. In J. V. Jordan, A. G. Kaplan, J. B. Miller, I. P. Stiver, and J. L. Surrey (Eds.), *Women's growth in connection* (pp. 11-26). New York: Guilford Press.

Miller, J. B. and Stiver, I. P. (1997). *The healing connection: How women form relationships in therapy and in life.* Boston: Beacon Press.

Millett, K. (1970). *Sexual politics.* Garden City, NY: Doubleday and Co.

Minuchin, S. (1984). *Family kaleidoscope.* Cambridge, MA: Harvard University Press.

Mirandé, W. and Enríquez, E. (1979). *La Chicana.* Chicago: University of Chicago Press.

Mitchell, J. (1969). Women: The longest revolution. In B. Roszak and T. Roszak (Eds.), *Masculine/Feminine: Readings in sexual mythology and the liberation of women* (pp. 160-173). New York: Harper Colophon Books.

Mitchell, J. (1974). *Psychoanalysis and feminism.* New York: Vintage Books.

Miyaji, N. and Lock, M. M. (1994). Monitoring motherhood: Sociocultural and historical aspects of maternal and child health in Japan. *Daedalus, 123*(4), 87-112.

Mohlman, J. (2000). Taking our housebound sisters to the mall: What can a feminist perspective add to CBT for panic and agoraphobia? *The Behavior Therapist, 23*(2), 30-34, 41.

Molony, B. (1995). Japan's 1986 equal employment opportunity law and the changing discourse on gender. *Signs, 20,* 268-302.

Moore, D. M. (1981). Assertiveness training: A review. In S. Cox (Ed.), *Female psychology: The emerging self* (Second edition) (pp. 402-416). New York: St. Martin's Press.

Moradi, B., Fischer, A. R., Hill, M. S., Jome, L. M., and Blum, S. A. (2000). Does "feminist" plus "therapist" equal "feminist therapist"? *Psychology of Women Quarterly, 24,* 285-296.

Moradi, B., Subich, L. M., and Phillips, J. C. (2002). Revisiting feminist identity development theory, research, and practice. *The Counseling Psychologist, 30,* 6-43.

Moraga, C. and Anzaldúa, G. (Eds.) (1983). *This bridge called my back.* New York: Kitchen Table/Women of Color Press.

Morawski, J. G. (1987). The troubled quest for masculinity, femininity, and androgyny. In P. Shaver and C. Hendrick (Eds.), *Sex and gender* (pp. 44-69). Newbury Park, CA: Sage.

Morawski, J. G. (1990). Toward the unimagined: Feminism and epistemology in psychology. In R. T. Hare-Mustin and J. Marecek (Eds.), *Making a difference* (pp. 150-183). New Haven, CT: Yale University Press.

Morawski, J. G. and Bayer, B. M. (1995). Stirring trouble and making theory. In H. Landrine (Ed.), *Bringing cultural diversity to feminist psychology: Theory, research, and practice* (pp. 113-138). Washington, DC: American Psychological Association.

Morgan, R. (1980). Theory and practice: Pornography and rape. In L. Lederer (Ed.), *Take back the night: Women on pornography* (pp. 134-140). New York: William Morrow.

Morgan, R. (Ed.) (1984). *Sisterhood is global: The international women's movement anthology.* Garden City, NY: Anchor Books.

Morrow, S. L. (2000). Feminist reconstructions of psychology. In M. Biaggio and M. Hersen (Eds.), *Issues in the psychology of women* (pp. 15-31). New York: Kluwer Academic/Plenum Publishers.

Morrow, S. L. and Hawxhurst, D. M. (1998). Feminist therapy: Integrating political analysis in counseling and psychotherapy. *Women and Therapy, 21*(2), 37-50.

Morrow, S. L. and Smith, M. L. (1995). Constructions of survival and coping by women who have survived childhood sexual abuse. *Journal of Counseling Psychology, 42,* 24-33.

Morton, S. B. (1998). Lesbian divorce. *American Journal of Orthopsychiatry, 68,* 410-419.

Moschkovich, J. (1983). "—But I know you, American woman." In C. Moraga and G. Anzaldúa (Eds.), *This bridge called my back* (Second edition) (pp. 79-84). New York: Kitchen Table/Women of Color Press.

Moya, P. M. L. (2001). Chicana feminism and postmodernist theory. *Signs: Journal of Women in Culture and Society, 26,* 441-483.

Muehlenhard, C. L. (1983). Women's assertion and the feminine sex-role stereotype. In V. Franks and E. D. Rothblum (Eds.), *The stereotyping of women: Its effects on mental health* (pp. 153-171). New York: Springer.

Murdock, N. L. (2004). *Theories of counseling and psychotherapy: A case approach.* Upper Saddle River, NJ: Prentice-Hall.

Myron, N. and Bunch, C. (Eds.) (1975). *Lesbianism and the women's movement.* Baltimore, MD: Diana Press.

National Organization for Women (1967/1970). Bill of rights. In R. Morgan (Ed.), *Sisterhood is powerful* (pp. 512-514). New York: Random House.

Neimeyer, R. A. and Stewart, A. E. (2000). Constructivist and narrative psychotherapies. In C. R. Snyder and R. E. Ingram (Eds.), *Handbook of psychological change: Psychotherapy processes and practices for the 21st century* (pp. 337-357). New York: Wiley.

Nelson, G. M. (1991). *Here all dwell free: Stories to heal the wounded feminine.* New York: Doubleday.

New York Radical Feminists (1973). Politics of the ego: A manifesto for New York Radical Feminists. In A. Koedt, E. Levine, and A. Rapone (Eds.), *Radical feminism* (pp. 379-383). New York: Quadrangle Books.

Noddings, N. (1984). *Caring: A feminine approach to ethics and moral education.* Berkeley: University of California Press.

Noguchi, M. G. (1992). The rise of the housewife activist. *Japan Quarterly, 39*(3), 339-352.

Nolen-Hoeksema, S. (2000). The role of rumination in depressive disorders and mixed anxiety/depressive symptoms. *Journal of Abnormal Psychology, 109,* 504-511.

Norgren, T. (2001). *Abortion before birth control: The politics of reproduction in postwar Japan.* Princeton, NJ: Princeton University Press.

Nutt, R. L., Rice, J. K., and Enns, C. Z. (2003). Annual report: Divisions 17 and 35 interdivisional task force to develop guidelines for psychological practice with girls and women. Unpublished report prepared for the executive boards of the American Psychological Association Societies of the Psychology of Women and Counseling Psychology.

Nutt, R. L., Rice, J. K., Enns, C. Z., and the American Psychological Association Interdivisional Task Force to Develop Guidelines for Counseling/Psychotherapy with Girls and Women. (2003). Guidelines for psychological practice with girls and women. Washington, DC: American Psychological Association, Division 17 (Counseling Psychology) and Division 35 (Psychology of Women). January 27 draft of the interdivisional task force.

Oakley, A. (1990). What is a housewife? In T. Lovell (Ed.), *British feminist thought* (pp. 71-76). Cambridge, MA: Basil Blackwell.

O'Brien, K. M. and Fassinger, R. E. (1993). A causal model of the career orientation and career choice of adolescent women. *Journal of Counseling Psychology, 40,* 456-469.

O'Connell, A. N. (1980). Karen Horney: Theorist in psychoanalysis and feminine psychology. *Psychology of Women Quarterly, 5,* 81-93.

Okun, B. F. (1992). Object relations and self psychology: Overview and feminist perspective. In L. S. Brown and M. Ballou (Eds.), *Personality and psychopathology: Feminist reappraisals* (pp. 20-45). New York: Guilford Press.

O'Neil, J. M. (1981). Patterns of gender role conflict and strain: Sexism and fear of femininity in men's lives. *Personnel and Guidance Journal, 60,* 203-210.

O'Neil, J. M., Good, G. E., and Holmes, S. (1995). Fifteen years of theory and research on men's gender role conflict. In R. F. Levant and W. S. Pollack (Eds.), *The new psychology of men* (pp. 164-206). New York: Basic Books.

Orr, C. M. (1997). Charting the currents of the third wave. *Hypatia, 12,* 29-45.

Ossana, S. M., Helms, J. E., and Leonard, M. M. (1992). Do "womanist" identity attitudes influence college women's self-esteem and perceptions of environmental bias? *Journal of Counseling and Development, 70,* 402-408.

O'Sullivan, E. (1976). What has happened to rape crisis centers? A look at their structures, members, and funding. *Victimology, 3*(1/2), 45-62.

Patterson, C. J. (1995). Families of the lesbian baby boom: Parents' division of labor and children's adjustment. *Developmental Psychology, 31,* 115-123.

Payne, C. W. (1973). Consciousness raising: A dead end? In A. Koedt, E. Levine, and A. Rapone (Eds.), *Radical feminism* (pp. 282-284). New York: Quadrangle Books.

Perkins, R. E. (1991a). Therapy for lesbians?: The case against. *Feminism and Psychology, 1*(3), 325-338.

Perkins, R. E. (1991b). Women with long-term mental health problems: Issues of power and powerlessness. *Feminism and Psychology, 1*(1), 131-139.

Perry, W. G. (1970). *Forms of intellectual and ethical development in the college years*. New York: Holt, Rinehart, and Winston.

Pesquera, B. M. and Segura, D. A. (1993). There is no going back: Chicanas and feminism. In N. Alarcón, R. Castro, E. Pérez, B. Pesquera, A. Sosa-Riddell, and P. Zavella (Eds.), *Chicana critical issues* (pp. 95-115). Berkeley, CA: Third Woman Press.

Peterson, V. S. and Runyan, A. S. (1999). *Global gender issues* (Second edition). Boulder, CO: Westview.

Peterson, Z. D. (2002). More than a mirror: The ethics of therapist self-disclosure. *Psychotherapy: Theory/Research/Practice/Training, 39,* 21-31.

Phillips, F. B. (1990). NTU psychotherapy: An Afrocentric approach. *The Journal of Black Psychology, 17*(1), 55-74.

Phillips, R. D. and Gilroy, F. D. (1985). Sex-role stereotypes and clinical judgments of mental health: The Brovermans' findings reexamined. *Sex Roles, 12,* 179-193.

Philpot, C. L., Brooks, G. R., Lusterman, D. D., and Nutt, R. L. (1997). *Bridging separate gender worlds: Why men and women clash and how therapists can bring them together*. Washington, DC: American Psychological Association.

Plant, J. (Ed.) (1989). *Healing the wounds: The promise of ecofeminism*. Philadelphia: New Society.

Pleck, J. (1984). Men's power with women, other men, and society: A men's movement analysis. In E. Carmen and P. P. Rieker (Eds.), *The gender gap in psychotherapy* (pp. 79-90). New York: Plenum.

Polster, M. (1974). Women in therapy: A Gestalt therapist's view. In V. Franks and V. Burtle (Eds.), *Women in therapy* (pp. 247-262). New York: Brunner/Mazel.

Pope, K. S. and Brown, L. S. (1996). *Recovered memories of abuse: Assessment, therapy, forensics*. Washington, DC: American Psychological Association.

Powers, P. S. (2002). Eating disorders. In S. G. Kornstein and A. H. G. Clayton (Eds.), *Women's mental health: A comprehensive textbook* (pp. 242-262). New York: Guilford Press.

Pratt, A. V. (1985). Spinning among field: Jung, Frye, Levi-Strauss and feminist archetypal theory. In E. Lauter and C. S. Rupprecht (Eds.), *Feminist archetypal theory* (pp. 93-136). Knoxville: University of Tennessee Press.

Prouty, A. M. and Bermúdez, J. M. (1999). Experiencing multiconsciousness: A feminist model for therapy. *Journal of Feminist Family Therapy, 11*(3), 19-39.

Radden, J. (2001). Relational individualism and feminist therapy. *Hypatia, 11*(3), 71-96.

Radicalesbians (1973). The woman identified woman. In A. Koedt, E. Levine, and A. Rapone (Eds.), *Radical feminism* (pp. 240-245). New York: Quadrangle Books.

Raja, S. (1998). Culturally sensitive therapy for women of color. *Women and Therapy, 21*(4), 67-84.

Rando, R. A., Rogers, J. R., and Brittan-Powell, C. S. (1998). Gender role conflict and college men's sexually aggressive attitudes and behavior. *Journal of Mental Health Counseling, 20*, 359-369.

Rave, E. J. and Larsen, C. C. (1990). Development of the code: The feminist process. In H. Lerman and N. Porter (Eds.), *Feminist ethics in psychotherapy* (pp. 49-76). Springfield, IL: Charles C. Thomas.

Rave, E. J. and Larsen, C. C. (Eds.) (1995). *Ethical decision making in therapy: Feminist perspectives.* New York: Guilford Press.

Rawlings, E. and Carter, D. (1977). Feminist and nonsexist psychotherapy. In E. I. Rawlings and D. K. Carter (Eds.), *Psychotherapy for women* (pp. 49-76). Springfield, IL: Charles C. Thomas.

Redstockings (1969). Redstockings Manifesto. In B. Roszak and T. Roszak (Eds.), *Masculine/feminine: Readings in sexual mythology and the liberation of women* (pp. 272-274). New York: Harper Colophon Books.

Reichert, E. (1994). Expressive group therapy with adult survivors of sexual abuse. *Family Therapy, 21*, 99-105.

Reid, P. T. and Kelly, E. (1994). Research on women of color: From ignorance to awareness. *Psychology of Women Quarterly, 18*, 477-486.

Reinelt, C. (1995). Moving onto the terrain of the state: The battered women's movement and the politics of engagement. In M. M. Ferree and P. Y. Yancey (Eds.), *Feminist organizations: Harvest of the new women's movement* (pp. 84-104). Philadelphia, PA: Temple University Press.

Resick, P. A. (2001). Cognitive therapy for posttraumatic stress disorder. *Journal of Cognitive Psychotherapy, 15*, 321-329.

Resick, P. A. and Schnicke, M. K. (1992). Cognitive processing therapy for sexual assault victims. *Journal of Consulting and Clinical Psychology, 60*, 748-756.

Resick, P. A. and Schnicke, M. K. (1993). *Cognitive processing therapy for rape victims: A treatment manual.* Thousand Oaks, CA: Sage.

Reynolds, A. L. and Pope, R. L. (1991). The complexities of diversity: Exploring multiple oppressions. *Journal of Counseling and Development, 70*, 174-180.

Rice, J. K. and Ballou, M. (2002). *Cultural and gender awareness in international psychology.* Washington, DC: American Psychological Association, Division 52, International Psychology, International Committee for Women.

Rice, J. K. and Rice, D. G. (1973). Implications of the women's liberation movement for psychotherapy. *American Journal of Psychiatry, 130*, 191-196.

Rich, A. (1976). *Of woman born: Motherhood as experience and institution.* New York: Norton.

Rich, A. (1979). *On lies, secrets and silence.* New York: Norton.

Rich, A. ([1980] 1989). Compulsory heterosexuality and lesbian existence. In L. Richardson and V. Taylor (Eds.), *Feminist frontiers II* (pp. 120-141). New York: McGraw-Hill.

Rich, A. (1986). *Blood, bread, and poetry: Selected prose, 1979-1985.* New York: Norton.

Richards, A. (1998). Body image: Third wave feminism's issue? In O. Edut (Eds.), *Adiós Barbie: Young women write about body image and identity* (pp. 196-201). Seattle, WA: Seal Press.

Richardson, M. and Johnson, M. (1984). Counseling women. In S. D. Brown and R. W. Lent (Eds.), *Handbook of counseling psychology* (pp. 832-877). New York: Wiley.

Riddiough, C. (1981). Socialism, feminism, and gay/lesbian liberation. In L. Sargent (Ed.), *Women and revolution* (pp. 71-90). Boston: South End Press.

Rigazio-DiGilio, S. A. (2000). Relational diagnosis: A coconstructive-developmental perspective on assessment and treatment. *Journal of Clinical Psychology: Psychotherapy in Practice, 56,* 1017-1036.

Riger, S. (1992). Epistemological debates, feminist voices: Science, social values, and the study of women. *American Psychologist, 47,* 730-740.

Rochlen, A. B. and O'Brien, K. M. (2002). The relation of male gender role conflict and attitudes toward career counseling to interest in and preferences for different career counseling styles. *Psychology of Men and Masculinity, 3,* 9-21.

Rogers, C. R. (1951). *Client-centered therapy: Its current practice, implications, and theory.* Boston: Houghton Mifflin.

Rogers, C. R. (1956). What it means to become a person. In C. E. Moustakas (Ed.), *The self* (pp. 195-211). New York: Harper Colophon.

Romaniello, J. (1992). Beyond archetypes: A feminist perspective on Jungian therapy. In L. S. Brown and M. Ballou (Eds.), *Personality and psychopathology: Feminist reappraisals* (pp. 46-69). New York: Guilford Press.

Romney, P. (1991). Perspectives on racism and the psychology of women. *Association for Women in Psychology Newsletter,* fall, 1-2.

Root, M. P. P. (1992). Reconstructing the impact of trauma on personality. In L. S. Brown and M. Ballou (Eds.), *Personality and psychopathology: Feminist reappraisals* (pp. 229-265). New York: Guilford Press.

Rose, H. (1983). Hand, brain, and heart: A feminist epistemology for the natural sciences. *Signs: Journal of Women in Culture and Society, 9,* 73-90.

Rose, S. (1996). Integrating lesbian studies into the feminist psychology classroom. In B. Zimmerman and T. McNaron (Eds.), *The new lesbian studies: Into the twenty-first century* (pp. 108-134). New York: The Feminist Press.

Rosen, R. (2000). *The world split open: How the modern women's movement changed America.* New York: Penguin Books.

Rosewater, L. B. (1990). Public advocacy. In H. Lerman and N. Porter (Eds.), *Feminist ethics in psychotherapy* (pp. 229-247). New York: Springer.

Rosewater, L. B. and Walker, L. E. A. (Eds.) (1985). *Handbook of feminist therapy: Women's issues in psychotherapy* (pp. 137-155). Norwood, NJ: Ablex.

Rothenberg, B. (2003). "We don't have time for social change": Cultural compromise and the battered woman syndrome. *Gender and Society, 17*(5), 771-787.

Rowland, S. (2002). *Jung: A feminist revision.* Oxford, England: Polity Press.

Rubin, G. ([1975] 1984). The traffic in women: Notes on the "political economy" of sex. In A. Jaggar and P. Rothenberg (Eds.), *Feminist frameworks* (pp. 155-171). New York: McGraw-Hill.

Rubin, L. and Nemeroff, C. (2001). Feminism's third wave: Surfing to oblivion? *Women and Therapy, 23*(2), 91-104.

Ruddick, S. (1989). *Maternal thinking: Toward a politics of peace.* New York: Ballantine Books.

Rudman, L. A. and Glick, P. (2001). Prescriptive gender stereotypes and backlash toward agentic women. *Journal of Social Issues, 57,* 743-762.

Rudy, K. (2001). Radical feminism, lesbian separatism, and queer theory. *Feminist Studies, 27*(1), 191-222.

Ruiz, V. L. (1998). *From out of the shadows: Mexican women in twentieth-century America.* New York: Oxford University Press.

Russ, J. (1998). *What are we waiting for?* New York: St. Martin's Press.

Russell, D. E. H. and Lederer, L. (1980). Questions we get asked most often. In L. Lederer (Ed.), *Take back the night: Women on pornography* (pp. 23-29). New York: William Morrow and Co.

Russo, A. (1987). Conflicts and contradictions among feminists over issues of pornography and sexual freedom. *Women's Studies International Forum, 10*(2), 103-112.

Sanchez-Hucles, J. and Hudgins, P. (2001). Trauma across diverse settings. In J. Worell (Ed.), *Encyclopedia of women and gender* (Volume 2) (pp. 1151-1168). San Diego, CA: Academic Press.

Sandoval, C. (1991). U.S. third world feminism: The theory and method of oppositional consciousness in the postmodern world. *Genders, 10,* 1-36.

Sandoval, C. (1998). Mestizaje as method: Feminists-of-color challenge the canon. In C. Trujillo (Ed.), *Living Chicana theory* (pp. 352-370). Berkeley, CA: Third Woman Press.

Santos de Barona, M. S. and Dutton, M. A. (1997). Feminist perspectives on assessment. In J. Worell and N. G. Johnson (Eds.), *Shaping the future of feminist psychology* (pp. 37-56). Washington, DC: American Psychological Association.

Sarachild, K. (1970). A program for feminist "consciousness raising." In S. Firestone and A. Koedt (Eds.), *Notes from the second year* (pp. 78-80). New York: Redstockings, Inc.

Sarachild, K. (1975). Consciousness-raising: A radical weapon. In Redstockings (Eds.), *Feminist revolution* (pp. 144-150). New York: Redstockings, Inc.

Sargent, L. (1981). New left women and men: The honeymoon is over. In L. Sargent (Ed.), *Women and revolution* (pp. xi-xxxi). Boston: South End Press.

Sato, Y. (1995). From the home to the political arena. In K. Fugimura-Fanselow and A. Kameda (Eds.), *Japanese women: New feminist perspectives* (pp. 365-372). New York: The Feminist Press.

Saulnier, C. F. (1996). *Feminist theories and social work.* Binghamton, NY: The Haworth Press.

Savin-Williams, R. C. and Esterberg, K. G. (2000). Lesbian, gay and bisexual families. In D. Demo, K. Allen, and M. Find (Eds.), *Handbook of family diversity* (pp. 197-315). New York: Oxford University Press.

Scarborough, E. and Furumoto, L. (1987). *Untold lives: The first generation of American women psychologists.* New York: Columbia University Press.

Schechter, S. (1982). *Women and male violence.* Boston: South End Press.

Scheel, K. R. (2000). The empirical basis of dialectical behavior therapy: Summary, critique, and implications. *Clinical Psychology: Science and Practice, 7,* 68-86.

Scher, M. (2001). Male therapist, male client: Reflections of critical dynamics. In G. R. Brooks and G. E. Good (Eds.), *The new handbook of psychotherapy and counseling with men,* Volume 2 (pp. 719-734). San Francisco: Jossey-Bass.

Schneir, M. (Ed.) (1972). *Feminism: The essential historical writings.* New York: Vantage Books.

Scott, J. W. (1988). Deconstructing equality-versus-difference: Or, the uses of poststructuralist theory for feminism. *Feminist Studies, 14*(1), 35-50.

Segura, D. A. (2001). Challenging the Chicano text: Toward a more inclusive contemporary causa. *Signs: Journal of Women in Culture and Society, 26,* 541-550.

Segura, D. A. and Pierce, J. L. (1993). Chicana/o family structure and gender personality: Chodorow, familism, and psychoanalytic sociology revisited. *Signs: Journal of Women in Culture and Society, 19,* 62-91.

Sharf, R. S. (2004). *Theories of psychotherapy and counseling: Concepts and cases* (Third edition). Pacific Grove, CA: Brooks/Cole.

Sharpe, M. J. and Heppner, P. P. (1991). Gender role, gender-role conflict, and psychological well-being in men. *Journal of Counseling Psychology, 38,* 323-330.

Sheared, V. (1994). Giving voice: A womanist construction. In E. Hayes and S. A. J. Colin III (Eds.), *Confronting racism and sexism in adult continuing education* (pp. 27-38). San Francisco: Jossey Bass.

Shepard, D. S. (2002). A negative state of mind: Patterns of depressive symptoms among men with high gender role conflict. *Psychology of Men and Masculinity, 3,* 3-8.

Sherman, J. A. (1980). Therapist attitudes and sex-role stereotyping. In A. Brodsky and R. T. Hare-Mustin (Eds.), *Women and psychotherapy* (pp. 35-66). New York: Guilford Press.

Shimomura, M. (1998). Too much Mommy-san [interview]. *New Perspectives Quarterly, 15*(3), 61-65.

Shorter-Gooden, K. and Jackson, L. C. (2000). The interweaving of cultural and intrapsychic issues in the therapeutic relationship. In L. C. Jackson and B.

Greene (Eds.), *Psychotherapy with African American women: Innovations in psychodynamic perspectives and practice* (pp. 15-32). New York: Guilford Press.

Siegel, D. (1997). The legacy of the personal: Generating theory in feminism's third wave. *Hypatia, 12,* 46-75.

Silverstein, L. B. and Goodrich, T. J. (Eds.) (2003). *Feminist family therapy: Empowerment in social context.* Washington, DC: American Psychological Association.

Simi, N. and Mahalik, J. R. (1997). Comparison of feminist versus psychoanalytic/dynamic and other therapists on self-disclosure. *Psychology of Women Quarterly, 21,* 465-483.

Singer, L. (1992). Feminism and postmodernism. In J. Butler and J. W. Scott (Eds.), *Feminists theorize the political* (pp. 464-475). New York: Routledge.

Smith, A. and Douglas, M. A. (1990). Empowerment as an ethical imperative. In H. Lerman and N. Porter (Eds.), *Feminist ethics in psychotherapy* (pp. 43-50). New York: Springer.

Smith, A. J. and Siegel, R. F. (1985). Feminist therapy: Redefining power for the powerless. In L. B. Rosewater and L. E. A. Walker (Eds.), *Handbook of feminist therapy* (pp. 13-21). New York: Springer.

Smith, B. (Ed.) (1983). *Home girls: A Black feminist anthology.* New York: Kitchen Table/Women of Color Press.

Smith, B. (1985). Some home truths on the contemporary black feminist movement. *Black Scholar, 16*(March/April), 4-13.

Solomon, L. J. and Rothblum, E. D. (1985). Social skills problems experienced by women. In L. L'Abate and M. A. Milan (Eds.), *Handbook of social skills training and research* (pp. 303-325). New York: Wiley.

Solomon, M. (1987). *Emma Goldman.* Boston: Twayne Publishers.

Sommers-Flanagan, J. and Sommers-Flanagan, R. (2004). *Counseling and psychotherapy theories in context and practice.* New York: Wiley.

Spelman, E. V. (1988). *Inessential woman.* Boston: Beacon Press.

Springer, K. (2001). The interstitial politics of Black feminist organizations. *Meridians: Feminism, race, transnationalism, 1*(2), 155-191.

Sprock, J. and Yoder, C. Y. (1997). Women and depression: An update on the report of the APA task force. *Sex Roles, 36,* 269-303.

Stanton, E. C. ([1848] 1972). Declaration of sentiments and resolutions, Seneca Falls. In M. Schneir (Ed.), *Feminism: The essential historical writings* (pp. 76-82). New York: Vantage Press.

Stanton, E. C. ([1860] 1972). Address to the New York Legislature, 1960. In M. Schneir (Ed.), *Feminism: The essential historical writings* (pp. 117-121). New York: Vantage Press.

Stanton, E. C. ([1865] 1881). Letter to the editor: "Year of the negro." In E. C. Stanton, S. B. Anthony, and M. J. Gage (Eds.), *History of woman suffrage,* Volume 2: 1861-1876 (pp. 94-95). Rochester, NY: Charles Mann.

Stanton, E. C. ([1891] 1968). The matriarchate. In A. S. Kraditor (Ed.), *Up from the pedestal* (pp. 140-147). Chicago: Quadrangle Books.

Stanton, E. C. ([1892] 1972). Solitude of self. In M. Schneir (Ed.), *Feminism: The essential historical writings* (pp. 157-159). New York: Vantage Books.

Stanton, E. C. (1895/1898). *The woman's Bible.* New York: European Publishing Co.

Stanton, E. C., Anthony, S. B., and Gage, M. J. (Eds.) (1881). *History of woman suffrage,* Volume 2. Rochester, NY: Charles Mann.

Starhawk (1989). Feminist, earth-based spirituality and ecofeminism. In J. Plant (Ed.), *Healing the wounds: The promise of ecofeminism* (pp. 174-185). Philadelphia, PA: New Society Publishers.

Steil, J. M. (1997). *Marital equality: Its relationship to the well-being of husbands and wives.* Thousand Oaks, CA: Sage.

Steil, J. M. (2001). Family forms and member well-being: A research agenda for the decade of behavior. *Psychology of Women Quarterly, 25,* 344-363.

Stein, A. (1997). *Sex and sensibility: Stories of a lesbian generation.* Berkeley: University of California Press.

Stere, K. L. (1985). Feminist assertiveness training: Self-esteem groups and skill training for women. In L. B. Rosewater and L. E. A. Walker (Eds.), *Handbook of feminist therapy* (pp. 51-61). New York: Springer.

Stillson, R. W., O'Neil, J. M., and Owen, S. V. (1991). Predictors of adult men's gender-role conflict: Race, class, unemployment, age, instrumentality-expressiveness, and personal strain. *Journal of Counseling Psychology, 31,* 3-12.

Stiver, I. P. (1991). The meanings of "dependency" in female-male relationships. In J. V. Jordan, A. G. Kaplan, J. B. Miller, I. P. Stiver, and J. L. Surrey (Eds.), *Women's growth in connection* (pp. 143-161). New York: Guilford Press.

Students for a Democratic Society (1969). National resolution on women. In B. Roszak and T. Roszak (Eds.), *Masculine/feminine: Readings in sexual mythology and the liberation of women* (pp. 254-258). New York: Harper and Row.

Sturdivant, S. (1980). *Therapy with women.* New York: Springer Publishing Co.

Sue, D. W. and Sue, D. (1999). *Counseling the culturally different: Theory and practice* (Third edition). New York: Wiley.

Surrey, J. L. (1991). The relational self in women: Clinical implications. In J. V. Jordan, A. G. Kaplan, J. B. Miller, I. P. Stiver, and J. L. Surrey (Eds.), *Women's growth in connection* (pp. 35-43). New York: Guilford Press.

Suyemoto, K. L. (2002). Constructing identities: A feminist, culturally contextualized alternative to "personality." In M. Ballou and L. S. Brown (Eds.), *Rethinking mental health and disorder: Feminist perspectives* (pp. 71-98). New York: Guilford Press.

Suzuki, K. (1996). Equal job opportunity for whom? *Japan Quarterly, 43*(3), 55-60.

Swim, J. K. and Cohen, L. L. (1997). Overt, covert, and subtle sexism. *Psychology of Women Quarterly, 21,* 103-118.

Tatum, B. D. (2002). *"Why are all the Black kids sitting together in the cafeteria?" And other conversations about race* (Revised edition). New York: Basic Books.

Tavris, C. (1992). *The mismeasure of woman.* New York: Simon & Schuster.

Taylor, M. (1999). Changing what has gone before: The enhancement of an inadequate psychology through the use of an Afrocentric-feminist perspective with African American women in therapy. *Psychotherapy, 36,* 170-179.

Tennov, D. (1973). Feminism, psychotherapy, and professionalism. *Journal of Contemporary Psychotherapy, 5,* 107-111.

Thase, M. E., Buysse, D. J., Frank, E., Cherry, C. R., Comes, C. L., Mallinger, A. G., and Kupfer, D. J. (1997). Which depressed patients will respond to interpersonal psychotherapy? *American Journal of Psychiatry, 154,* 502-509.

Thase, M. E., Reynolds, C. F., Frank, E., Simons, A. D., McGeary, J., Fasiczka, A. L., Garamoni, G. G., Jennings, J. R., and Kupfer, D. J. (1994). Do depressed men and women respond similarly to cognitive behavioral therapy? *American Journal of Psychiatry, 151,* 500-505.

Thomas, A. J. (1998). Understanding culture and world view in family systems: Use of the multicultural genogram. *Family Journal, 6,* 24-32.

Thomas, A. J. (2001). African American women's spiritual beliefs: A guide for treatment. *Women and Therapy, 23*(4), 1-12.

Thomas, C. (1985). The age of androgyny: The new views of psychotherapists. *Sex Roles, 13,* 381-392.

Thompson, A. (1998). Not the color purple: Black feminist lessons for educational caring. *Harvard Educational Review, 68,* 522-554.

Thompson, B. W. (1994). *A hunger so wide and so deep.* Minneapolis: University of Minnesota Press.

Thompson, C. (1971). *On women.* New York: New American Library.

Thompson, J. K., Heinberg, L. J., Altabe, M., and Tantleff-Dunn, S. (1999). *Exacting beauty: Theory, assessment, and treatment of body image disturbance.* Washington, DC: American Psychological Association.

Tolman, R. M., Mowry, D. D., Jones, L. E., and Brekke, J. (1986). Developing a profeminist commitment among men in social work. In N. Van Den Bergh and L. B. Cooper (Eds.), *Feminist visions for social work* (pp. 61-79). Silver Springs, MD: National Association of Social Workers.

Tomm, W. (1992). Ethics and self-knowing: The satisfaction of desire. In E. B. Cole and S. Coultrap-McQuin (Eds.), *Explorations in feminist ethics* (pp. 125-130). Bloomington: Indiana University Press.

Tong, R. (1993). *Feminine and feminist ethics.* Belmont, CA: Wadsworth.

Tong, R. (1998). *Feminist thought: A comprehensive introduction* (Second edition). Boulder, CO: Westview Press.

Trotman, F. K. (2000). Feminist and psychodynamic psychotherapy with African American women: Some differences. In L. C. Jackson and B. Greene (Eds.), *Psychotherapy with African American women: Innovations in psychodynamic perspectives and practice* (pp. 251-274). New York: Guilford Press.

True, R. H. (1990). Psychotherapeutic issues with Asian American women. *Sex Roles, 22,* 477-486.

Trujillo, C. (1991). Chicana lesbians: Fear and loathing in the Chicano community. In C. Trujillo (Ed.), *Chicana lesbians: The girls our mothers warned us about* (pp. 186-194). Berkeley, CA: Third Woman Press.

Trujillo, C. (Ed.) (1998). *Living Chicana theory.* Berkeley, CA: Third Woman Press.

Truth, Sojourner ([1867] 1972). Keeping the things going while things are stirring. In M. Schneir (Ed.), *Feminism: The essential historical writings* (pp. 128-131). New York: Vantage Press.

Turner, C. W. (1997). Clinical applications of the Stone Center theoretical approach to minority women. In J. V. Jordan (Ed.), *Women's growth in diversity: More writings from the Stone Center* (pp. 74-90). New York: Guilford Press.

Ueno, C. (1997). Are the Japanese feminine? Some problems of Japanese feminism in its cultural context [interview]. In S. Buckley (Ed.), *Broken silence: Voices of Japanese feminism* (pp. 272-301). Berkeley: University of California Press.

Unger, R. K. (1993). The personal is paradoxical: Feminists construct psychology. *Feminism and Psychology, 3,* 211-218.

Van Velsor, P. and Cox, D. L. (2001). Anger as a vehicle in the treatment of women who are sexual abuse survivors: Reattributing responsibility and accessing personal power. *Professional Psychology: Research and Practice, 32*(6), 618-625.

van Wormer, K. (1989). Co-dependency: Implications for women and therapy. *Women and Therapy, 8*(4), 51-63.

Vasquez, M. J. T. (1994). Latinas. In L. Comas-Díaz and B. Greene (Eds.), *Women of color: Integrating ethnic and gender identities in psychotherapy* (pp. 114-138). New York: Guilford Press.

Vaz, K. M. (1992). A course on research issues on women of color. *Women's Studies Quarterly, 20*(1/2), 70-85.

Vogel, S. R. (1979). Discussant's comments symposium: Applications of androgyny to the theory and practice of psychotherapy. *Psychology of Women Quarterly, 3,* 255-258.

Wade, M. E. (2001). Women and salary negotiation: The costs of self-advocacy. *Psychology of Women Quarterly, 25,* 65-77.

Walker, A. (1983). *In search of our mothers' gardens: Womanist prose.* New York: Harcourt, Brace, Jovanovich.

Walker, L. (1979). *The battered woman.* New York: Harper and Row.

Walker, L. (1984). *The battered woman syndrome.* New York: Springer.

Walker, L. E. A. (1989). Psychology and violence against women. *American Psychologist, 44,* 695-702.

Walker, L. E. A. (1991). Post-traumatic stress disorder in women: Diagnosis and treatment of battered woman syndrome. *Psychotherapy, 28,* 21-29.

Walker, L. E. A. (1994). *Abused women and survivor therapy.* Washington, DC: American Psychological Association.

Walker, L. E. A. (1999). Psychology and domestic violence around the world. *American Psychologist, 54,* 21-29.

Walker, L. E. A. and Dutton-Douglas, M. A. (1988). Future directions: Development, application, and training of feminist therapies. In M. Douglas and L. E. Walker (Eds.), *Feminist psychotherapies: Integration of therapeutic and feminist systems* (pp. 276-300). Norwood, NJ: Ablex.

Walker, R. (Ed.) (1995). *To be real*. New York: Anchor Books/Doubleday.

Walters, M. (1993). The codependent Cinderella and Iron John. *Family Therapy Networker, 17*(2), 60-65.

Ward, M. C. (1998). *A world full of women*. Boston: Allyn & Bacon.

Warren, K. J. (2000). *Ecofeminist philosophy: A Western perspective on what it is and why it matters*. Lanham, MD: Rowman and Littlefield.

Warren, L. W. (1976). The therapeutic status of consciousness-raising groups. *Professional Psychology: Research and Practice, 7*, 132-140.

Watanabe, K. (1999). Trafficking in women's bodies, then and now: The issue of military "comfort women." *Women's Studies Quarterly, 27*(1/2), 19-31.

Waterhouse, R. L. (1993). "Wild women don't have the blues": A feminist critique of "person-centred" counselling and therapy. *Feminism and Psychology, 3*, 55-72.

Waugh, P. (1998). Postmodernism and feminism. In S. Jackson and J. Jones (Eds.), *Contemporary feminist theories* (pp. 177-193). New York: New York University Press.

Way, N. (1995). "Can't you see the courage, the strength that I have?": Listening to urban adolescent girls speak about their relationships. *Psychology of Women Quarterly, 19*, 107-128.

Weed, E. (1997). Introduction. In E. Weed and N. Schor (Eds.), *Feminism meets queer theory* (pp. vii-xiii). Bloomington: Indiana University Press.

Wehr, D. S. (1987). *Jung and feminism: Liberating archetypes*. Boston, MA: Beacon Press.

Wei, W. (1993). *The Asian American movement*. Philadelphia, PA: Temple University Press.

Weingourt, R., Maruyama, T., Sawada, I., and Yoshino, J. (2001). Domestic violence and women's mental health in Japan. *International Nursing Review, 48*, 102-108.

Weisstein, N. ([1968] 1993). Psychology constructs the female; or the fantasy life of the male psychologist. *Feminism and Psychology, 3*, 195-210.

Weitzman, L. M. (1994). Multiple-role realism: A theoretical framework for the process of planning to combine career and family roles. *Applied and Preventive Psychology, 3*, 15-25.

West, C. M. (1995). Mammy, Sapphire, and Jezebel: Historical images of Black women and their implications for psychotherapy. *Psychotherapy: Theory, Research, and Practice, 32*, 458-466.

West, C. M. (2000). Developing an "oppositional gaze" toward the images of Black women. In J. Chrisler, C. Golden, and P. D. Rozee (Eds.), *Lectures on the psychology of women* (Second edition) (pp. 221-233). Boston: McGraw-Hill.

West, C. and Zimmerman, D. G. (1987). Doing gender. *Gender and Society, 1*, 125-151.

Wester, S. R. and Vogel, D. L. (2002). Working with the masculine mystique: Male gender role conflict, counseling self-efficacy, and the training of male psychologists. *Professional Psychology: Research and Practice, 33,* 370-376.

Whalen, M. (1996). *Counseling to end violence against women: A subversive model.* Thousand Oaks, CA: Sage.

White, M. (1987). The virtue of Japanese mothers: Cultural definitions of women's lives. *Daedalus, 116*(3), 149-163.

White, M. (1992). Home truths: Women and social change in Japan. *Daedalus, 121*(4), 61-82.

White, M. (1995). *Re-authoring lives: Interviews and essays.* Adelaide, Australia: Dulwich Centre Publications.

White, M. B. and Tyson-Rawson, K. J. (1995). Assessing the dynamics of gender in couples and families: The gendergram. *Family Relations, 44,* 253-260.

Wijeyesinghe, C. L. (2001). Racial identity in multiracial people: An alternative paradigm. In C. L. Wijeyesinghe and B. W. Jackson III (Eds.), *New perspectives on racial identity development: A theoretical and practical anthology* (pp. 129-152). New York: New York University Press.

Wilfley, D. E. and Cohen, L. R. (1997). Psychological treatment of bulimia nervosa and binge eating disorder. *Psychopharmacology Bulletin, 33,* 437-454.

Wilkinson, S. (2001). Theoretical perspectives on women and gender. In R. Unger (Ed.), *Handbook of the psychology of women and gender* (pp. 17-28). New York: Wiley.

Williamson, D. A. and Netemeyer, S. B. (2000). Cognitive-behavior therapy. In K. J. Miller and J. S. Mizes (Eds.), *Comparative treatments for eating disorders* (pp. 61-81). New York: Springer.

Willis, E. (1975). The conservatism of *Ms.* In Redstockings (Eds.), *Feminist Revolution* (pp. 170-171). New York: Random House.

Willis, E. (1984). Radical feminism and feminist radicalism. In S. Sayres, A. Stephanson, S. Aronowitz, and F. Jameson (Eds.), *The 60s without apology* (pp. 91-118). Minneapolis: University of Minnesota Press.

Wilson, E. (1990). Psychoanalysis: Psychic law and order? In T. Lovell (Ed.), *British feminist thought: A reader* (pp. 211-226). Cambridge, MA: Basil Blackwell Ltd.

Wilson, G. T. and Fairburn, C. G. (1998). Treatments for eating disorders. In P. E. Nathan and M. M. Gorman (Eds.), *Treatments that work* (pp. 501-530). New York: Oxford University Press.

Wilson, G. T., Fairburn, C. C., Agras, W. S., Walsh, B. T., and Kraemer, H. (2002). Cognitive-behavior therapy for bulimia nervosa: Time course and mechanisms of change. *Journal of Consulting and Clinical Psychology, 70,* 267-274.

Wilson, G. T., Loeb, K. L., Walsh, B. T., Labouvie, E., Petkova, E., Liu, X., and Waternaux, C. (1999). Psychological versus pharmacological treatments of bulimia nervosa: Predictors and processes of change. *Journal of Consulting and Clinical Psychology, 67,* 451-459.

Wing, A. K. (Ed.) (2000). *Global critical race feminism: An international reader.* New York: New York University Press.

Wing, A. K. (Ed.) (2003). *Critical race feminism: A reader* (Second edition). New York: New York University Press.

Winslade, J., Crocket, K., and Monk, G. (1997). The therapeutic relationship. In G. Monk, J. Winslade, K. Crocket, and D. Epston (Eds.), *Narrative therapy in practice: The archaeology of hope* (pp. 53-81). San Francisco: Jossey-Bass.

Wisch, A. F. and Mahalik, J. R. (1999). Male therapists' clinical bias: Influence of client gender roles and therapist gender role conflict. *Journal of Counseling Psychology, 46,* 51-60.

Wisch, A. F., Mahalik, J. R., Hayes, J. A., and Nutt, E. A. (1995). The impact of gender role conflict and counseling technique on psychological help seeking in men. *Sex Roles, 33,* 77-89.

Withorn, A. (1980). Helping ourselves: The limits and potential of self help. *Radical America, 14*(3), 25-39.

Wolfe, J. L. (1995). Rational emotive therapy women's groups: A twenty year retrospective. *Journal of Rational-Emotive and Cognitive-Behavior Therapy, 13,* 153-170.

Wolfe, J. L. and Fodor, I. G. (1975). A cognitive/behavioral approach to modifying assertive behavior in women. *The Counseling Psychologist, 5,* 45-59.

Wolfe, J. L. and Fodor, I. G. (1977). Modifying assertive behavior in women: A comparison of three approaches. *Behavior Therapy, 8,* 567-574.

Wolfe, J. and Kimerling, R. (1997). Gender issues in the assessment of posttraumatic stress disorder. In J. P. Wilson and T. M. Keane (Eds.), *Assessing psychological trauma and PTSD* (pp. 192-237). New York: Guilford Press.

Wollstonecraft, M. ([1792] 1972). A vindication of the rights of woman. In M. Schneir (Ed.), *Feminism: The essential historical writings* (pp. 6-16). New York: Vantage Books.

Wong, N. (1991). Socialist feminism: Our bridge to freedom. In C. T. Mohanty, A. Russo, and L. Torres (Eds.), *Third world women and the politics of feminism* (pp. 288-296). Bloomington: Indiana University Press.

Wong, N. (2000). The art and politics of Asian American women. In F. Ho, C. Antonio, D. Fujjino, and S. Yip (Eds.), *Legacy to liberation: Politics and culture of revolutionary Asian Pacific America* (pp. 235-242). San Francisco: Big Red Media.

Woo, M. (1983). Letter to Ma. In C. Moraga and G. Anzaldúa (Eds.), *This bridge called my back* (pp. 140-147). New York: Kitchen Table/Women of Color Press.

Woolger, J. B. and Woolger, R. J. (1989). *The goddess within: A guide to the eternal myths that shape women's lives.* New York: Fawcett Columbine.

Worell, J. (2001). Feminist interventions: Accountability beyond symptom reduction. *Psychology of Women Quarterly, 25,* 335-343.

Worell, J. (2002). Guidelines for psychological practice with girls and women: Update. *The Feminist Psychologist, 29*(3), 8,10.

Worell, J. and Johnson, N. G. (Eds.) (1997). *Shaping the future of feminist psychology: Education, research, and practice.* Washington, DC: American Psychological Association.

Worell, J. and Remer, P. (2003). *Feminist perspectives in therapy: Empowering diverse women* (Second edition). New York: Wiley.

Wright, E. O., Baxter, J., and Birkelund, G. E. (1995). The gender gap in workplace authority: A cross-national study. *American Sociological Review, 60,* 407-435.

Wyche, K. F. (1993). Psychology and African-American women: Findings from applied research. *Applied and Preventive Psychology, 2,* 115-121.

Wyche, K. F. and Rice, J. K. (1997). Feminist therapy: From dialogue to tenets. In J. Worell and N. G. Johnson (Eds.), *Shaping the future of feminist psychology* (pp. 57-71). Washington, DC: American Psychological Association.

Wyckoff, H. (1971). Radical psychiatry in women's groups. In J. Agel (Ed.), *The radical therapist* (pp. 181-187). New York: Ballantine Books.

Wyckoff, H. (1977a). Radical psychiatry for women. In E. I. Rawlings and D. K. Carter (Eds.), *Psychotherapy for women* (pp. 370-391). Springfield, IL: Charles C Thomas.

Wyckoff, H. (1977b). Radical psychiatry techniques for solving women's problems in groups. In E. I. Rawlings and D. K. Carter (Eds.), *Psychotherapy for women* (pp. 392-403). Springfield, IL: Charles C Thomas.

Yamasaki, E. W. (2000). Perspective of a revolutionary feminist. In F. Ho, C. Antonio, D. Fujjino, and S. Yip (Eds.), *Legacy to liberation: Politics and culture of revolutionary Asian Pacific America* (pp. 47-51). San Francisco: Big Red Media.

Yoder, J. D. (2003). *Women and gender: Transforming psychology* (Second edition). Upper Saddle River, NJ: Prentice-Hall.

Yoder, J. D. and Kahn, A. S. (1993). Working toward an inclusive psychology of women. *American Psychologist, 48,* 846-850.

Yoshihama, M. and Sorenson, S. B. (1994). Physical, sexual, and emotional abuse by male intimates: Experiences of women in Japan. *Violence and Victims, 9,* 63-77.

Young-Eisendrath, P. (1984). *Hags and heroes: A feminist approach to Jungian psychotherapy with couples.* Toronto, Canada: Inner City Books.

Zeldow, P. B. (1984). Sex roles, psychological assessment, and patient management. In C. S. Widom (Ed.), *Sex roles and psychopathology* (pp. 355-374). New York: Plenum.

Ziemba, S. J. (2001). Therapy with families in poverty: Application of feminist family therapy principles. *Journal of Feminist Family Therapy, 12*(4), 205-237.

Zimmerman, J. L. and Dickerson, V. C. (1994). Using narrative metaphor: Implications for theory and clinical practice. *Family Process, 33,* 233-245.

Zweig, M. (1971). Is women's liberation a therapy group? In J. Agel (Ed.), *The radical therapist* (pp. 160-163). New York: Ballantine Books.

Index

Order a copy of this book with this form or online at:
http://www.haworthpress.com/store/product.asp?sku=5092

FEMINIST THEORIES AND FEMINIST PSYCHOTHERAPIES
Origins, Themes, and Diversity, Second Edition

_____ in hardbound at $69.95 (ISBN: 0-7890-1807-1)

_____ in softbound at $39.95 (ISBN: 0-7890-1808-X)

Or order online and use special offer code HEC25 in the shopping cart.

COST OF BOOKS_____

POSTAGE & HANDLING_____
(US: $4.00 for first book & $1.50
for each additional book)
(Outside US: $5.00 for first book
& $2.00 for each additional book)

SUBTOTAL_____

IN CANADA: ADD 7% GST_____

STATE TAX_____
(NY, OH, MN, CA, IL, IN, & SD residents,
add appropriate local sales tax)

FINAL TOTAL_____
(If paying in Canadian funds,
convert using the current
exchange rate, UNESCO
coupons welcome)

☐ **BILL ME LATER:** (Bill-me option is good on
US/Canada/Mexico orders only; not good to
jobbers, wholesalers, or subscription agencies.)
☐ Check here if billing address is different from
shipping address and attach purchase order and
billing address information.

Signature_____

☐ **PAYMENT ENCLOSED: $**_____

☐ **PLEASE CHARGE TO MY CREDIT CARD.**

☐ Visa ☐ MasterCard ☐ AmEx ☐ Discover
☐ Diner's Club ☐ Eurocard ☐ JCB

Account # _____

Exp. Date_____

Signature_____

Prices in US dollars and subject to change without notice.

NAME_____

INSTITUTION_____

ADDRESS_____

CITY_____

STATE/ZIP_____

COUNTRY_____ COUNTY (NY residents only)_____

TEL_____ FAX_____

E-MAIL_____

May we use your e-mail address for confirmations and other types of information? ☐ Yes ☐ No
We appreciate receiving your e-mail address and fax number. Haworth would like to e-mail or fax special
discount offers to you, as a preferred customer. **We will never share, rent, or exchange your e-mail address
or fax number.** We regard such actions as an invasion of your privacy.

Order From Your Local Bookstore or Directly From
The Haworth Press, Inc.
10 Alice Street, Binghamton, New York 13904-1580 • USA
TELEPHONE: 1-800-HAWORTH (1-800-429-6784) / Outside US/Canada: (607) 722-5857
FAX: 1-800-895-0582 / Outside US/Canada: (607) 771-0012
E-mailto: orders@haworthpress.com

For orders outside US and Canada, you may wish to order through your local
sales representative, distributor, or bookseller.
For information, see http://haworthpress.com/distributors

(Discounts are available for individual orders in US and Canada only, not booksellers/distributors.)
PLEASE PHOTOCOPY THIS FORM FOR YOUR PERSONAL USE.
http://www.HaworthPress.com   BOF04